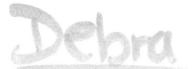

Working with Serious Mental Illness

Especially for John

For Baillière Tindall

Senior Commissioning Editor: Jacqueline Curthoys
Project Development Manager: Karen Gilmour
Project Manager: Jane Shanks
Design Direction: George Ajayi

Working with Serious Mental Illness

A Manual for Clinical Practice

Edited by

Catherine Gamble BA(Hons) RGN RMN RNT
Director, Thorn Mental Health Programme, RCN Institute, London, UK

Geoff Brennan BSc(Hons) RNMH RMN
Head of Nursing Practice, Oxleas NHS Trust, Bexley, UK

Foreword by

Julian Leff BSc MD FRCPsych MRCP MFPHM
Professor of Social and Cultural Psychiatry,
Institute of Psychiatry, London, UK

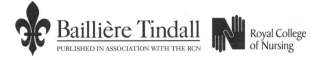

Baillière Tindall
PUBLISHED IN ASSOCIATION WITH THE RCN

Royal College
of Nursing

EDINBURGH LONDON NEW YORK PHILADELPHIA ST LOUIS SYDNEY TORONTO 2000

BAILLIÈRE TINDALL
An imprint of Harcourt Publishers Limited

© Harcourt Publishers Limited 2000

 is a registered trademark of Harcourt Publishers Limited

The right of Catherine Gamble and Geoff Brennan to be identified as
editors of this work has been asserted by them in accordance with the
Copyright, Designs and Patents Act 1988

First published 2000
 Reprinted 2000
 Reprinted 2001
0 7020 2446 5

British Library Cataloguing in Publication Data
A catalogue record for this book is available from the British Library

Library of Congress Cataloging in Publication Data
A catalog record for this book is available from the Library of Congress

Note
Medical knowledge is constantly changing. As new information
becomes available, changes in treatment, procedures, equipment and
the use of drugs become necessary. The editors, contributors and the
publishers have, as far as it is possible, taken care to ensure that the
information given in this text is accurate and up to date. However,
readers are strongly advised to confirm that the information, especially
with regard to drug usage, complies with the latest legislation and
standards of practice.

The
publisher's
policy is to use
**paper manufactured
from sustainable forests**

Printed in China by RDC Group Limited

Contents

SECTION 2 ASSESSMENTS: CHOOSING AND USING

SECTION 4   CONSIDERATIONS FOR EFFECTIVE PRACTICE

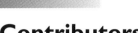

Contributors

Dinesh Bhugra MA MSc MBBS FRCPsych MPhil PhD
Dr Bhugra is currently a Senior Lecturer in Psychiatry at the Department of
Psychiatry in the Institute of Psychiatry, London. He has written extensively
on cross-cultural psychiatry, social psychiatry, religion and mental health and
sexual dysfunction. As an Honorary Consultant at the Maudsley Hospital, he
runs a community-based team for patients with severe illness. He is also
Chairman of the Faculty of General and Community Psychiatry at the Royal
College of Psychiatrists.

Geoff Brennan BSc(Hons) RNMH RMN
Geoff Brennan is Northern Irish and a registered Nurse in Learning
Disabilities and Mental Health. Geoff works in education, practice
development and maintains a clinical caseload with regard to family
interventions. He has recently taken the post of Head of Nursing Practice,
Oxleas NHS Trust.

Paddy Conroy RMN RGN ENB 650 Cog Skills Course
Paddy Conroy is a Registered Mental Nurse, who has specialised in Cognitive
Behavioural Psychotherapy having trained as a therapist at the Maudsley
Hospital and Institute of Psychiatry, London. After working as a Cognitive
Behavioural Psychotherapist at City & Hackney NHS Trust, he worked as a
Trainer and Research Fellow in South Australia. This involved training health
professionals in cognitive behavioural strategies for use with people with
long term illnesses and evaluating the outcomes. He currently works as a
Senior Psychotherapist with Liverpool Psychotherapy and Consultation
Service, North Mersey NHS Trust. This role involves clinical work with severe
and complex cases, consultation, training and supervision.

TF Chan BPharm(Hons) DipClinPharm MRPharmS
TF Chan is Chief Pharmacist for Camden and Islington Community Health
Services NHS Trust in London. After gaining his Bachelor of Pharmacy at the

University of London in 1986, he worked at various London hospitals as a clinical pharmacist before specialising in Mental Health in 1993. His work includes direct client work, research in discharge planning and education and training. TF teaches psychopharmacology on the THORN programme for the RCN and runs workshops for the College for Pharmacist Postgraduate programme.

Tom KJ Craig MB BS PhD FRCPsych
Tom Craig is the Professor of Community Psychiatry at Guy's, King's and St Thomas' School of Medicine, Dentistry and Biomedical Sciences. He has researched and published widely on the influence of social deprivation on the onset and course of psychiatric disorder including studies of homeless young people and other disadvantaged populations in the inner city. His clinical interests concern the development and dissemination of innovative community-based psychiatric services. These programmes have included residential alternatives to the hospital asylum, the development of clinical case management models for severe mental illness, and the establishment and evaluation of pan-London psychiatric services for homeless mentally ill people.

Sharon Dennis BSc RMN Dip Family Therapy CMS RNT
Sharon Dennis is Deputy Director of Nursing at South London & Maudsley NHS Trust. Her mental health nursing career was motivated by the desire to work in a therapeutic capacity. Her clinical career focused predominantly on acute inpatient wards and she has published articles related to practice in this field. She reviews both potential articles and books for the journal *Mental Health Care*. Sharon has contributed to the development of national mental health policies and was recently elected onto the steering committee of the Royal College of Nursing's Mental Health Forum, which represents the interests of the profession.

Jayne Fox RMN ENB 650
Jayne Fox is a Registered Mental Nurse, who has specialised in Cognitive Behavioural Interventions. She trained in this area at the Maudsley Hospital, London and from there contributed to the delivery and development of the Thorn Initiative Training programme at the Institute of Psychiatry. In 1996 she took up a clinical research position in Adelaide, South Australia. This research project was funded by the Australian Government and involved developing coordinated clinical care for people with long term and complex illnesses. In addition, this role involved developing and delivering training programmes to health professionals working in this area. Jayne is now working in the Wirral and West Cheshire NHS as a cognitive–behavioural

psychotherapist for people with serious mental illness. This role combines clinical work, supervision and service development.

Catherine Gamble BA(Hons) RGN RMN RNT
Catherine Gamble is the course director for the Thorn Programme in problem centred interventions for people with serious mental illness, based at the Royal College of Nursing Institute. This innovative programme equips mental health practitioners with a variety of psychosocial interventions to help mental health service users and their carers. In 1991, Catherine took the lead responsibility for developing and implementing the inaugural Thorn programme at the Institute of Psychiatry in London, UK, and has subsequently used this experience to set up the first mental health degree programme for the RCN. Her knowledge and expertise in schizophrenia family work in particular, has resulted in her being asked to disseminate the approach to mental health professionals both in the UK and abroad. As users and their carers are searching for recognition, support and practical help, her main line of interest lies in ensuring that these skills and interventions are routinely used in clinical practice. This book reflects this interest.

Sue Kerr RMN Thorn 2/3
Sue Kerr is a Psychiatric Nurse. Her interest and commitment are to the severe and enduring mentally ill, and she considers herself as a 'born again nurse' since completing her studies with the Thorn Initiative. Sue teaches part time on the Thorn course at the Institute of Psychiatry and Cambridge, and works with individuals and their families in Suffolk eagerly attempting to mitigate the impact and distress caused by mental illness.

Avie Luthra MBChB BSc(Hons) MRCP MRCPsych
Avie Luthra is completing his registrar training at the Bethlem and Maudsley Hospital. He has been actively involved in research at the Institute of Psychiatry. His research interests include stigma and public attitudes to mental illness.

Kenny Midence BSc MPhil DClinPsy CPsychol AFBPsS
Dr Kenny Midence is a Principal Clinical Psychologist working in Adult Mental Health in Gwynedd, Wales. He has carried out research in different psychological and medical conditions, and has published extensively, including experimental and theoretical papers, and books.

Jem Mills RMN ENB 650 PgDip CT (Contact email jemmills@globenet.co.uk)
Jem Mills works as a cognitive behavioural psychotherapist and training consultant in both NHS and private healthcare settings. He first gained

experience of CBT in Salisbury during RMN training. He completed the ENB 650 at the University of Brighton and undertook cognitive therapy training at Oxford University. He is currently involved with the innovative development of rehabilitation services within Eastbourne and County Healthcare NHS Trust. Previously he was responsible for the CBT component of the Thorn course and remains an Honorary Tutor at the Institute of Psychiatry, London.

Paula Morrison BSc(Hons) RMN
Paula Morrison is the Clinical Governance Facilitator for Oxleas NHS Trust which is a Community Trust providing Mental Health, Learning Disabilities, Forensic and Community Nursing Services in three London Boroughs. Paula has worked in mental health services for many years with experiences in both acute and community areas in Northern Ireland and London. Paula also worked at the King's Fund for 4 years and had responsibility for Nursing Development Units in Mental Health and Learning Disabilities throughout England. Paula's current role involves taking the lead within Oxleas on clinical governance.

Sally Goldspink BSc(Hons) SROT
Sally Goldspink is an Occupational Therapist, and after completing her degree Sally worked in London, focusing mainly on group work. Sally is one of the new breed of occupational therapist who focus on individuals' cognitive disabilities, therefore providing individual plans that work with clients' assessed difficulties using the Allen model of Occupational Therapy. Sally now works full time with clients and carers. Sally is committed to clients with severe and enduring mental illness and is a colleague in arms in the battle against mental illness.

Cliff Roberts BSc(Hons) RGN PGDE MSc
For the past 6 years Cliff Roberts has been teaching on nursing degrees at the RCN Institute in London. He is the module leader for the Clinical Skills in Psychopharmacology module in the Thorn programme at the RCN Institute. His past and current research background is in the area of neuroscience, particularly interactions between stress, the brain and peripheral hormones. His professional background as a nurse is in critical care. Cliff worked at Barnet General Hospital in the Intensive Care Unit for 10 years. This diverse background has given him the knowledge and motivation to encourage nurses to explore neuroscience in an endeavour to enhance their understanding and care of their clients.

Paul Rogers RMN Cert ENB 650 Dip Behav Psych MSc
Paul Rogers has worked in secure environments for over 10 years. He

completed the ENB 650 (Adult Behavioural Psychotherapy) course at the Maudsley Hospital in 1995 since when he has worked in his role as a Clinical Nurse Specialist in Behavioural Psychotherapy at the Caswell Clinic, South Wales Forensic Psychiatric Service. Paul has written a number of articles on Cognitive–Behaviour Therapy, Clinical Supervision and Postraumatic Stress Disorder. He is an elected member of the Royal College of Nursing Forum: The Development of Mental Health Practice, and is on the editorial advisory board of *Mental Health Practice*. Paul is an external reviewer for forensic mental health for The Health Advisory Service 2000.

Iain Ryrie BScNursing DipNursing RMN

Iain Ryrie is a lecturer in research in Health and Social Care Section at King's College, University of London. He has specialised in the substance misuse field for over 10 years and maintains an active research portfolio in this area. He is also responsible for a 4-year mental health nursing degree course and leads a programme of practice development in local NHS provider units.

Andrew Vidgen MA(Hons) MSc

Since graduating from Aberdeen University with a degree in psychology, Andrew has worked in a variety of settings including health, social services and the voluntary sector. At present he is undertaking training in clinical psychology and maintains an active interest in psychological approaches to psychoses, offending and forensic issues.

Foreword

The community psychiatric nurse (CPN) is the backbone of the community mental health team. This is not to minimise the important roles of psychologists, occupational therapists, psychiatrists, social workers, support workers and others, but CPNs are not only the most numerous professionals, they are the ones who spend most of their time in the patients' homes. The development of the CPN service was initiated by the introduction of depot preparations of antipsychotic drugs. Clinics were set up in hospitals and in outpatient facilities to deliver the depot injections, which were given by psychiatric nurses. Psychiatrists did not consider it necessary to see the patients every time they came for an injection, so that the nurses took increasing responsibility for monitoring the patients' mental state and response to medication. Of course there were some patients who failed to turn up for their scheduled appointment. Since the efficacy of prophylactic antipsychotic medication had been firmly established, it was considered vital for non-attenders to be actively pursued. The clinic nurses started visiting the defaulters in their homes to give them their injections in time to prevent a relapse. One could say that psychiatric nurses rode out into the community on their syringes!

When I was a medical student learning obstetrics, I used to go out with the Flying Squad, as it was called, to difficult deliveries in the home. My eyes were opened to the conditions under which people lived, and since then I have given great importance to seeing patients in their home environments. The understanding which comes from appreciation of family relationships and the social and economic milieu of our patients cannot be overemphasised. It was this understanding that the psychiatric nurses gained when they began to visit patients in their homes. They realised that there was much more they could do than simply giving an injection. In time their therapeutic activities were formalised by the creation of the specialty of community psychiatric nursing. This development has not occurred uniformly in western countries. It was facilitated in Britain by the long tradition of home visiting by general practitioners (GPs). In the USA home visiting by doctors had virtually disappeared by the middle of the century. Therefore it became necessary to reinvent the idea of professionals leaving their offices and travelling to see patients. This practice was dignified by the name of Assertive Community Treatment. Some European countries, such as Italy, have adopted the outreach approach, while in others, such as Belgium, the work of psychiatric nurses is confined to the hospital.

Once CPNs were firmly established in the community in Britain, liaison with GPs became desirable since these two groups of professionals were often looking after the same patients. GPs saw the advantage of having a CPN attached to their practice and relationships became very close. The focus of many CPNs shifted from the hospital to the general practice, and the nature of their client group also altered. This was also true of CPNs working in the community mental health centres which were beginning to spread over the country at the time. One of the spurs to this shift in the client groups treated by CPNs was the development of cognitive and behavioural techniques for anxiety and depression. CPNs were excited by the prospect of becoming therapists, and obtained training in the necessary skills. It was more rewarding to treat patients with neuroses, who usually responded relatively quickly and were more grateful for the attentions of the CPNs than the average person with a chronic psychosis. As a result patients with serious mental illnesses were often neglected in favour of those with neuroses. A survey of the clientele of community mental health teams by Patmore and Weaver (1992) revealed great variation in the client mix. Some teams were treating predominantly psychotic patients, while others saw very few patients of this kind. The Department of Health became understandably alarmed by the neglect of the severely mentally ill and attempted to redress the balance with various directives. People can be pressurised to do work they are not attracted to, but they generally do not perform well. It is a more effective strategy to make the work challenging and rewarding. Fortunately, exciting therapeutic developments in the past two decades have transformed clinical work with serious mental illness, and have prompted the writing of this book. The first social treatment for serious mental illness to achieve prominence during this period was work with families. Once it became clear from a number of randomised controlled trials that, when used in conjunction with antipsychotic medication, this form of intervention was efficacious in reducing the relapse rate of schizophrenia, I worked with Elizabeth Kuipers and Dominic Lam to establish a course to teach the necessary skills. We thought of the trainees as being CPNs since they were already visiting the patients' families. We had in mind a cascade model of training in order to make the skills available nationally. Therefore we hoped that some of our trainees would demonstrate an ability to become trainers themselves. This did indeed prove to be the case for two of the trainees on the first course. They were Catherine Gamble and Geoff Brennan, the editors of the volume.

More recently the introduction of cognitive therapy for psychotic experiences has given new hope to people whose symptoms are poorly controlled with medication. Training in these skills was incorporated with family work training and case management in a national training programme known as the Thorn Initiative, which is based in two centres in London and Manchester. The aim is to generate satellite training centres throughout Britain, and six of these are already operating successfully. The training programme has expanded to include modules on medication management, dual diagnosis disorder, and forensic issues. All these topics are covered in this book, while many of the contributors teach on the Thorn Initiative or have assisted in its development. The training was never considered to be exclusively for CPNs and indeed a social worker attended our first family work course. More recently trainees from a whole range of disciplines have been accepted on the course, as the recognition has grown that what is taught is relevant to any professional working with the seriously mentally ill. The development of community psychiatry has blurred the boundaries between the disciplines and all can profit from the knowledge and experience offered in these pages.

London, 2000   Professor Julian Leff

 References

Patmore C, Weaver T 1992 Improving community services for serious mental disorders. Journal of Mental Health 1: 107–115

Acknowledgements

We wish to acknowledge the many people without whose help this book would not have been produced.

First, to all the users and carers who have taught us how to be practitioners.

Jacqueline Curthoys, who found us in the first place and remained a friend despite it all.

Karen Gilmour for professional but considerate harassment.

The contributors for maintaining contact, their patience and hard work.

All the students we have had the privilege to teach and learn from.

On a personal note, Rachel, Sam, Hannah, Freddie and Ella for keeping us sane. All the people we have neglected over the past 2 years (you know who you are) and, finally, Sarah Gamble for doing the cover.

Introduction

Mental health care is changing and evolving. The traditional medical model is being augmented and modified by the influence of newer disciplines, such as clinical psychology and humanistic models of care. The change in philosophy can be seen in recent social policy and mental health care provision and with the implementation of the Community Care Act. The basis of this change is to improve the quality of life of the user of services. Consequently, there is a need for all practitioners to place greater emphasis on working with users, using skills that have a sound theoretical basis.

The underlying aim of this book is to guide practitioners through this process and deconstruct any patriarchal attitudes that can alienate individual clients. Although it is acknowledged that this alienation has occurred through ignorance rather than malice, there is no longer any justification for it. Clients have long been aware that their needs were and are not being met. Fortunately, their voice is now gaining strength. But there is a potential that it may still be heard as angry and resentful.

In order to reduce the likelihood of such emotions being induced, practitioners need to continually address their own attitudes. To replace patriarchal assumptions, which justifiably induce negative emotions, alternative practices and beliefs must be adopted. Practitioners are attempting to correct these past errors. Indeed, rather than trusting to intuitive ideas or blindly following charismatic leaders and their individual philosophies, they are beginning to challenge and scientifically analyse their treatment methods. Nevertheless, in this scientific quest (so-called 'evidence-based analysis') it should not be forgotten that the best evidence is the personal experience of the user. Collaboration and inclusion should therefore always be the cornerstone of current and future practice.

It is the adaptation of evidence-based treatment methods to suit the individual that is the concern of this book. There are many publications aimed at either exploring the theoretical implications for change in service delivery or focusing on an in-depth analysis of specific clinical interventions. There is, however, a gap with regard to how practitioners comprehensively amalgamate theory with practice. This book seeks to guide, plan and suggest down to earth treatment ideas for individuals on a day to day basis.

To assist the reader, the book is divided into four distinct sections.

Section 1: Manifestations of serious mental illness

The opening section is designed to promote reflection on how serious mental illness (SMI) is perceived and treated. Within this section, particular notice should be given to the first chapter, 'A view from within'; it is an eyewitness account and therefore is as truly 'evidence based' as possible. Chapter 2 of this section introduces the practitioner to how the treatment methods used within this book have been developed and evaluated. Such approaches fit neatly with the concept of stress vulnerability and the diagnostic process; the final chapters cover these areas.

Section 2: Assessments: choosing and using

Assessment is the cornerstone of successful interventions. This section focuses on the assessment process and how to choose and use some of the tools available. It identifies specific skills in focusing this information towards clients' goals and identifying risk factors.

Section 3: Interventions

This forms the main body of the book. To get the best use from this section it is advised that practitioners first examine their own beliefs, attitudes and assumptions and consider their overall treatment aim and their relationship with clients. Chapter 8 will help the reflection of these issues.

Subsequent chapters concern direct interventions and practitioners should match the chapters to the individuals they wish to work with. For example, if your client is hearing voices and/or experiencing strange thoughts then Chapter 9 will be of most relevance. Many individuals will have complex needs and it is worth reading the other chapters that pertain to their presentation, such as negative symptoms, family issues, dual diagnosis, anger, offending behaviour and medication issues.

Section 4: Considerations for effective practice

The chapters in this section are issues that although they appear to stand alone, often frame the potential success or failure of interventions. They aim to guide practitioners to reflect further on issues outside their relationship with service users. These issues are: cultural, ethical and professional considerations.

Section 1

Manifestations of serious mental illness

1

Serious mental illness: a view from within

EDITORS' NOTE

In many ways, this chapter is written by the book's truest expert. 'A view from within' is a clear, no-nonsense account of a personal journey through serious mental illness by someone who has come out the other side. It does not seek to prescribe or direct practitioners to particular interventions, attitudes or knowledge, but merely asks the reader to 'walk in the footsteps' of a person who has a lot to teach us.

There were several things that influenced my illness:

I was a clumsy child who suffered from dyspraxia.
I was the eldest of four girls and was jealous of my sister who was 18 months younger than me.
I found a few things physically difficult, e.g. riding a bike and knitting.
I had nightmares and sleepwalked.
I had a fixation about death.
I always wanted to please and was very sensitive.
I was a diligent reader and from the age of three I had a vivid imagination.
I had a difficult birth, was paralysed down one side for a few weeks and was shortsighted – I have often asked myself 'Could this have led to brain changes?'
I was picked on at school at the age of 14 and not invited to peers' parties.
I wanted to be a nurse from the age of 12 to help others.
I failed my English A level and was bitterly disappointed.
I did achieve my ambition and started nurse training – unfortunately there were problems straight away.

I experienced two people dying while I was giving them bed baths. I remember being 'sent for a coffee break', shocked and upset, as a means of coping.

Another time I spent several hours talking to a young girl who was 18 years old like me. She had leukaemia and died. The next day I had a panic attack.

During my psychiatric placement there were two incidents that particularly upset me. First a lesbian woman made a pass at me, which shocked me as I was only 19. I didn't know how to deal with this. Secondly I was looking after this gay young man who I became involved with. It all became too much and I completely flipped. I was hysterical, but no one did anything about it. I feel I should have been counselled or offered supervision. Basically the work had stimulated past experiences in my life and this, with other experiences in my nurse training, should have made me give up the training as it was affecting me badly. I continued for another 8 years.

Another factor was I worked on a cancer ward and witnessed lots of deaths including those of young people. As this went on I became scared of death, which led me to become phobic.

At the age of 24, I started local philosophy classes after I had seen the course advertised on the bus. It was run by an organisation called the School of Economic Science. I did not know this was an undercover cult. I attended 17 sessions. I can't really remember them clearly, as we were encouraged to clear our minds of everything and not to tell people, especially our family, what was going on and what we heard. As a consequence I became cut off from my family. My family, however, knew something was wrong.

Eventually a housemate alerted me to the fact that the classes were run by a cult. Luckily I got out, but I became paranoid and frightened that someone from the cult was following me. At this point I became psychotic and suspicious of everyone. I moved in with friends who were into buddhism and the occult. They lived in a flat decorated in black. At the time I thought nothing of it, but my family were growing more concerned as they didn't know where I was.

I began meditating. I stayed up all night and all day. I starved myself. Around this time, my boyfriend left for Mexico. I began isolating myself and staying in my room. Friends and family rang, but I didn't come out. I started reading books about black magic and the occult. I listened to tapes and heard messages and I experienced double meanings in the books I was reading. Things came to a head when I saw myself on the television conducting an orchestra. I ran to the TV and turned it off. My flatmate didn't know what was happening. He asked 'What do you think you're doing?' I couldn't tell him.

I was left at home on my own. When someone came round I thought they were from the cult and I wouldn't let them in. That was it – I was totally paranoid. I thought I had to get away. In desperation I telephoned my gran and said I was in trouble. This prompted my family to start searching for me. They knew something was very wrong. I wandered around the city with the words 'Come out of the dark, walk into the light' ringing in my head. I thought the cult were following me and I was going to be sacrificed. Throughout the day I tried to call home but I couldn't get through. I thought the city had been shut down by occult means, and my home town no longer existed. I felt I couldn't use any money as I thought the money had been changed.

I then decided I would find my boyfriend. I got on a train to the airport. Once there I went up to one of the ticket desks and asked for a ticket to Mexico. The attendant told me that there were no flights to Mexico from this particular airport and I didn't have my passport on me. I decided to go to a sea port as, coincidentally, I had enough money. On the train I threw all my possessions away. During the journey I was hallucinating. I thought I was on a train to heaven. I remember looking at all the people on the train and deciding if they were going to heaven or hell based on their possessions. For example, I saw people using mobile phones, Filofaxs or Walkmans and these had separate meanings. Eventually I arrived at the sea port, which I had previously visited with a friend, on our way abroad. I queued up at passport control but of course I had no passport or ticket so I was not allowed on the boat.

I also thought I was there to be a martyr and I was to be sacrificed. I began wandering around. I was having visual and auditory hallucinations. I came to a bridge. There were seagulls on either side of me and I thought I was walking into heaven. Suddenly I heard voices and turned to find the police. It was about two in the morning. The police picked me up and took me back to the station. It was terrifying as I thought all men were witch doctors. I kept trying to run out of the room as I thought I was going to be sacrificed. Somehow I remembered my parents' telephone number and the police phoned them. By now it was 4 a.m. Eventually my parents arrived. I was very anxious and scared of my dad as I felt he was also a witch doctor. It took them quite a while to persuade me to get in the car. I was disorientated and frightened. When we got home I had to have a shower. I think my Mum thought I had been sexually assaulted. I was shown to my parents' bed, as they thought this would help me get some sleep but, as I lay down, I felt an electric shock and refused to get back in. I was crying and screaming hysterically as I still thought my father was a witch doctor and was going to sacrifice me.

I had other psychotic thoughts. I thought all men were in the cult and that my family were part of an undercover species who came to life at night and went into hibernation during the winter. I would not drink tap water because I thought it was poisoned. I felt people with various eye colours were good or bad: blue was good, brown was bad.

Later that morning the general practitioner (GP) came round; I was totally disorientated. I thought I had died and gone to heaven. The doctor said I had to be admitted to the local psychiatric hospital as soon as possible. I didn't want to go but my gran came. Gran was the only one who could persuade me.

An ambulance was eventually called and mum came with me. During the journey my mind was racing and I was reliving my childhood life and memories. I thought I had become a child again. We arrived at the hospital, where I was shown into a small room with a clock on the wall and a female doctor was sitting in front of me. I thought it was a concentration camp and my parents were interned with me. The doctor stupidly asked my parents if they wanted to take me home for the weekend. They refused. It had taken all their strength to get me there and they were exhausted.

I remained disorientated and confused. A nurse was assigned to me for 24 hour observations. I was shown to the first bed in a dormitory. I was examined and a blood test was taken. I screamed and shouted, thinking I was being attacked. My parents left to get me some toiletries and clothes. I was alone and I was scared.

I remember sitting in bed on the first night with a nurse by my side, thinking I was going to die. I was very frightened and needed lots of reassurance. I told her I was a Catholic and she said she was one too. I remember drifting off to sleep as the medicine made me drowsy. I woke up next morning and there was tea at the hatch on the main ward. I still had a nurse with me; it was 6 a.m. in the morning. The women in the beds adjacent to me starting talking and reassuring me that I would get well and not to be frightened. I became like a small child, vulnerable and quiet.

In the early days, I can remember sitting in the lounge with a nurse by my side. I was experiencing hallucinations. I thought I was in a plane and I was flying to heaven. I suppose I must have started taking Largactil to help with my symptoms. The days began to drift into each other as I had many hallucinations and delusions and remained disorientated. I remember thinking I was a princess and was going to get married. When my family came to see me I thought the hospital was my palace and I was receiving my family. I then used to go to the kitchen and make them a pot of tea.

I became muddled up with past friends. A young man who was a friend became my fiancee in my mind. He came to see me a few times. I thought my dad was my bodyguard and was there to protect me. He would come and see me every day and take me out for drives. My mum used to find it hard to see me suffering and would often burst into tears. My sisters used to come and visit and tried to get some normality into my existence.

I continued to see and hear messages so the medication was increased and increased. Eventually my body began to be affected. I was stiff. I had pains in my legs. My mouth was dry. I shook and could not keep still, so I spent hours pacing the ward. I paced so much that the nurses used to say I would wear the carpet out.

In spite of this, the suspicious thinking continued. I still felt I was being watched and that some patients were in the occult. I also saw myself on TV again. I continued to believe I was in heaven and the hospital was heaven. I also thought that the hospital was the home of the cult and I had been imprisoned by a relative who was a high teacher within the occult.

My days comprised of getting up at 6 a.m. and having tea, then a wash, breakfast, watching TV and walking around the hospital. There was a library, shop, coffee, drop-in and lots of grounds. I used to put on my Walkman and go walking. I found this helped to lift my mood. It also helped when I thought the hospital was my palace.

I continued to experience side-effects of medication. I could smell rotting flesh, I had severe headaches and was affected by anything electrical. I also saw strange things like the water flowing in the opposite direction when I ran the tap. Of course all this was very frightening. Because of all these symptoms I began to think I was dying. I became even more restless and anxious. I was then prescribed drugs for my side-effects. I began to be so anxious I could not sleep. I would wander around the ward all night or would lie on my bed and writhe. I could not keep still. I did not sleep for 2 weeks. I just wanted to be given an injection to knock me out. It was terrible, truly awful.

After this my medication was changed completely. I started on Stelazine. Then I collapsed as my blood pressure dropped too fast. I hit my head and was allowed to spend the morning in bed. They also tried me on antidepressants as they thought I was depressed, but these made me more depressed and I eventually refused to take them.

Interspersed with all this I attended OT (occupational therapy) daily. This was truly an escape from the hell of the ward. In OT I used to do things like word games, typing, cooking, puzzles, relaxation and brass rubbing. I used to enjoy this time and the OTs really encouraged me.

After about 6 weeks I was discharged. Unfortunately things did not work out and I ended up in back in hospital three times in 3 months. Lots of my nursing friends came to see me. They were not impressed with the hospital; they thought it was old and run down and did not have a nice atmosphere.

One day I decided I had had enough, so I walked off the ward in my nightie and bare feet. I walked through reception. I walked down the steep slope to the main road and tried to run into the traffic. Luckily a distraught woman rescued me and took me back to the ward. There was a man with me. I think he was a policeman. I remember he was furious and told the nurses to 'lock me up'. The staff and my parents were very surprised at what I had done. My clothes were taken off me for 24 hours.

On another occasion, when I was at home and I felt I could not bear the pains in my head any more, it was so bad I took an overdose. My younger sister found me and couldn't understand why I had done it. 'We love you so much' she said. My stomach was pumped, I was admitted to another hospital and then sent back to the original one.

After all these incidents my family decided I should be transferred to a more renowned psychiatric hospital. A top nurse had been in touch with the consultant there and he agreed to take me on. My room was cleared and I moved the next day. I arrived on the ward with my dad. I was shown into the quiet room. I remember feeling upset and disillusioned as I thought I was never going to get better. I now had the diagnosis of 'paranoid schizophrenic'.

I was shown into my room. It was quite nice. I remember my dad gave me a hug and said 'I like this place. I think this place will help you.' I met my primary nurse and we had a chat. I told him I thought my brain was dead and that there was no hope for me. I didn't know what he must have thought. Things were very different at this hospital. I met the consultant and had to go into the ward round to tell them all about me. As I came out I was told I had done very well. I was started on clozapine 200 mg. With this I needed weekly blood tests. This drug was to help me a lot in the future.

I still had delusions. I had nightmares. One night I thought I was being executed. I saw myself flying on the ceiling. I felt my soul left me.

Every day I spent 15 minutes with my morning nurse and time later with my afternoon nurse. Because I was convinced my brain was dead a scan was arranged for me. It was normal. I began OT again and this really helped. I did such things as typing, creative art, pottery, stress management, cookery, gym, swimming, writing and craft. Each ward had its own OT and mine used to spend an hour counselling me, which really helped.

I began going home at weekends. I found it hard to sleep and I often felt anxious. My parents took me out at weekends for drives in the country. I began to relive my childhood again and had nightmares and fears. These lessened when I returned to the ward.

I was on the ward 9 months. My room became a haven. I put up artwork, psalms, books by my bed and so on. Many other patients would come into my room and be mesmerised. Then they would calm down as they sat on my bed.

Eventually the delusions drifted away and I became more positive. I would go for my daily walk around the grounds. Many friends visited me and my family remained very supportive. I was now ready to leave. But I had nowhere to live so I moved to a hostel. After 3 months a flat was found for me – it was a few minutes away from my parents. I was seen as an outpatient for 6 months.

One side-effect was I had put on a lot of weight, which knocked my confidence. I still have regular blood tests, which means I will always have a tie to the hospital. I developed a feeling of blackness and deadness, which has stayed with me; to this day I have felt I have died inside. I have lost all my inner energy and because of this I have thought I am going to die, which is very frightening.

When I first got discharged I got a job at Dillons book shop, which I found difficult because my medication made me so drowsy. I did this for 18 months. I then got involved in the voluntary services and started a job at a playgroup for children with special needs. I worked there for $4\frac{1}{2}$ years and really enjoyed it. I also became involved in a Clubhouse rehabilitation scheme. I worked in the office, kitchen, took part in meetings and did a 3 week training in America. I spent $4\frac{1}{2}$ years at the Clubhouse.

I am now an education project officer for our local user group on a part time basis. I run seminars, give presentations and talks to school children and train nurses about mental health issues. My job carries responsibility and I find it challenging and empowering. I am also involved in a women's Clubhouse. I am on the management committee. In this I do a lot of outreach work, going into the community and meeting women in psychiatric wards or in day centres. I also take part in a 'schizophrenia roadshow' where I travel around the country talking about and sharing my experiences.

I still need medication, and see a psychiatrist. But I feel some good has come out of my illness. I am working and functioning. I am part of the community.

There *is* life after schizophrenia.

2

An introduction to and rationale for psychosocial interventions

Kenny Midence

KEY ISSUES

◆ Social skills training.
◆ Family interventions.
◆ Cognitive–behavioural therapy.
◆ Community psychiatric nurses.

INTRODUCTION

Psychosocial treatments for schizophrenia are not new in the research literature. Since the 1970s, researchers have been investigating the potential contribution of psychosocial treatments to help patients suffering from serious mental illness (e.g. Trower, Bryant & Argyle 1978). Despite all the research available providing evidence of their effectiveness, these approaches have not been well recognised or accepted into routine clinical practice (Slade & Haddock 1996). It is now clear, however, that psychosocial interventions are necessary to help patients cope with their condition, and improve their quality of life. These interventions are also beneficial to relatives, and are effective in improving the quality of the family environment (Penn & Mueser 1996). Psychosocial interventions are aimed at empowering patients, and, as Slade & Haddock (1996) have pointed out, 'since the 1980s, the task of the therapist was no longer to "change the behaviour of the patient" but rather to "help the client to change their own behaviour, if they wish to do so"'.

This chapter provides an overview of the psychosocial interventions available including social skills training, family interventions and cognitive–behavioural therapy (CBT) for psychotic symptoms, and the role of community psychiatric nurses in the implementation of these approaches. The aim is not to provide a comprehensive academic review of psychosocial interventions for serious mental illness. Instead, it is to give the reader an overview of the state of research and developments of recent research studies. This chapter also tries to condense the available evidence to help health care professionals to get a general outlook of these exciting and promising new approaches. Recommended empirical, theoretical, or review papers, and books (in asterisks), are provided in the reference section for those readers who want a comprehensive description of the theoretical and empirical research of these interventions.

SOCIAL SKILLS TRAINING

Schizophrenia is characterised by a deficiency in social functioning associated with poor prognosis and low quality of life. People who suffer from serious mental illness have social skills deficits, and relatives report that negative symptoms are the most difficult behaviours to cope with (Leff & Vaughn 1985). Recent findings have shown that up to two-thirds of patients show deficits in assertiveness and symptom management. Trower, Bryant & Argyle (1978) suggested that the lack of social skills in patients hindered the development of supportive social networks, and decreased the ability to cope with stressors leading to a deterioration of patients' prognosis and quality of life. This, in turn, leads to poor community functioning and social isolation (Halford & Haynes 1995). There is also evidence that premorbid social functioning is a strong predictor of long term functioning, and recent research suggests that cognitive deficits including social perception (e.g. self-awareness), and problem-solving skills (e.g. appraisal of situations) can determine the level of social skill in patients.

Social skills training (SST) has been available to patients over the last two decades to help them develop social competencies, and its effectiveness has been studied since the early 1970s. Originally, it included instruction, modelling, role playing and homework tasks. Early studies showed some evidence that patients could learn social skills in suitable environments. Researchers, however, were concerned about the generalisation of trained social skills, and the effectiveness of training in improving social functioning. Furthermore, Smith, Bellack & Liberman (1996) have made a distinction between social competence and social adjustment, which can have important implications for practitioners. They describe social competence as 'a subjective, evaluative term representing the individual's overall ability to impact favourably on the social environment through the application of specific skills in particular environmental settings'. Social adjustment 'refers to the actual meeting of instrumental and affiliative needs that is the natural consequence of social competence'. These subtle differences are important in any social skills training programme. Social skills also involves a widely accepted three process model, which includes 'receiving information' (e.g. social perception), 'processing information' (e.g. problem solving) and 'sending a response' (e.g. response topography), and any social skills training programme should include these three aspects (Liberman et al 1986).

How effective is social skills training?

There is good evidence that social skills training can be beneficial to patients suffering from schizophrenia. We know that patients with schizophrenia suffer from prevalent and persisting deficits in social and instrumental skills that can be overcome only by highly structured and intensively focused training (Bellack & Mueser 1986), and there is good evidence that patients can learn new skills using social skills training, which can be maintained after training. Social skills training can increase patients' comfort in social situations and improves social skills in the training setting (Halford & Hayes 1991). Moreover, social skills can be generalised to other inpatient settings (e.g. hospital wards), but the evidence of its effectiveness in community settings is less clear.

Previous research has produced different results about the effectiveness of social skills training on patients' community functioning. More recently, Hayes, Halford & Varghese (1995) investigated the effect of 36 sessions of social skills training on patients' improvement in social skills, social functioning, and reduction in positive and negative symptoms and relapse rate compared with a control group. Measures included social skills and anxiety, patients' skills in initiating conversation, community functioning, severity of psychopathology, activities and quality of life. Negative symptoms and relapse were assessed before and after treatment, and at 6 months follow-up. The training included instructions, modelling, behaviour rehearsal, feedback, homework tasks, conversational skills and assertion, social problem solving, and identifying activities to practise skills. Results showed that patients who received social skills training had a greater improvement in social skills, but there were no other significant differences between the conditions. Both groups of patients showed improvement on quality of life and reduced psychopathology, and the effect of social skills training had limited effect on community functioning. It has been suggested that patients' social environment (e.g. hostels) does not provide them with the opportunities to practise their skills, and generalisation of these skills can be achieved only when environments that promote and reinforce socials skills are provided (Smith, Bellack & Liberman 1996).

The techniques used in social skills training have included speech and non-verbal behaviour, independent living skills, conversation, dating, job seeking, and social perception skills, stress management, affect regulation, assertiveness and conversation skills, recreational, interpersonal, and social problem-solving skills, symptom and medication management. Comparison groups have included drama and group discussion, day hospital treatment, holistic health treatment, social milieu treatment (supportive discussion, exercise and activity groups), family psychoeducation, discussion groups and supportive group therapy. The duration of social skills training has ranged from two to four sessions per week and a duration from 7 weeks to 6 months or 12 months with reduced sessions a week. Outcome assessment has included role plays for speech and non-verbal behaviours, role play, self-report rating of skill, level of depression, symptomatology, family perceptions, social and occupational functioning, relapse rates, skill levels, social adjustment, family burden, interpersonal skills and social adjustment.

Overall, research findings supporting the effectiveness of social skills training have provided strong evidence for the acquisition and maintenance of social skills, moderate evidence for the generalisation of social skills and social adjustment, and weak evidence for reduction of symptoms and relapse and hospitalisation (Smith, Bellack & Liberman 1996). The effectiveness of social skills training on patients' vocational adjustment and quality of life is less clear. Results from studies also suggest that this kind of intervention is effective especially if it is intensive (e.g. more than two sessions per week), and of sufficient duration (e.g. at least 6 months) (Smith, Bellack & Liberman 1996).

FAMILY INTERVENTIONS

Early research on Expressed Emotion (EE) carried out in the last 20 years by researchers in the MRC Social Psychiatry Unit at the Institute of Psychiatry, London, provided evidence of the negative impact of high EE families on the course of schizophrenia. According to Leff & Vaughn (1985), these high EE families not only experienced distress in coping with the condition, but they also showed behaviours that were either extremely critical or hostile, or both, and emotionally overinvolved with the relative with schizophrenia. These early findings led to the development of family intervention programmes to reduce the effects of schizophrenia on patients (e.g. relapse, hospitalisation), to increase patients' social functioning, and to reduce family burden and improve the quality of life of sufferers and their families (Tarrier & Barrowclough 1995). Family interventions are based on broad psycho-educational and/or behavioural approaches, and research examining the effectiveness of these approaches has been mainly carried out by Falloon and colleagues, and Hogarty and colleagues in the USA; and Vaughan and colleagues in Australia. In the UK, research has been conducted by Leff and colleagues in London, and Tarrier, Barrowclough and colleagues in Manchester.

What are the components of family intervention?

According to Kavanagh (1992), the components of family intervention include engagement of families, education, communication training, goal setting, problem solving, cognitive–behavioural self-management, increasing family well-being and maintenance of skills. Bellack & Mueser (1993) have suggested that four main aspects of the psychosocial treatment of patients should be emphasised. These are the need for a comprehensive and long term treatment including drugs, individually tailored treatment programmes, an active participation by patients and relatives and the acknowledgement of patients' cognitive limitations. According to Lam (1991), family approaches include the following components:

◆ a genuine working relationship
◆ a structured and stable intervention plan with additional contacts if necessary
◆ a focus on improving stress and coping in the here and now
◆ interpersonal boundaries within the family
◆ information about the biological nature of schizophrenia
◆ the use of behavioural techniques
◆ improving communication between family members.

Lam (1991) has also identified three possible mechanisms underlying the better outcome of patients who receive family therapy:

◆ lower negative family affect (i.e. EE)
◆ improved patient adherence with medication
◆ better patient monitoring by the treatment team.

The techniques used in these family intervention approaches have been published by the researchers responsible for their development (e.g. Anderson, Reiss & Hogarty 1986, Barrowclough & Tarrier 1992, Falloon 1995, Kuipers, Leff & Lam 1992). The techniques involved include initial assessment of relatives' and patients' needs, educating families, stress management and coping responses, issues about engaging and maintaining the family involvement, dealing with violence and suicide risk, assessment of psychotic symptoms, and coping strategies (cognitive and behavioural) (e.g. Barrowclough & Tarrier 1992). Family intervention by Kuipers, Leff & Lam (1992) includes assessing the relative and their family, engaging the family, education about schizophrenia, improving communication, identification of stressors, setting realistic goals, dealing with emotional issues (e.g. anger, conflict, rejection), dealing with overinvolvement, getting everyone in the family involved, employment, cultural issues, special issues (e.g. substance abuse, suicide, incest) and running a relatives' group.

How effective are family interventions?

The positive results of the studies on family interventions have provided strong evidence for the effectiveness of these psychosocial approaches. Overall, research findings indicate that these approaches are more effective than routine treatment, and are beneficial for patients and their relatives. Family interventions are effective in reducing EE in relatives, family burden and relapse rate in patients over 1 to 2 years, and in improving patients' social functioning, especially when families change from high to low EE. Moreover, long term family intervention seems to reduce patients' relapse rate, and treatment gains are stable and can be maintained for as long as 2 years. The duration of the treatment is related to the outcome of the intervention, and this means that the longer the treatment the better is the outcome; short term interventions show less beneficial effect on relapse rate. Furthermore, the financial savings to the mental health service in providing family intervention for 9 months has been reported to be as high as 27%, including less social work contact and hospital admission (Tarrier, Lowson & Barrowclough 1991).

Fadden's (1998) review of family interventions showed the effectiveness of these approaches. She points out that 'family interventions have been shown to result in at least a fourfold reduction in relapse rates at one year post-intervention, and even though relapse increases in the second year, the rates are still only half what they are when no such intervention is provided'. However, we still do not know which family intervention model provides the best benefits for patients and their families, what aspects of family intervention are most effective, and the characteristics of patients and their families who do not benefit from family intervention. Furthermore, not all families are willing to engage in family intervention. The difficulty in engaging relatives in family work has been investigated by McCreadie et al (1991). In their study, half of the families invited to take part refused the treatment (almost half were low EE families), the main reasons given included 'things are fine at the moment', 'it is the patient who needs help, not me', and 'the patient doesn't want anyone else to know he has been ill'. The STEP clinical team in Wales found that 26% of families did not take part in the family intervention (Hughes et al 1996).

According to Smith & Birchwood (1990), between 7 and 21% of families tend to refuse family intervention, the range of families withdrawing from treatment range between 7 and 14%, and between 8 and 35% of families do not adhere to the treatment.

Implementing family intervention in routine clinical practice

Using family intervention for schizophrenia in routine clinical practice is a difficult task. Leff & Gamble (1995) have identified four main obstacles to implement this approach. First, research on family intervention has been carried out on high EE families using the Camberwell Family Interview (CFI) to assess families; this, of course, is not a practical assessment that can be used in routine clinical practice. However, Leff & Gamble (1995) have suggested that families most in need can be identified by the following criteria: frequent arguments between patient and relatives, inability to contain conflict, high relapse rate and relatives' frequent contact with staff for information and reassurance. Barrowclough & Tarrier (1992) have addressed this problem by designing the Relative Assessment Interview (RAI) for routine clinical use; this assessment is based on the CFI. Secondly, the nature of family intervention requires training manuals, which need to be learnt over a period of time, and the set of family intervention skills needs to be used in a flexible way. Thirdly, training places are limited because they involve intensive clinical supervision, and only a minority of CPNs are trained to deliver this service to a large number of families in need. Fourthly, the main problem is to persuade health authorities to buy the training course, and provide the support and conditions needed to implement family intervention. Unfortunately, health authorities seem to be more interested in how costly this service is rather than in its effectiveness, and in the help that patients and families can gain from this intervention. Fortunately, researchers on family intervention have been addressing this issue in order to persuade purchasers that this seems to be the best way to help patients and their families in the long term.

To the author's knowledge, the only research paper reporting the implementation of family intervention as part of a routine clinical service rather than as a funded research project is that of the STEP team in Wales (Hughes et al 1996). The STEP team was established in 1985 and has seen over 200 families. During clinical practice, the team begins by administering the CFI to obtain information about the family's perception of schizophrenia and attitude towards the relative with schizophrenia. After the initial introductory sessions, the team introduces an information package on schizophrenia. During the next stage, clarification of specific behavioural goals for continuing intervention is reviewed, and if family intervention is to be offered, the treatment focuses on problem solving, encouraging active involvement in local service, reinforcing advice previously given, discussing coping strategies, setting goals to promote rehabilitation and monitoring early signs of relapse. Although communication training is not part of the STEP programme, attempts are made to encourage family members to consider how they relate to each other, and to develop more effective strategies for resolving conflict and communication difficulties. The STEP intervention is normally provided for 1 year, and one main emphasis of this approach is the development of a long term strategy for rehabilitation.

Budd & Hughes (1997) have reported that, according to the families involved in family intervention, the most helpful aspects of the intervention include: knowledge/understanding of schizophrenia, feeling supported, reassured and encouraged, and having someone to call in emergencies. Families also said that the intervention had helped them to become more tolerant of their relative's behaviour, and to improve communication between family members. Although the papers by Hughes et al (1996) and Budd & Hughes (1997) do not provide data about the effectiveness of its approach, Hughes and colleagues have provided some evidence of the practical implication and difficulties of implementing family intervention in routine clinical practice. For example, the team has encountered a culture of benign neglect rather than active opposition from management. Another problem refers to other professionals professing that 'they are already doing family work' even when these professionals have not been trained in psychosocial intervention for schizophrenia. They have pointed out that 'it is much simpler to incorporate new drugs into clinical practice than it is to incorporate family intervention service as part of the routine clinical service' (Hughes et al 1996).

In conclusion, there is no doubt that the effectiveness of family interventions is well established. The most recent review paper of the effectiveness of family intervention has concluded that family intervention is highly effective when it is provided for at least 9 months (Penn & Mueser 1996). Despite the overwhelming evidence regarding the effectiveness of family intervention, however, Anderson & Adams (1996) have rightly pointed out that this psychosocial intervention is not being used to its full potential in clinical practice. Implementation of family intervention continues to be a problem because not enough health care professionals are being trained, and those who are trained do not receive the support needed to implement this psychosocial intervention. Finally, Hughes et al (1996) have also pointed out that 'it is necessary to provide interventions which are tailored to the individual needs of sufferers and their families and which take into account the family's history and construction of the problem. This requires skilled clinicians who have a solid understanding of family processes and serious mental illness and who are able to work in a structured, problem-focused behavioural way with families.'

COGNITIVE–BEHAVIOURAL APPROACHES FOR PSYCHOSIS

The previous sections of this chapter have provided an overview of the significant and effective contribution of social skills training, and especially family intervention approaches. Psychosocial treatments for schizophrenia have been available for the last two decades, but the development and refinement of these treatments have led to an increasing interest in investigating their effectiveness and implementation. This section looks at the contribution and effectiveness of cognitive–behavioural treatment (CBT) for psychotic symptoms. Psychosocial approaches have normally aimed at improving the functioning deficits of patients rather than the symptoms of psychosis. We know that the effectiveness of medication for psychotic symptoms is limited. Although patients may have adequate medication, some receive little or no benefit from it, and almost half of patients experience psychotic symptoms and suffer relapse. More recently, clinical psychologists have been conducting research investigating the effectiveness of CBT in the management of patients' psychotic symptoms, and schizophrenia more generally. Research findings suggest that CBT for psychosis is a promising intervention that can effectively help patients to cope with their psychotic symptoms.

The aim of CBT is to help patients gain knowledge about schizophrenia and its symptoms, to overcome hopelessness, to reduce distress from psychotic symptoms, to reduce dysfunctional emotions and behaviour and to help them analyse and modify dysfunctional beliefs and assumptions (Slade & Haddock 1996). Since the 1970s, researchers have tried to modify psychotic symptoms using cognitive–behavioural techniques including psychoeducation, coping responses, delusional belief modification, relabelling psychotic experiences, dealing with dysfunctional assumptions, and goal setting. Effective treatment, however, may depend on the patient's motivation, the distress associated with positive symptoms, the type and structure of the symptoms and the patient's cognitive deficits (Sellwood et al 1994).

The available literature on psychological treatments for positive psychotic symptoms is mainly in the form of individual case studies or series of case studies, and few large, controlled trials have been compared with traditional or routine treatments. The majority of treatment reports have been on the treatment of hallucinations or delusions including operant procedures, counterstimulation (e.g. distraction), use of ear plugs, thought stopping, focusing (e.g. content and beliefs about voices) and systematic desensitisation.

The treatment interventions of some researchers have focused on particular symptoms rather than addressing all the psychotic symptoms experienced by patients (e.g. Bentall, Haddock & Slade 1994, Chadwick & Birchwood 1994). Cognitive–behavioural intervention for psychotic symptoms can be summarised into two main groups: cognitive rehabilitation and content approaches (Penn & Mueser 1996).

Cognitive rehabilitation proposes that relapse could be prevented by addressing the cognitive deficits of patients, and it aims at the remediation of basic information-processing skills. Most of the research on cognitive rehabilitation has focused on remediation through repeated practice or related techniques. A number of case studies have suggested that this approach is associated with improved attention, greater cognitive flexibility and reduced paranoia. Studies have a number of characteristics in common, all focused on a specific cognitive deficit (e.g. vigilance) and training was conducted on an individual basis. The studies to date have not provided any consistent conclusions regarding the efficacy of cognitive rehabilitation (Penn & Mueser 1996).

Content approaches focus on residual positive symptoms (i.e. hallucinations and delusions) and stress management of these symptoms. These approaches aim at changing the nature of the content of dysfunctional thoughts and the patient's response to these thoughts by modifying thoughts or beliefs associated with delusions (e.g. that one's thoughts are being broadcast to others), and teaching ways to cope with auditory hallucinations (e.g. listening to music) (Penn & Mueser 1996).

There are various techniques used in CBT including 'coping strategy enhancement', which is aimed at building on the coping strategies that patients already have when they experience residual symptoms (Tarrier et al 1990, 1993). The procedures to help patients cope with these symptoms include explaining the treatment rationale, describing each psychotic symptom through a structured interview, assessing the frequency, duration, antecedents and consequences, assessing the interference of the symptoms, and the patient's beliefs and preoccupation; assessing the coping methods already used by the patients; identifying a target symptom and appropriate coping strategy; practising coping strategy during sessions; homework; and reassessment of the symptoms. Results from case studies suggest that coping strategy enhancement is effective in improving residual auditory hallucinations (Tarrier et al 1990). Coping strategy enhancement and problem-solving therapy have also been found to be superior in reducing positive symptoms compared with waiting list controls (Tarrier et al 1993).

Bentall, Haddock & Slade (1994) have used a different approach to deal with psychotic symptoms by looking at the fundamental cognitive bias underlying hallucinations (i.e. misattribution of internally generated events to an external source). Results of their studies have shown a reduction in the frequency and distress of auditory hallucinations in patients.

The cognitive–behavioural approach for psychosis used by Fowler, Garety & Kuipers (1995) includes improving coping responses, psychoeducation and belief modification. The main goals include the reduction of the distress and interference that arises from the experience of persistent psychotic symptoms, increasing the patient's understanding of psychotic disorders and fostering motivation to engage in self-regulation behaviour; and reducing the occurrence of dysfunctional emotions and self-defeating behaviour arising from feelings of hopelessness, negative self-image or perceived psychological threat (Kuipers, Garety & Fowler 1996). Research by Garety and colleagues is still ongoing, and preliminary results are promising. Haddock & Slade (1996) have maintained that patients' distress is related to their beliefs about the origin and content of their voices. Chadwick & Lowe (1990, 1994) have used non-confrontational verbal challenge and reality testing to reduce delusional beliefs. Delusions are assessed based on the available information including interpretation of the beliefs, and behavioural experiments to invalidate the delusions. Results suggest that CBT reduces patients' conviction in and preoccupation with delusional beliefs. Moreover, there is evidence that some patients may reject their delusional beliefs completely (Chadwick et al 1994).

More recently, Nelson (1997) has provided a comprehensive practical manual to guide clinicians in their work with patients with schizophrenia. This manual provides information about treatment strategies with delusions including assessment, lessening the impact/distress of delusional ideas, promoting insight, modifying and challenging delusions, and long term strategies. Treatment strategies with hallucinations include assessment and setting the goals of therapy, practical ways of reducing the voices, promoting insight, CBT with non-psychotic beliefs, disempowering the voices, modifying and challenging the delusional beliefs about the voices, and long term strategies. However, despite the encouraging findings of these studies, some patients can be reluctant to engage in therapy because of their strong beliefs and feelings about their voices. Fortunately, some researchers have developed a number of techniques to deal with the resistance shown by some patients by looking at the connections between the perceived benevolence or malevolence and resistance and engagement in relation to the voices (Chadwick & Birchwood 1996). In conclusion, the results from studies on psychotic symptoms have provided strong evidence of the effectiveness of CBT in helping patients to cope with psychotic symptoms (Haddock & Slade 1996). However, some of these benefits may be temporary, and patients may need continued intervention to maintain any improvements.

THE ROLE OF COMMUNITY PSYCHIATRIC NURSES (CPNs) IN THE MANAGEMENT OF SCHIZOPHRENIA

The important role of CPNs in the management of mental illness has been widely acknowledged, especially when they have more contact with patients than any other healthcare professionals including psychiatrists and clinical psychologists (Midence & Gamble 1995). Although the evidence of the effectiveness of psychosocial interventions for schizophrenia is well established, this evidence is based on treatment interventions carried out mainly by clinical psychologists in clinical research trials. More recently, however, researchers have been investigating the potential role of CPNs in the treatment of psychosocial treatments for schizophrenia. For example, CPNs are being trained in family intervention in London and Manchester, and various studies have provided promising results. Furthermore, recent developments in the treatment of patients have encouraged the development of family intervention training courses for CPNs to meet the needs of patients with schizophrenia and their families.

Overall, training in family intervention includes an overview of schizophrenia (e.g. diagnosis, assessment, medication, etc.); assessment of patient and family; education; a problem-solving approach to care planning; coping strategies; assessment of psychotic symptoms and intervention; and clinical supervision (Lancashire et al 1997). The training course in London is clinically based, and lasts for about 1 year. During the first 3 months of training the focus is mainly on the theoretical aspect of family intervention, and learning clinical skills to deal with criticism, overinvolvement, relatives' needs, and problem solving including problem-oriented case management, psychosocial intervention, psychological management of psychotic symptoms, implementation of family intervention, and clinical supervision. The second part of training includes supervision of casework, clinical analysis and peer supervision groups (Gamble 1997).

The effectiveness of family intervention training in improving CPNs' attitude to and knowledge of schizophrenia has been reported by previous studies (e.g. Gamble, Midence & Leff 1994, Midence & Gamble 1995). Furthermore, Midence et al (1995) have also shown similar results even when the CPN trainers had been trained by a first generation of CPNs who had trained in family intervention. The results of these studies suggests that CPNs can become trainers of other healthcare professionals (Leff & Gamble 1995). Preliminary studies have also shown that family intervention can be effective when implemented by CPNs. For example, a study by Brooker et al (1994) looked at the effect of trained CPNs on patients and their families. The training included assessment, engagement with patient and family, assessment, family education, communication skills, problem-solving skills, adherence to medication, crisis management, social skills training, and cognitive–behavioural strategies. Results of their study showed that patients' positive and negative symptoms and their social functioning improved significantly. For relatives, there was a decrease in mental health problems, and an increase in knowledge about medication. Preliminary results by Lancashire et al (1997) also showed that, although negative symptoms were not reduced, family intervention implemented by CPNs significantly decreased affective and positive symptoms, and there was an increase in social functioning in patients with schizophrenia.

The research evidence clearly shows that CPNs can be trained to carry out family intervention. However, family intervention for schizophrenia can be very difficult to implement owing to lack of facilities and resources. For example, CPNs have reported very little support from their service managers (e.g. Brooker & Butterworth 1991). Brennan & Gamble (1997) found that CPNs trained in family intervention had difficulties in including this approach within their responsibility at work. Trained CPNs also had difficulty in having access to consultation or supervision, and allowance of time from the service to do the intervention. Kavanagh et al (1993) have also reported that the main difficulties experienced by health care professionals in implementing family intervention included integrating family work with their other responsibilities, allowance of time from the service, availability of appropriate patients, clash of research needs and clinical needs of patients or families, availability of time in lieu or overtime for appointments, long term commitment to a specific patient and family, access to supervision and lack of support from managers. More recently, Fadden's (1997) survey of 86 therapists trained in family intervention showed that, although 70% of therapists were using the approach in their work, the mean number of families seen was only 1.7, and 40% of families were seen by only 8% of therapists.

Finally, Haddock & Slade (1996) have rightly pointed out that the number of clinical psychologists working with patients suffering from schizophrenia is still very small, and, given that there is strong evidence that psychosocial interventions are effective for managing psychotic symptoms, there is a need to train other health care professionals to carry out these psychological interventions under the guidance of clinical psychologists. Preliminary findings, as mentioned before, have shown that CPNs are in a strong position to implement psychosocial interventions providing that they have the appropriate training and supervision (Haddock et al 1994). Oppong-Tutu & Price (1997) have suggested that 'the CPN embarking on working with families must have the knowledge and training in the skills required to work with families, and be motivated to provide family members with their expertise and time'. Finally, Tarrier (1996) has suggested that 'the potential for family interventions to become standard practice requires two conditions: first, the availability of quality training in family intervention methods, and second, radical organisational change to accommodate family and psychosocial management as the core management approach for psychosis'.

CONCLUSIONS

It is interesting to note that Mueser, Wallace & Liberman (1995) have pointed out that:

> ...for 30 years, anti-psychotic medication has been considered to be effective despite the need to provide it on a long-term, maintenance basis. Psychosocial treatments, on the other hand, have been considered effective only if they could produce enduring benefits with time-limited administration. The social skills training studies suggest that it is the time to re-evaluate this assumption, and organise clinical trials of psychosocial treatments that are provided on a long-term, maintenance basis.

Unfortunately, a recent document by the American Psychiatric Association (APA) (1997) ignored the evidence about the effectiveness of psychosocial approaches to help patients and their families, and did not include psychosocial interventions in their guidelines for better treatment for schizophrenia.

Despite the lack of interest of some psychiatrists who believe that pharmacological treatment is the only solution to help patients and their families, coordinated clinical efforts to improve the quality of life of patients are being carried out with promising results. Comprehensive, biopsychosocial interventions designed to improve the community functioning of patients are in progress combining training in community living or assertive community treatment, and psychoeducation or family intervention. The programme described by McFarlane, Stastny & Deakins (1992) includes community functioning (e.g. integration of the patient's life into the community, in vivo teaching of coping and problem-solving skills, prevention of relapse and crisis interventions, support and education of community members) and multi-family group treatment (engagement, goal setting and family education). Vaccaro et al (1992) described another clinical research programme that includes case management, goal setting and treatment and rehabilitation planning, psychopharmacological treatment and social skills training. Liberman (1992) argues that rehabilitation needs to offer a wide range of skills training across areas including medication and symptom management, social skills training, family psychoeducation, recreation and leisure skills and basic community survival skills, and the offerings need to be tailored according to the patients' needs. The significant evidence about the effectiveness of all these psychosocial interventions suggests the need to think about how to integrate these treatments to provide a comprehensive treatment package for patients and their families (Penn & Mueser 1996).

Finally, psychosocial interventions for serious mental illness need to be implemented in general clinical practice, otherwise all the work of researchers would be fruitless (Gamble 1997). McKeown, McCann & Bentall (1997) have rightly pointed out that:

Delivering training within the ward environment in a way which involves all staff is much more likely to lead to systematic adoption of the psychosocial model, so that good practice becomes part of the ward routine, not the isolated activity of a small group of specialist practitioners. Such an approach necessitates a system of training which focuses on whole teams, with the trainers committed to a full-time presence on the ward for an appreciable length of time.

These psychosocial approaches can also be implemented in the community, and it is about time that this knowledge is put into practice to help clients and their families.

Cross references

For Practical Strategies and Implementation ideas see Chapters:

- ◆ 9 Dealing with voices and strange thoughts
- ◆ 10 Lack of motivation, confidence and volition
- ◆ 11 Working with families and informal carers
- ◆ 13 Working with people with serious mental illness (SMI) who are angry

References

American Psychiatric Association 1997 APA guideline for treating adults with schizophrenia. Medscape Mental Health 2(5) (Internet website www.medscape.com/medscape/psychiatry/journal/1997)

Anderson C, Reiss D, Hogarty G E 1986 Schizophrenia in the family: a practical guide. Guilford, New York

Anderson J, Adams C 1996 Family intervention in schizophrenia. British Medical Journal 313:232–236

*Barrowclough C, Tarrier N 1992 Families of schizophrenic patients: cognitive behavioural intervention. Chapman & Hall, London

Bellack A, Mueser K T 1986 A comprehensive treatment program for schizophrenia and chronic mental illness. Community Mental Health Journal 22:175–189

Bellack A S, Mueser K T 1993 Psychosocial treatment for schizophrenia. Schizophrenia Bulletin 19(2):317–336

Bentall R P, Haddock G, Slade P D 1994 Psychological treatment for auditory hallucinations: from theory to therapy. Behaviour Therapy 25:51–66

References (cont'd)

Brennan G, Gamble C 1997 Schizophrenia family work and clinical practice. Mental Health Nursing 17(4):12–15

Brooker C, Butterworth C 1991 Working with families caring for a relative with schizophrenia: the evolving role of the community psychiatric nurse. International Journal of Nursing Studies 28(2):189–200

Brooker C, Falloon I, Butterworth A, Goldberg D, Graham-Hole V, Hillier V 1994 The outcome of training community psychiatric nurses to deliver psychosocial intervention. British Journal of Psychiatry 165:222–230

Budd R, Hughes I 1997 What do relatives of people with schizophrenia find helpful about family intervention? Schizophrenia Bulletin 23(2):341–347

Chadwick P, Birchwood M 1994 The omnipotence of voices. A cognitive approach to auditory hallucinations. British Journal of Psychiatry 164:190–201

Chadwick P, Birchwood M 1996 Cognitive therapy for voices. In: Haddock G, Slade P D (eds) Cognitive-behavioural interventions for psychotic disorders. Routledge, London, pp 71–85

Chadwick P D J, Lowe C F 1990 Measurement and modification of delusional beliefs. Journal of Consulting and Clinical Psychology 58:225–232

Chadwick P D J, Lowe C F 1994 A cognitive approach to measuring and modifying delusions. Behaviour Research Therapy 32:355–367

Chadwick P D J, Lowe C F, Horne P J, Higson P J 1994 Modifying delusions: the role of empirical testing. Behaviour Therapy 25:35–49

Fadden G 1997 Implementation of family interventions in routine clinical practice following staff training programmes: a major cause for concern. Journal of Mental Health 6(6):599–612

*Fadden G 1998 Family intervention. In: Brooker C, Repper J (eds) Serious mental health problems in the community: policy, practice and research. Baillière Tindall, London, pp 159–183

*Falloon I R H 1995 Family management of schizophrenia. Johns Hopkins University Press, Baltimore

Fowler D, Garety P, Kuipers L 1995 Cognitive behaviour therapy for people with psychosis: a clinical handbook. John Wiley, Chichester

Gamble C 1997 The Thorn nursing programme: its past, present and future. Mental Health Care 1(3):95–97

Gamble C, Midence K, Leff J 1994 The effects of family work training on mental health nurses' attitude to and knowledge of schizophrenia: a replication. Journal of Advanced Nursing 19:893–896

Haddock G, Slade P D 1996 Implications for services and future research. In: Haddock G, Slade P D (eds) Cognitive–behavioural interventions for psychotic disorders. Routledge, London, pp 265–275

Haddock G, Sellwood W, Tarrier N, Yusupoff L 1994 Developments in cognitive behaviour therapy for persistent psychotic symptoms. Behaviour Change 11(4):200–212

Halford W, Hayes R 1991 Psychological rehabilitation of chronic schizophrenic patients: recent findings on social skills training and family psychoeducation. Clinical Psychology Review 23:23–44

Halford W, Hayes R 1995 Social skills in schizophrenia: assessing the relationship between social skills, psychopathology, and community functioning. Social Psychiatry and Psychiatric Epidemiology 30:14–19

Hayes R, Halford W, Varghese F 1995 Social skills training with chronic schizophrenic patients; effects on negative symptoms and community functioning. Behaviour Therapy 26:433–449

Hughes I, Hailwood R, Abbati-Yeoman J, Budd R 1996 Developing a family intervention service for serious mental illness: clinical observations and experiences. Journal of Mental Health 5(2):145–159

References (cont'd)

Kavanagh D J 1992 Family intervention for schizophrenia. In: Kavanagh D J, (ed) Schizophrenia: an overview and practical handbook. Chapman & Hall, London, pp 407–423

Kavanagh D J, Piatkowska O, Clark D et al 1993 Application of cognitive behavioural family intervention for schizophrenia in multidisciplinary teams: what can the matter be? Australian Psychologist 28(3):181–188

*Kuipers L, Leff J, Lam D 1992 Family work for schizophrenia: a practical guide. Gaskell, London

Kuipers E, Garety P, Fowler D 1996 An outcome study of cognitive–behavioural treatment for psychosis. In: Haddock G, Slade P D (eds) Cognitive–behavioural interventions for psychotic disorders. Routledge, London, pp 116–136

Lam D 1991 Psychosocial family intervention in schizophrenia: a review of empirical studies. Psychological Medicine 21:423–441

Lancashire S, Haddock G, Tarrier N, Baguley I, Butterworth C, Brooker C 1997 Effects of training in psychosocial interventions for community psychiatric nurses in England. Psychiatric Services 48(1):39–41

Leff J, Vaughn C 1985 Expressed emotion in families: its significance for mental illness. Guilford, New York

Leff J, Gamble C 1995 Training of community psychiatric nurses in family work for schizophrenia. International Journal of Mental Health 24(3):76–88

Liberman R 1992 Handbook of psychiatric rehabilitation. Macmillan, New York

Liberman R, Mueser K, Wallace C, Jacobs H, Eckman T, Massel H 1986 Training skills in the psychiatrically disabled: learning coping and competence. Schizophrenia Bulletin 12:631–647

McCreadie R, Phillips K, Harvey J, Waldron G, Stewart M, Baird D 1991 The Nithsdale schizophrenia surveys. VIII: do relatives want family intervention, and does it help? British Journal of Psychiatry 158:110–113

McFarlane W R, Stastny P, Deakins S 1992 Family-aided assertive community treatment: a comprehensive rehabilitation and intensive case management approach for persons with schizophrenic disorders. New Directions for Mental Health Services 53:43–53

McKeown M, McCann G, Bentall R 1997 Time for action: a new system for training mental health practitioners. Mental Health Care 1(5):158

Midence K, Marshall L, Bell R, Leff J 1995 Community psychiatric nurses: their role as trainers in schizophrenia family work. Journal of Clinical Nursing 4:335–336

Midence K, Gamble C 1995 Family work and attitudes to schizophrenia. Nursing Times 290:12

Mueser K T, Wallace C, Liberman R P 1995 New developments in social skills training. Behaviour Change 12(1):31–40

*Nelson H 1997 Cognitive behavioural therapy with schizophrenia. Stanley Thornes, Cheltenham

Oppong-Tutu A, Price V 1997 Working with the mentally ill and their families. Mental Health Nursing 17(4):8–10

*Penn D L, Mueser K T 1996 Research update on the psychosocial treatment of schizophrenia. American Journal of Psychiatry 153(5):607–617

Sellwood W, Haddock G, Tarrier N, Yusupoff L 1994 Advances in the psychological management of positive symptoms of schizophrenia. International Review of Psychiatry 6:201–215

Slade P D, Haddock G 1996 A historical overview of psychological treatments for psychotic symptoms. In: Haddock G, Slade P D (eds) Cognitive–behavioural interventions for psychotic disorders. Routledge, London, pp 28–44

References (cont'd)

Smith J, Birchwood M 1990 Relatives and patients as partners in the management of schizophrenia: the development of a service model. British Journal of Psychiatry 156:654–660

*Smith T E, Bellack A S, Liberman R P 1996 Social skills training for schizophrenia: review and future directions. Clinical Psychology Review 16(7):599–617

Tarrier N 1996 Family interventions for schizophrenia. In: Haddock G, Slade P D (eds) Cognitive–behavioural interventions for psychotic disorders. Routledge, London, pp 212–234

Tarrier N, Barrowclough C 1995 Family interventions in schizophrenia and their long-term outcomes. International Journal of Mental Health 24(3):38–53

Tarrier N, Harwood S, Yusopoff L, Beckett R, Baker A 1990 Coping strategy enhancement (CSE): a method of treating residual schizophrenic symptoms. Behavioural Psychotherapy 18:283–293

Tarrier N, Lowson K, Barrowclough C 1991 Some aspects of family interventions in schizophrenia. II: financial considerations. British Journal of Psychiatry 159:481–484

Tarrier N, Beckett R, Harwood S, Baker A, Yusopoff L, Ugareburu I 1993 A trial of two cognitive–behavioural methods of treating drug-resistant residual psychotic symptoms in schizophrenic patients, I: outcome. British Journal of Psychiatry 162:524–532

Trower P, Bryant B, Argyle M 1978 Social skills and mental health. Methuen, London

Vaccaro J, Liberman R, Wallace C J, Blackwell G 1992 Combining social skills training and assertive case management: the social and independent living skills program of the Brentwood Veterans Affairs Medical Center. New Directions for Mental Health Services 53:33–41

Annotated further reading

Fadden G 1998 Family intervention. In: Brooker C, Repper J (eds) Serious mental health problems in the community: policy, practice and research. Baillière Tindall, London

This chapter provides a comprehensive and up-to-date review of the research literature on family intervention.

Nelson H 1997 Cognitive behavioural therapy with schizophrenia. Stanley Thornes Publishers, Cheltenham

This is an excellent book for anyone who wants to develop an understanding of CBT in the management of psychosis.

*Haddock G, Slade P G 1996 Cognitive–behavioural interventions for psychotic disorders. Routledge, London

3

Stress vulnerability model of serious mental illness

Geoff Brennan

KEY ISSUES

◆ Prevalance of serious mental illness.
◆ Analysis of vulnerability factors.
◆ Stress and life events.
◆ Coping: relevance for practitioners.

INTRODUCTION

Let us imagine a world in which mental illness is as well defined as a medical condition such as measles or diabetes. A practitioner in this world would have a definitive test for mental illness. More than likely this would involve a superior scan or chemical analysis. It would be evidence based and valid. We could show people definitive pictures or numbers denoting the definite presence of … something. From this we could accurately diagnose the condition, administer the recommended treatment and, eventually, cure the ailment. If we are all honest, we would all like to live and work in this world – a world of definites.

In this world, how easy it would be to say to an individual 'We know that you have this form of illness, but don't worry, take this medication, change your diet, wear this plaster. In 1 year's time your symptoms will have completely disappeared, and we won't need to see you again' or 'You have schizophrenia type A, which means that you will suffer from voices for several years. We know that medication X will reduce these voices and let you function as normal, but the voices will persist.' No matter how many claims are made that this world is soon to be discovered (and the progress in clarification and diagnosis), all practitioners, clients and carers know we do not live in this ideal world. Moreover, if we go back and look closer at the medical world we would find that diagnosing some physical ailments, for example meningitis, is not that clear cut either. Indeed, many physical illnesses are also influenced by factors discussed in this chapter.

This would appear to be a depressing way to begin an exploration of the manifestation of mental illness, and yet the above paragraph highlights the mistakes in thinking that many practitioners make. This mistake is summed up by a desire to make mental illness a disease of the body. The first flaw in this conceptualisation is the misconception that the client, the patient, the sufferer, Mr or Ms X, is a person 'to be cured'. The practitioner's drive to 'cure' is a battle between them and illness. The practitioner, however, is not the person with the illness. Only by considering the person, and what constitutes illness and health for this individual, can we set realistic treatment objectives and measure outcomes.

In order to achieve this we need to reinstate the person within the explanation of serious mental illness. In doing this we should beware of alienating the individuals who manifest symptoms. This is because symptoms are not separate phenomena that manifest themselves in an isolated population. Having said this, the population of individuals diagnosed with serious mental illness do have unique experiences, which should be seen as an aspect of the continuum of human experience. In this case, however, difference does not equate to deviance. Consider the following two descriptions.

Mr A is a schizophrenic, first diagnosed 6 years ago. His first admission involved being arrested by the police and treated under Section 3 of the Mental Health Act. He is now maintained on medication and been well for 2 years.

Mr B is a happily married man with one child. Six years ago he suffered a breakdown following the death of his mother. Only in the past 2 years has Mr B felt life is worth living again. He works part time and is able to support his family. He is interested in writing about his experiences and is active within his church.

Given that Mr A and Mr B are the same person, it is interesting the differing impressions we get from the short descriptions. The first, Mr A, reduces our understanding and is focused around psychiatric terminology. This results in a distorted picture of who this person is and what his capabilities are. It is what I call 'practitioner speak' and is related to reducing Mr A to the essentials that are an import for the clinical world. If we look closely we will see that the description reduces Mr A to the manifestation itself: 'Mr A is a schizophrenic'. We begin to think of Mr A and others who share such experiences as 'them', the 'other', not like 'us', someone else. This is because all his experiences, as described, are outside of our understanding. We do not know what it is like to be labelled 'schizophrenic', to be arrested when experiencing psychotic symptoms, detained under the Mental Health Act, or to have 2 years of health after a psychotic relapse.

An example of this reduction of the person can also be explained by the continuing use of the label 'schizophrenic', as described by Haghighat & Littlewood (1995): 'Another important aspect of the semantics of labels relates to adjectives used as nouns. An adjective used as a noun, e.g. a schizophrenic, may rob the individual of his other aspects as it subsumes personhood and agency into illness'. From here it is a short step to thinking of the individual ('the schizophrenic', 'the manic depressive') as less than us, not equal, subhuman, tainted. If we accept this, it is up to us, the 'more able', to dictate to the 'poor sufferer', to take on the burden of care, to alleviate the suffering, to administer our services for the good of the poor afflicted. The reduction of people to stereotypical labels is the cornerstone of all prejudice, as has been shown throughout human history.

So how can practitioners begin the difficult path of addressing treatment of serious mental illness without reducing individuals' personhood or being patronising? How should we begin to conceptualise the process that will best address the challenges that the position of practitioner holds?

There are no definitive answers to these questions, but a beginning would be to find a way to view serious mental illness from the individuals' point of view. This may be easier said than done. As mentioned, it requires us to view individuals in their unique circumstances without shirking the difficult reality that they are experiencing phenomena we find alien to our own experience. One means of aiding this process is to view the manifestation of the difference – serious mental illness – within the explanatory model of stress vulnerability.

COMPONENTS OF STRESS VULNERABILITY

The concept of stress vulnerability is essentially simple. In it we think of the person's health as influenced by several factors that interact. As the title suggests, it is the interface and relationship between stress and vulnerability that are the main determinants of the model.

To begin with, let's take a brief look at these components.

Stress

Stress is a fairly modern concept, yet has become fully incorporated into our language. It is a word that is used in a myriad of situations and has various meanings. The physical and psychological effects of excessive exposure to stress are recognised as anxiety, agitation, insomnia, irritability, low motivation, anger, frustration, poor concentration and difficulties in decision making. In this situation, stress means a force that acts upon the system in such a way as to place it under strain. It is important to remember that stressors can be either negative factors such as boredom and inactivity, or pleasant events such as marriage, birth or promotion, as the latter can also put strain on an individual.

Within the stress vulnerability model there is an understanding that stress is a variable that influences the manifestation of symptoms. To understand its impact fully we need to consider the differing forms that stress can take.

Ambient stress

All individuals have stressors in their lives. To live is to be under strain. We are directly aware of this in our own lives. If you stop for a second and begin to think about your own stressors you will realise that there are always things that cause concern. Maybe you haven't paid a bill, your cat/child/ partner/plant is ill, your job is not all it could be, you've got a headache, you have to write an essay and are bored reading this chapter. All these things can cause you strain, no matter how small. This type of strain is what constitutes 'ambient stress'. As with vulnerability, these levels can vary from person to person. The ambient stress of junior doctors going through the years of over-work and late hours may be high, while the ambient stress of retired people on a comfortable pension may be quite low. Alternatively, junior doctors may love their job and feel a low level of ambient stress, while retired people may be suffering major ambient stress due to losing self-worth, being under-stimulated, etc. (In addition, retirement itself can be seen as a life event, as we shall see.) As with beauty, stress is in the eye of the beholder.

The emotional atmosphere within families can be a cause of variable ambient stress and has been shown to be influential in people's levels of health. Expressed Emotion (or EE) is a means by which the family management of the psychosis can be judged as working to exacerbate symptoms or alleviate them. Families who cope better (and in some cases extremely well) manage to create a climate of tolerance that balances asking too much or too little of the individual with the symptoms and so reduces the latter's ambient stress. These families fall into what is known as the 'low Expressed Emotion' category. Families who find the illness difficult to accept or adjust to can become critical of the ill person as they are unaware of the effects of the illness or extremely frustrated with the challenges they have to deal with. They can also overcompensate for the illness and can infringe the person's autonomy in an attempt to ensure the person is cared for. These families fall into what is known as the 'high Expressed Emotion' category and can unwittingly increase the level of ambient everyday stress for the individual (Leff & Vaughn 1985).

The comments above also apply to professionals as we can increase the ambient stress of our clients if we deal with them in ways that denote criticism of them as people, or overcompensate and patronise them.

Life event stress

All people go through episodes or events that cause specific and high levels of stress. These episodes or events can be recognised as common experiences that most people report as placing them under high stress. Table 3.1 shows a rating for life experiences.

It has been acknowledged that many people who undergo a psychotic experience for the first time have recently experienced a traumatic life event (Ambelas 1987), such as a death in the family, or losing their job. What is also recognised is that some people will have short-lived psychotic experiences that are strongly linked to a life event. A good example of this is when people hear the voice of a loved one who has recently died. As we shall see below, this is not necessarily indicative of a psychosis.

Vulnerability

An individual's vulnerability is the disposition of the person to manifesting

Table 3.1 Ranking of life events in order of perceived severity (Ambelas 1987)

Rank	Life event
1	Death of a child
2	Death of a husband/wife
3	Being sent to gaol
4	Death of a close family member
5	Serious financial difficulty
6	Miscarriage or stillbirth
7	Court appearance for serious offences
8	Business failure
9	Marital separation due to arguments
10	Unwanted pregnancy
11	Divorced
12	Fired
13	Death of a close friend
14	Serious illness of family member
15	Unemployed for 1 month
16	Serious personal physical illness

Box 3.1 Components of vulnerability

Inborn vulnerability
◆ Genetically determined
◆ Reflected in the neurophysiology of the organism

Acquired vulnerability
◆ Specific to individual life experience
◆ Can include: specific disease, perinatal complications, family experience, adolescent peer interactions, previous life events

Source: Adapted from Zubin & Spring (1977)

---

symptoms of serious mental illness. At present, vulnerability is thought to be dependent on two components (see Box 3.1).

In other words, our vulnerability is determined by a combination of nature and nurture, as further demonstrated by Figure 3.1.

Within this hypothesis there will be a range of vulnerabilities within the population, with some people having vulnerability factors that place them at high probability of developing symptoms, whilst others will have a low probability with all levels in between.

One implication of this hypothesis is that it potentially challenges the concept that serious mental illness is confined to those diagnosed with psychosis. As Zubin & Spring (1977), in their seminal article on stress vulnerability with regard to schizophrenia, write: '… whether such vulnerability extends to all of mankind and whether it is the same sort that predisposes an individual to disorders other than schizophrenia remains an open question.' This would appear to be reinforced by the fact that some symptoms that are the corner-stone of diagnostic criteria are found in people who are not diagnosed. If

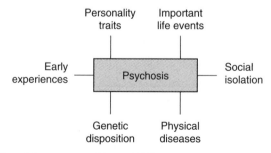

Figure 3.1 Vulnerability to stress (Honig 1993).

hallucinations are taken as an example, the percentage of the population who report visions or hear voices is greater than that of people diagnosed with a serious mental illness (Slade & Bentall 1988). Indeed, when consideration is given to individuals who hear their dead relatives in the early stages of bereavement or those who believe in the power of divine intervention, clairvoyance, telepathy, tarot cards and horoscopes, etc. we can see that one person's 'symptom' is another person's coping strategy, belief system or normal reaction to abnormal events.

This further adds to a deconstruction of our understanding of serious mental illness by means of the diagnostic process alone. Indeed, the stress vulnerability concept suggests that there is a potential that *any person* can develop and experience transient psychotic symptoms.

MANIFESTATION OF ILLNESS WITHIN THE STRESS VULNERABILITY MODEL

So why don't more people get diagnosed with serious mental illness? Well, there is a wide range of vulnerability factors and stress levels. The more stress people have, the more their health is placed under a strain, and the higher the probability they will reach a level where the vulnerability will be expressed. Perhaps most people have certain internal and external protective mechanisms to guard them against stress and therefore never reach the level of vulnerability necessary to develop psychosis. Horowitz (1986) has this to say in writing about stress response:

> *Additional evidence regarding the duration of stress responses and the frequency of occurrence of stress symptoms arose from the most deplorable circumstances imaginable. Studies of concentration camp victims indicated that profound and protracted stress may have chronic or permanent effects no matter what the predisposition of the pre-stress personality. This evidence was found in the decades of studying the survivors of the Nazi concentration camps ... Study after study ... confirm the occurrence of stress response syndromes, persisting for decades, in major proportions of those populations who survived ... As just one example 99% of the 226 Norwegian survivors of a Nazi concentration camp ... had some psychiatric disturbance when intensively surveyed years after their return to normal life.*

Concentration camp survivors must have undergone some of the most stressful experiences known to humans. With regard to this exploration, what is interesting is the conception that victims were not protected by their coping skills or their personality in the face of this overwhelming stress. What is less clear is how many of the 'psychiatric disturbances' noted would be classified as psychotic symptoms. Indeed, Lifton, cited by Horowitz (1986), outlines the experiences of Hiroshima victims who talked of 'pictures in their mind' and 'people walking with their skin peeling off'. These vivid portrayals were still present 17 years after the event. Others who have experienced less famous, but still significant, traumas have described intrusive thoughts, flashbacks, nightmares and depression. From such descriptions it would appear necessary to reconsider further the supposition that psychotic experience is isolated to a few individuals.

Psychosis: a unique experience

What should also be considered is that individuals who describe psychotic symptoms are more vulnerable to stress. These individuals will not have single, isolated experiences that are explainable in reference to recent life events, specific biological changes such as happen through illicit drug use and thyroid gland malfunction, but have a capacity either to experience complex psychotic symptoms for a long period of time or have frequent episodes of recurring symptoms. The differences between the individual who will be diagnosed with a serious mental illness and the individual who will experience specific phenomena such as auditory hallucinations is the basis of psychiatry.

COPING

The discussion so far has perceived the individual as a passive recipient of life's traumas. In reality, of course, the individual has personal attributes that influence their reaction to stressors. This reaction is termed 'coping'.

In common usage, coping seems to have a positive value judgement (in the same way that 'stress' tends to have a negative value judgement). This means that the word 'coping' seems to be used in positive instances. In actual fact, there is positive coping and negative coping.

Positive coping is the ability to ameliorate the strain and reduce stressors, whereas negative coping is where the stress or resultant strain is intensified. Often, coping strategies may give an immediate sense of relief, but in the long term will result in harm to the individual. These should be considered to be negative coping strategies. An example of this would be an individual who takes street drugs to alleviate symptoms, does experience some relief in the short term, but has an increase in symptoms in the long term (De Quardo, Carpenter & Tandon 1994).

Within the stress vulnerability model, coping can influence not only the possible onset of psychotic symptoms, but also the course and prognosis of the illness. Some commentators have argued that individuals who develop serious mental illness had limited positive coping skills prior to the illness, but this is a debatable issue. In this regard it would be well to remember the findings from concentration camp victims in that not being able to deal with stress in certain circumstances is not only understandable, but should be expected.

An individual's coping abilities are affected by many factors including: personality, culture, family experience and education, but it is one of the areas where health professionals can help or hinder individuals. Historically, for example, practitioners have been taught and advised to ignore clients when they reported voices and delusions (Hamilton 1984). Whilst the philosophy behind this was non-collusion with symptoms, as this may reinforce them, individuals experienced this attitude as a negation of their experiences. This negation actually increased stress for many.

The notion of not acknowledging the experience appears to relate to the utopian world, previously described, where the aim of treatment is total eradication of symptoms. Subsequently, it was perceived that the manner in which individuals cope with psychosis, irrespective of whether they had a positive or negative effect upon their quality of life, was irrelevant. It is only recently that people have begun to realise that there are more ways to treat and cope with psychosis than medication alone. There is still much to learn from those who experience and cope with psychotic symptoms. Investigations into coping strategies have helped to identify that some people have developed very positive relationships with their voices. As a direct consequence a number of diverse coping strategies have been successfully cultivated. These range from diverting attention from the voices to acknowledging them rather then denying them (for examples see Carr 1988, Falloon & Talbot 1981, Nelson, Thrasher & Barnes 1991, Tarrier 1987). Indeed, the predominate work of Romme & Esher (1993) has helped us to:

1. uncover the important concept of coping
2. understand the advantages enjoyed by those who succeed, despite all the odds, in coping well with their experiences, environment and vulnerability.

Coping and prognosis

If we accept that coping can ameliorate the symptoms of mental illness, it would follow that interventions should promote positive coping. A reality is that many individuals find the illness blocks or hinders effective coping (as will be discussed with regard to negative symptoms). What should also concern us is the possibility that society and, indeed, the mental health system itself, can also block good coping or increase the stress on individuals.

Warner (1994) identifies the following factors that can influence relapse in the individual:

1. drug use
2. stressful family environment
3. labelling and stigma
4. social isolation or reintegration
5. social role rehabilitation
6. patterns of institutional care.

If the above are explored it is possible to question whether the mental health system is effective in reducing the negative aspects of these factors. While drug use and family environment are discussed in later chapters, the other issues remain a constant area of concern. Services do little to address negative stereotypes such as whether clients are employable, have a role in or are perceived as valued members of society. If we take a fresh look at relapse and the so-called 'revolving door client' we may begin to notice that these individuals have the greatest blocks to effective coping. In these cases we need to look for creative means to restore the individual's sense of role. This requires us to do more than alleviate symptoms, but also address political issues such as exclusion from employment, education, and indeed all areas of human life.

CONCLUSIONS

Stress vulnerability is a model which has opened up the area of mental illness. It has moved us from seeing individual sufferers as being alien to viewing them as people with extraordinary experiences. We must continue to see mental illness as a normal aspect of human experience. The work of the mental health practitioner is to join with individuals who have these extraordinary experiences and reintegrate them and their experiences into society.

 Cross references

Chapter 1: gives an insight into how stress, life events and coping can influence the manifestation and outcomes for an individual. It should be read prior to or in conjunction with this chapter

Chapters 4 and 9: from an assessment and intervention standpoint contain references to stress vulnerability; however, it should be pointed out that all of Section 2 content derives and is influenced by the model

References

Ambelas A 1987 Life events and mania: a special relationship? British Journal of Psychiatry 150:135–240

Carr V 1988 Patients techniques for coping with schizophrenia: an exploratory study. British Journal of Medical Psychology 61:339–352

De Quardo J R, Carpenter C F, Tandon R 1994 Patterns of substance abuse in schizophrenia: nature and significance. Journal of Psychiatric Research 28(3):267–275

Falloon I R H, Talbot R E 1981 Persistent auditory hallucinations: coping mechanisms and implications for management. Psychological Medicine 11:329–339

Haghighat R, Littlewood, R 1995 What should we call patients with schizophrenia? A sociolinguistic analysis. Psychiatric Bulletin 19:407–410

Hamilton M 1984 Fish's schizophrenia, 3rd edn. Wright, Bristol

Honig A 1993 Medication and hearing voices. In: Romme M, Escher S (eds) Accepting voices. Mind, London, p 237

Horowitz M D 1986 Stress response syndromes. Aronson, New Jersey

Leff J, Vaughn C 1985 Expressed emotion in families. Guilford, New York

Nelson H E, Thrasher S, Barnes T R E 1991 Practical ways of alleviating auditory hallucinations. British Medical Journal 302:6772, 327

Romme M, Esher S (eds) 1993 Accepting voices. Mind, London

Slade P D, Bentall R P 1988 Sensory deception: a scientific analysis of hallucination. Croom Helm, London

Tarrier N 1987 An investigation of residual psychotic symptoms in discharged schizophrenic patients. British Journal of Clinical Psychology 26:141–143

Warner R 1994 Recovery from schizophrenia: psychiatry and political economy, 2nd edn. Routledge, London

Zubin J, Spring B 1977 Vulnerability: a new view of schizophrenia. Journal of Abnormal Psychology 86:260–266

Annotated further reading

Kingdon D G, Turkington D 1995 Cognitive behaviour therapy of schizophrenia. Guildford Press, London

Chapters 3 and 4 of this book, 'Vulnerability and life events' and 'Suggestibility,' contain a valuable, in-depth summary of the issues raised within this chapter. It is a concise, user friendly account of manifestation of illness.

Zubin J, Spring B 1977 Vulnerability: a new view on schizophrenia. Journal of Abnormal Psychology 86:103–126

Although the author recognises that this is an old reference, the article itself is a seminal work that still has relevance to today's practitioners. The article summarises various views on the manifestation of illness prior to the stress vulnerability model.

4

Severe mental illness: symptoms, signs and diagnosis

Tom K J Craig

INTRODUCTION

This chapter describes the phenomenology of severe mental illness, starting with definitions of abnormal experiences and closing with a brief overview of current diagnostic guidelines for schizophrenia and the major affective disorders. It is aimed at non-medical members of the multidisciplinary team who need to carry out front-line assessments and to undertake sophisticated psychosocial interventions that call for precision in assessing the abnormal experiences of their clients.

Consider, for example, the assessment of a young man who has been referred with a 3 month history of anxiety and depression during his first term at university. The assessment proceeds slowly as his account is vague and rambling. He says that he has always been a loner who has difficulty making friends. He has not settled into university life, and has fallen out with another student after complaining about a radio that was playing all night. He has subsequently heard this student referring to him as a 'poofter' though the student denied having said any such thing. The noises continue to keep him awake and he is convinced that this is deliberate. The more he thinks about it, the more certain he is that something unpleasant is going on, involving spreading rumours about his sexuality to other students who are now avoiding him.

The questions asked by the assessor from this point on are crucial. One might be dealing with a shy young man with a rather prickly, sensitive personality who has been unlucky enough to have been placed next door to an extroverted insomniac. But it is also possible that his story reflects an altogether more sinister process. Schizophrenia, arguably the most serious mental illness, may begin in just this way – anxiety and perplexity associated with vague persecutory ideas. While the first explanation might be resolved by a change in residence and his shyness helped by counselling, this is unlikely to be enough for a major mental illness. Equally, one would not wish to recommend drug treatment without first obtaining more definite evidence of mental illness. But how to continue? What questions are most helpful? What answers should we look for?

AN ORGANISATIONAL FRAMEWORK FOR ASSESSMENT

Mental disorders affect individuals' cognitive processes, their beliefs, perceptions and outward behaviour. Many of the phenomena of mental disorders lie on a continuum that include everyday experiences, making it quite difficult to decide when an experience should be labelled abnormal. A useful rule of thumb is that experiences are likely to be abnormal when they are involuntary, out of proportion to any situation that precipitated them and cannot be turned off or greatly reduced by conscious effort.

A fundamental principle in describing and classifying these abnormal experiences is the distinction of *form* from *content*. Content refers to what people describe as their mental experiences. It is unique to the individuals concerned and influenced by previous experiences and the culture and society in which they dwell. Form, on the other hand, is a codified description of the common threads of these experiences that are recognisable across individuals. For example, consider two young men, both of whom are suffering from schizophrenia. One, in a small village in Upper Egypt, states that he is possessed by a djinni that has resisted all efforts at exorcism. As evidence for this possession, he says that the djinni is able to take over his will and can cause him to shout out even when he tries to keep silent. At times he hears the djinni laughing at him and passing rude remarks about his appearance. The other young man has spent all his life in London. He also believes his will has been replaced by an alien power but attributes this to a microchip that has been implanted in his ear while he was asleep. This chip receives signals from a computer some miles away and the controllers can make him shout out when he tries to keep silent. They often laugh at his reactions to their torments. They also pass disparaging remarks about the clothes he is wearing and his personal hygiene. While the specific *content* of the experiences of these two men clearly reflect their different social origins, the *form* of experience is similar – both report that their will has been replaced by an alien power and both hear voices that comment on their actions.

A basic schema outlining the forms taken by common mental symptoms and observed behaviour is given in Table 4.1. The framework is a useful starting point for a discussion of the assessment of an individual's mental state.

1. Assessing mood

This is often an early step in the assessment although it is usual to refine initial impressions as the interview proceeds.

Tension symptoms

Questions include:

◆ Have there been times lately when you have been worried, tense or anxious?
◆ Have you had difficulties relaxing?
◆ Have you been very tired and exhausted for no particular reason?

This first group of symptoms include complaints of worry, apprehension, restlessness, muscular tension, irritability and excessive tiredness or fatigue.

Table 4.1 Overview of a schema for the assessment of mental state

Topic	Subjective experience (symptoms, complaints)	Observed behaviour (signs)
Mood (affect)	**Tension:** worry, nervous tension, muscular tension, tiredness, restlessness	Tense, fidgety, pacing
	Anxiety: free-floating anxiety, anxious foreboding, panic attacks, phobic avoidance	Anxious tense appearance, sweaty, shaky, shallow rapid breathing
	Irritability	Irritability/impatience
	Depression: loss of interests, tedium vitae, hopelessness, suicide, guilt, self-depreciation	Sad expression, tearful, frozen gloom
	Elation: expansive mood, excitement, grandiose thoughts	Euphoria, excitement, irritation/hostility
		Perplexity Incongruity Blunting or flattening Suspiciousness
Body functions	**Sleep problems:** delayed sleep, early waking, middle insomnia	
	Appetite and weight change **Altered levels of activity:** subjective slowing or excitement	Psychomotor retardation, excitement, stupor
Thinking	Thought flow and structure, thought echo, withdrawal, loud thoughts Thought content (delusions) Replacement of the 'will'	Incoherence, neologisms, thought blocking
Perception	Heightened/diminished perception Depersonalisation/derealisation Hallucinations	Behaves as though hallucinating
Cognition	Orientation, concentration, memory	Consciousness, orientation, concentration, memory

These occur on a continuum with normality, can occur singly or with each other and are seen in most disorders. Although they are non-specific, they are good indicators of the severity of distress.

Anxiety with autonomic nervous system arousal

Questions include:

◆ Have there been times lately when you have been very panicky or frightened?
◆ Do you ever get fearful that something terrible is about to happen?
◆ Have you ever been so frightened you simply had to stop what you were doing?

If any of these are endorsed:

◆ When you have felt like that, did you also have palpitations/butterflies in your stomach/sweating/giddiness/difficulty in breathing?

As with symptoms of tension, just about everyone will have been anxious at some time. It is pathological when it is out of proportion to the circumstances that provoked it and when it persists against all efforts at self-control for hours at a time. Anxiety is distinguished from tension by the presence of one or more physical sensations of autonomic nervous system arousal, such as fluttering sensations in the abdomen ('butterflies'), palpitations, sweating, tremor and urinary urgency. While anxiety is often triggered by a worrying thought or by some phobic situation, it can also arise out of the blue (*free-floating anxiety*) or be associated with an apprehension that something dreadful is about to occur (*anxious foreboding*). *Panic attacks* are discrete episodes of marked fearfulness, beginning abruptly and rising rapidly to a crescendo that may last up to an hour after which the anxiety gradually abates, leaving the sufferer feeling exhausted, drained and shaky. The attacks may be associated with escape responses – for example, the agoraphobic who rushes out of a supermarket or off a crowded bus. Common generalised phobias, which result in significant social impairment, include agoraphobia and social phobia.

Depression

Questions include:

◆ Have you been depressed or low spirited?
◆ Have you lost interest in work/hobbies/seeing friends/appearance?
◆ How do you see the future? Has life ever seemed not worth living?
◆ What opinion do you have of yourself compared with others?
◆ Have you been feeling particularly guilty or blaming yourself at all?
◆ Do you get the feeling others are blaming you for things?

The complaint of depressed mood can have many different expressions (e.g. sadness, low spirits, gloom or an incapacity to enjoy anything). Tearfulness may be a clue to severity but very severe depression may also be a frozen misery that is subjectively beyond tears. A reduction in the usual reactivity of mood to day to day events is a fairly good guide to severity. When the mood is very low, the sufferer's mind will be almost totally absorbed by gloomy topics. The syndrome of depression will typically also include non-specific 'tension' symptoms as well as poor concentration, sleep disturbance, appetite disturbance and loss of interests. In addition there may be a loss of hope for the future that may extend to a feeling that life holds nothing of interest and little to live for (*tedium vitae*) and even to suicidal thoughts or acts. The depressed mood may show a characteristic diurnal variation, being worst during the early part of the day. Depressed people lose confidence in their day to day dealings with other people, withdraw from social contact and feel inferior or worthless (*self-depreciation*). Feelings of lassitude and general ill health can result in *hypochondriacal* preoccupations with some imagined and often fearful physical disease. *Pathological guilt* refers to overconcern with actions that most people would not take very seriously. The sufferer recognises that this guilt is exaggerated but cannot help feeling it all the same. This symptom can intensify to the point where individuals blame themselves for almost everything that goes wrong. A similar experience is that of *guilty ideas of reference*, in which sufferers feel they are accused of some blameworthy act, which they may not actually have committed.

Elation

Questions include:

◆ Have there been times when you felt particularly cheerful without any reason?
◆ Have you felt very full of energy or full of exciting ideas?
◆ Have you felt especially healthy?
◆ Have you any special talents or abilities?

People with pathologically elevated mood are euphoric and elated, excited, irritable and impatient with those around who seem slower in their bodies and wits than themselves. When euphoric, the mood often has an infectious quality. Linked with these changes in mood are various alterations in speech and motor activity that can be observed in the assessment. Sufferers are typically overtalkative and difficult to interrupt. Concentration is often objectively impaired yet sufferers experience the opposite, feeling themselves to be full of exciting ideas and of above average ability and intelligence. Self-esteem is exaggerated and they may be excessively optimistic about the future, feeling that nothing can stand in their way. There may be marked motor overactivity with a decreased need for sleep and increased sexual drive.

Reckless actions are common – inappropriate shopping sprees, reckless driving, quarrels and generally foolish behaviour that is out of character. The changes in mood and activity may also be linked to *grandiose beliefs* – for example, that the sufferer is of extraordinarily high intellect or is a gifted inventor.

2. Assessing thought processes

Questions include:

❖ Can you think clearly? Have you any difficulty in concentrating?
❖ Is there any interference with your thinking?

Difficulties in concentrating, making decisions and feeling muddled are common accompaniments of most mental illnesses, but there are some changes in thinking processes that are linked to more specific disorders.

Obsessional ruminations and compulsions

Questions include:

❖ Do you have to keep checking things you know you have already done?
❖ Do you have to spend a lot of time on personal cleanliness?
❖ Do you get awful thoughts coming into your mind even when you try to keep them out?

These are experienced as the patient's own thoughts, yet are intrusive, unwanted and irresistible or incapable of being stopped for any length of time. The intrusive thoughts may be associated with compulsive rituals involving checking, counting or cleaning. *Obsessional incompleteness* involves the intrusive need to get everything right before a task can be considered complete. Sufferers may, for example, rehearse an event in their mind over and over again in order to convince themselves that they can remember every detail.

Many other symptoms can easily be confused with obsessions. For example, neglect of everyday tasks while brooding over unhappy events may be mistaken for obsessional incompleteness and hypochondriacal fears of contracting a disease may be confused with the obsessional fear of contamination though the former carry no subjective sense of resistance. The experience of the intrusion of the unwanted thoughts against conscious resistance, coupled with the awareness that the thoughts are their own, are the key features for distinguishing obsessional ruminations. Even when resistance has waned after years of struggle, patients seldom forget the power of their initial reactions.

Abnormalities in the possession of thought

These include a variety of experiences through which individuals come to believe that the innermost secret workings of their mind are accessible to outsiders. These experiences are indicative of a psychotic illness. Questions include:

◆ **Thought echo**: Do you ever hear your thoughts repeated or echoed?

Sufferers experience an immediate repetition of their last thought. They are aware that these are their own thoughts that are echoed but are unable to control the experience.

◆ **Thought broadcasting**: Have you ever heard your thoughts spoken aloud, so that someone standing nearby could hear them?

With this symptom, the usually silent process of thinking is experienced 'aloud' so that someone standing nearby would be able to hear the thoughts. Sometimes this is elaborated so that sufferers feel that others can hear their thoughts even when they are not in the same room. The experience of hearing thoughts aloud differs from auditory hallucinations, in that sufferers are aware they are 'hearing' their own thoughts. Both thought echo and loud thoughts differ from the ruminations seen in obsessional disorders in the relative lack of consistency or theme to the content of the thoughts and by the fact that obsessional ruminations do not have the 'aloud' quality.

◆ **Thought insertion:** Are thoughts put into your mind that are not your own?

Here there is the loss of the normal sense of ownership of thoughts. This experience is almost always accompanied by a delusional explanation, for example, that the thoughts have been placed there by telepathy or X-rays. The quality of 'alienness' is crucial. These thoughts are not simply unwanted as might be the case with, say, wicked thoughts that are 'blamed' on the devil or intrusive obsessional ruminations where people acknowledge ownership of the thoughts even if they blame some outside influence for leading them to think that way.

◆ **Thought block and withdrawal**: Do your thoughts ever stop abruptly so that there are none left in your mind? Are your thoughts ever taken out of your head, as though some outside force were removing them?

Sufferers experience sudden stoppage of all thoughts. The experience is passive but abrupt. Thoughts were flowing quite freely before and there is no sense of the individual searching for their thoughts as, for example, happens when one loses ones train of thought at times of stress. In thought withdrawal, the experience is elaborated by a delusion that the thoughts have been withdrawn by someone or something. The experience goes beyond the simple delusion that thoughts are being read in that clients experience the physical removal of their thoughts.

◆ **Abnormalities in the possession of a 'will'**: Do you feel under the control of some force or power as though you were a robot or a zombie without a will of your own … does this ever make your movements without your willing it or use your voice or your handwriting?

This is perhaps the most dramatic of all symptoms of severe mental illness and also one of the most difficult to elucidate accurately. The essential element is that the sufferer's will is taken over or replaced by some external force or agency and that this is not under the sufferer's control. There are dozens of different ways this may be experienced, for example, the replacement of handwriting, voice, bodily movements and decision making (will). Sufferers often believe they are victims of possession, having been turned into a zombie or puppet of the higher being or force. This is a very different experience from believing that one's life is determined by fate or that God ultimately controls everything. It is not that one's choices are constrained but rather that one has no capacity to choose at all, that any feeling of personal intentions has been replaced by the alien will. The only 'normal' situation in which this is seen may be in socially sanctioned trance states – for example the automatic writing reported by some spiritualists or the shaman who induces a possession state to communicate with the gods.

Abnormalities in the content of thought (delusions)

A delusion is a belief that is held with absolute and compelling conviction, is not amenable to modification by experience or argument, is largely idiosyncratic, impossible, incredible or false and described clearly by the sufferer and not simply assented to following a leading question. The idiosyncratic nature of delusional beliefs helps to distinguish delusions from eccentric beliefs that are part of belonging to a particular religious, political or other social group (e.g. accounts of alien abduction).

Delusions are typically subclassified according to their basis in abnormal mood (e.g. delusions concerning sinfulness, catastrophe, guilt in severe depression and grandeur in mania). Such delusions are said to be 'mood congruent' in contrast to 'incongruent' delusions that have no such basis and are thought to be more typical of schizophrenia.

Some commonly encountered delusions include:

◆ Delusions of *reference*, in which sufferers are convinced that people are saying things with a double meaning or that items in newspapers, on the TV or advertisements refer to themselves and that people are tracking them, spying on them or checking up on them in some way.

◆ In delusions of *misidentification,* innocent bystanders seem to be members of the Mafia or the secret police, doctors and nurses are impostors, and even family or friends have been replaced by look-alikes (*Capgras syndrome*).

◆ Delusions of *persecution* are perhaps the most commonly encountered delusions and involve someone or some organisation on a campaign to harm, defame or destroy the sufferer.

Other fairly common delusions include *grandiose identity* (beliefs that the sufferer is of royal blood, Christ, etc.); *grandiose ability* (e.g. chosen for a special mission in life, a mathematical genius, etc.); *guilt, catastrophe, depersonalisation* and *hypochondriacal* delusions.

Some delusions appear as primary experiences in themselves. Their content cannot be explained by other delusions and seem to arise from some very ordinary perception. For example, one patient had a sudden insight that he was God when a traffic light turned from amber to green; another 'knew' the devil was inside his daughter at the instant of a flash of lightning. These experiences are called 'primary delusions' and are thought to be strongly suggestive of schizophrenia. They sometimes occur after a period of perplexity in which the sufferer is vaguely aware that something strange is going on – familiar surroundings seem changed in some way, and there is an ominous or threatening atmosphere (*delusional mood*).

3. Assessing perceptions

Questions include:

◆ Is there anything unusual about the way things sound, or look, or smell, or taste?

Perceptual experiences can be diminished, heightened or distorted by severe mental illnesses.

Diminished perceptions

These include the subjective experience of sounds being dull, colours lifeless and tastes bland. Heightened perceptions include sounds that are unnaturally clear, a vivid intensity of colours and an intrusive perception of patterns in everyday objects.

Hallucinations

Questions include:

◆ Do you ever hear noises or voices when there is no one around to explain it?
◆ What does the voice say?
◆ Do you ever hear several voices talking about you?
◆ Does the voice(s) comment on what you are doing?
◆ Do they speak directly to you? Do they give you orders?
◆ Do you ever have visions or seen things that others could not see?
◆ Have you ever noticed smells that other people seem not to notice?

Hallucinations are false perceptions in the sense that there is usually no adequate external stimulus to account for the experience. However, some may be triggered as, for example, the young man who heard the police talking about him while listening to a record. Hallucinations can occur in any sense (i.e. hearing, smell, touch, etc.). Hallucinations do not necessarily imply mental illness. For example, fleeting hallucinations are fairly common following bereavement. Those affected see the lost person in some familiar setting (e.g. sitting in their favourite chair); may hear the loved one saying some familiar phrase, feel a comforting pat on the shoulder or catch a whiff of a familiar scent.

Pathological hallucinations are typically grouped according to the sensory modality affected – auditory, visual, tactile, gustatory (taste) and olfactory. They may be highly invasive, frequent and interfere with virtually all normal function or may occur largely in the background with little apparent impact on ordinary functioning.

Auditory hallucinations. These may involve noises such as the sound of an engine running, electrical hums or rumbling. There may be voices speaking directly to sufferers (second person auditory hallucinations) or talking about them, either commenting on their behaviour, what they are wearing, etc., or having a conversation with another 'voice' (third person auditory hallucinations). The nature of the 'voice' may be congruent with mood, so, for example tending to be deprecatory with depressive delusions (e.g. 'you are a sinner and will burn in hell').

Visual hallucinations. These may be fleeting and fragmentary (e.g. flashes of light), formed objects or even vivid and complex scenes. Visual hallucinations are particularly associated with organic brain diseases such as temporal lobe epilepsy and delirium but also occur in schizophrenia and other functional psychoses.

Olfactory hallucinations. These include simple hallucinations of perfume or burning, and others with delusional elaboration such as patients who can smell the poison gas pumped into the room by their persecutors.

Tactile hallucinations. These include feelings of touch as well as of more noxious insertions of wires or needles into the body.

Gustatory hallucinations. These include tastes of poison in food. For example, one man claimed to be able to distinguish two varieties of cyanide in the food at a local café – one the 'usual' cyanide poison and the other a special ingredient put in the food by the hospital and designed to be helpful in building a resistance to the toxic effects of the former.

4. Assessing appearance, speech and behaviour

So far, we have dealt with the multitude of complaints that people with severe mental illness may express at interview, either spontaneously or in response to questioning. In addition, their behaviour during the interview holds important clues.

General appearance

This concerns fairly obvious abnormalities – poor self-care, bizarre appearance and dress and evidence of self-neglect or injury. More specific abnormalities include the presence of mannerisms, posturing and stereotypies. *Mannerisms* are odd stylised movements that suggest a special meaning or purpose (e.g. saluting, twirling); *posturing* is the assumption of an uncomfortable posture for hours at a time and *stereotypies* are repetitive movements such as rocking, nodding and grimacing. There may also be one or more inappropriate behaviours: for example giggling, behaving as if hallucinating, acting in an exaggerated, embarrassing or irreverent manner.

Observed abnormalities in speech/thinking

In addition to non-specific changes to the tone, pitch and volume of speech, a number of changes are characteristically associated with severe mental illness. These include *pressure of speech* (a rush of words that can be interrupted only with difficulty), *flight of ideas* (the patient skips from topic to topic with frequent punning and sound associations, though the logic of the associations is usually apparent), *rambling* in a vague and muddled way, *perseveration* (in which a particular theme is repeated over and over so as to be meaningless) and frank *incoherence* (in which there is no logical connections between one part of a sentence and another – e.g. 'I've seen the end of the circles of the moon through the miracle working of the prophets'). *Poverty of speech* describes a severe form of rambling in that the patient speaks freely but so vaguely that no information is conveyed. This differs from restricted quantity of speech when the patient repeatedly fails to answer at all, requiring repeated prompting, in extreme form ending in mutism.

Observed abnormalities of affect

This includes observed anxiety, depression, elation and hostile irritability or suspiciousness at interview. More difficult states to identify reliably include *perplexity*, in which patients look puzzled and cannot provide adequate explanations for their abnormal experiences. *Lability of mood* describes frequent and abrupt changes in mood – that is, at one moment fearful, at the next elated and at another tearful. *Blunted (flattened) affect* involves a global reduction in the usual emotional expressions seen in social interactions. There is little facial expression and speech is flat and emotionless. Apparently distressing topics may be discussed with indifference. *Incongruous affect* refers to a state where the range of emotional expression is normal or even increased but in the opposite direction to that expected (e.g. laughter on hearing distressing news or when discussing a sad event).

Objective orientation, concentration and memory

Finally, it is customary to check out the important cognitive functions of orientation, concentration and memory. Can respondents account for themselves and are they aware of where they are and the date? Is concentration (typically assessed by counting backwards from 100 in steps of 7) and short term memory (tested by recall of a fictitious name and address at 5 minutes) intact? Any suggestion of impairments in these areas would call for a more specialised assessment that is beyond the scope of this chapter (but see Kopelman 1994 for an excellent review).

DIAGNOSIS: THE 'TOP-DOWN' APPROACH

To this point we have provided working definitions of the common symptoms of severe mental illness and some suggested questions for accessing these. The next step involves an exploration of how these symptoms cluster together and an outline of modern clinical diagnostic systems as they apply to the functional psychoses. The approach favoured has been described as the 'empirical' approach to diagnosis. It begins with the astute observations that certain complaints or observations tend to occur in a pattern that is recognisable between sufferers and over time. These patterns, borrowing from medical roots, are often referred to as 'diagnoses', even though it is accepted that the conditions they describe may not represent diseases in the usual biological model of medicine.

All diagnostic systems in current use have to cope with three facts:

1. A small number of disorders are known to be the result of brain injury or disease.
2. People suffering from these organic brain disorders can experience any of the symptoms described earlier. So people with temporal lobe epilepsy may experience auditory hallucinations; those with brain tumours may present with symptoms that are entirely indistinguishable from schizophrenia; and some people in the early stages of dementia may experience severe depression.
3. Similarly, many symptoms, including hallucinations, thought disorder and delusions, can be caused by the ingestion of psychoactive substances.

All classification systems, therefore, distinguish 'organic' and 'functional' disorders and are arranged hierarchically so that it is only possible to end up with a label of say, schizophrenia, after organic brain disease has been excluded. Many classification systems also apply these hierarchical rules to distinguish functional psychoses from neurotic disorders. The term 'psychotic' is used as a shorthand expression for a disorder in which people's capacity to recognise reality, their thinking processes, judgements and communications are seriously impaired, together with the presence of delusions and hallucinations. For example, schizophrenia takes precedence in diagnosis over bipolar psychoses if criteria for both are present and affective psychoses in turn take precedence over simple depression and anxiety. Thus each disorder tends to manifest the symptoms of those lower down the hierarchy but not higher up (Foulds 1965, Sturt 1981).

With the exception of the handful of conditions for which a cause is known, most classification systems are descriptive and reflect a consensus between experts as to which symptoms and signs should be put together under one diagnostic grouping. The ICD-10 classification of mental and behavioural disorders (1992), for example, brought together experts from around the world, in order to identify those aspects of mental disorders that were commonly encountered across cultures and for which some consensus could be obtained. The broad result of their deliberations are outlined in Box 4.1. These broad categories are further broken down into a large number of separate conditions, each of which is defined in terms of the commonly encountered symptoms, typical course and the cause of the disorder if this is known. Two of these broad categories are of particular concern to this chapter.

1. Schizophrenia, schizotypal and delusional disorders

Schizophrenia

The concept of schizophrenia owes much to two psychiatrists working at

---

Box 4.1 ICD-10 classification of mental and behavioural disorders

F00–F09 Organic mental disorders (dementia, delirium, organic amnesia)
F10–F19 Psychoactive substance use (intoxication, harmful use, dependency, withdrawal)
F20–F29 Schizophrenia, schizotypal and delusional disorders
F30–F39 Mood (affective) disorders
F40–F48 Neurotic, stress-related and somatoform disorders (phobic disorder, obsessive compulsive disorder, stress reactions, somatoform disorder)
F50–F59 Behavioural syndromes (eating disorder, sleep disorder, sexual dysfunction)
F60–F69 Disorders of adult personality
F70–F79 Mental retardation
F80–F89 Disorders of psychological development (speech disorders, autism)
F90–F98 Behavioural disorders in childhood (hyperkinetic disorder, conduct disorder, emotional disorder, tics, etc.)
F99 Mental disorder not classified elsewhere

---

the turn of the century. Emil Kraepelin (1896) noticed the characteristic disturbances in thinking and behaviour that typify the disorder which he labelled 'dementia praecox'. He went on to distinguish this disorder from others that had recurring or periodic episodes involving mania and depression. His view of the disorder was a generally gloomy one, seeing it as having clear biological origins and an almost universally deteriorating course. Few psychiatrists have found the course quite as gloomy as suggested by Kraepelin, though the underlying belief in a largely incurable and progressive disease continues to influence classification systems to this day. The term 'schizophrenia' was introduced by Eugen Bleuler in 1911 to describe a disorder that encompassed most of the features of Kraepelin's dementia praecox together with some important additional observations. Bleuler maintained the separation from manic depressive psychosis but pointed out that affective symptoms could also occur in schizophrenia. His concept was based on the identification of a small number of primary symptoms, which occurred in all cases. The most important of these were a form of thought disorder (loosening of associations), an autistic withdrawal from reality, ambivalence and incongruous or restricted emotional expression. He regarded hallucinations and delusions as secondary to these primary defects. He had a more optimistic view of the outcome of the illness that partially reflected the tendency of his diagnostic approach to include a broader range of conditions but also may well have reflected a genuine improvement in the outcome of the disorder in Switzerland at that time.

Most modern approaches to the diagnosis of schizophrenia can be traced to one or both of these 'founding fathers' with variations on the way symptoms are packaged together. A possibly helpful distinction has been to distinguish 'positive' and 'negative' symptoms of the illness. Another German psychiatrist, Kurt Schneider (1959), is responsible for what has come to be the definitive list of positive symptoms. These 'symptoms of the first rank' include abnormalities in the possession of thoughts (loud thoughts, thought echo, withdrawal, broadcast, insertion or alien thoughts); auditory hallucinations in the 'third person'; passivity experiences; delusional mood and delusional perception. They carry no special theoretical or prognostic significance but most psychiatrists will diagnose schizophrenia when these symptoms are present and there is no organic brain disease or recent history of drug abuse to explain them. These positive symptoms can be distinguished from the 'negative' symptoms of apathy, slowness, incoherence and poverty of speech. Negative symptoms are particularly important markers of prognosis: those in whom negative symptoms are prominent tend to do badly in terms of future social function and adjustment. Environmental conditions of understimulation appear to amplify the manifestation of negative symptoms while overstimulation can trigger positive symptoms.

The ICD-10 diagnostic criteria for schizophrenia are set out in Box 4.2. The diagnosis is characterised by distortions in thinking and perception and by inappropriate or blunted affect. Characteristically, individuals' sense of self is eroded so that they come to believe that their most intimate thoughts and feelings are known by others, while mysterious forces seem to be able to influence their actions. Hallucinations are common and perception is usually disturbed in other ways. Thinking becomes vague, obscure and speech may be incomprehensible. Breaks in the train of thought are common and thoughts may appear to be withdrawn by some outside agency. Mood is typically shallow, incongruous or blunted. The onset may be sudden but is more typically gradual with the slow emergence of odd ideas and behaviour. The course of the condition is variable.

Subtypes of the disorder are widely recognised. The most common are as follows.

1. **Paranoid**: the clinical picture is dominated by stable persecutory delusions and hallucinations (usually auditory) with only minor changes in affect, volition and speech. Negative symptoms may be present but do not dominate the clinical picture.

2. **Hebephrenic**: affective symptoms are the most prominent with only fleeting or fragmentary hallucinations and delusions. Behaviour is often

---

Box 4.2 ICD-10 classification of mental and behavioural disorders: schizophrenia

Any one of (a) to (d) or any two of (e) to (h) for 1 month or more, on most days and not due to organic brain disease or alcohol or drug intoxication, dependence or withdrawal.

a. Thought echo, insertion, withdrawal or broadcasting.

b. Delusions of control, influence or passivity, clearly referred to body or limb movements or specific thoughts, actions or sensations; delusional perception.

c. Third person auditory hallucinations, either running commentary on actions or discussing the patient among themselves.

d. Persistent delusions that are culturally inappropriate and completely impossible.

e. Persistent hallucinations when accompanied by fleeting or half-formed delusions without clear affective content, or by persistent overvalued ideas or when occurring every day for weeks or months on end.

f. Breaks or interpolations in the train of thought, incoherence, irrelevant speech or neologisms.

g. Catatonic behaviour.

h. 'Negative' symptoms of apathy, paucity of speech and blunting or incongruity of affect, usually resulting in social withdrawal. Not due to depression or neuroleptic medication.

---

irresponsible and unpredictable and mannerisms are common. The mood is often shallow or incongruous, accompanied by giggling or self-absorbed smiling, grimaces and vague hypochondriacal complaints. Thought is disorganised and speech rambling and incoherent. 'Negative' symptoms of blunted affect and loss of volition are prominent. This form of schizophrenia usually starts between the ages of 15 and 25 years and tends to have a poor prognosis because the loss of drive leaves patients aimless and devoid of purpose in life.

3. **Catatonic**: psychomotor symptoms dominate the clinical picture. The patient may alternate between the extremes of excitement and stupor, adopt constrained attitudes and postures that are maintained for hours at a time. Other features, of negativism, rigidity, waxy flexibility and command automatism may also be present. Catatonia is now very rarely seen in Western industrialised society. This has led some to speculate that catatonic symptoms are a somatic expression of delusions of possession, symbolic thinking and

fear, much as bodily symptoms of hysteria are conversion symptoms for anxiety. Both catatonia and hysteria have receded in the West as the population has developed a capacity for expressing emotions in psychological rather than purely bodily terms.

Persistent delusional disorders

Sometimes, the only abnormality encountered comprises a long-standing delusion or set of related delusions that are not congruent with any obvious mood disorder. Often these are persecutory but they may also involve jealousy, be hypochondriacal, or comprise beliefs that parts of the body are misshapen or give off an unpleasant smell. The content of the delusion can often be related to the individual's life situation. Depression may be present intermittently and a few cases develop limited olfactory or tactile hallucinations. However, more classical schizophrenic symptoms such as marked blunting of affect or the experience of passivity symptoms are not seen. Onset is commonly in middle age (except for beliefs about having a misshapen body, which tend to begin in early adult life). The ICD-10 diagnostic criteria require symptoms to be present for at least 3 months in the absence of brain disease and clear schizophrenic symptoms.

Acute, transient psychotic disorders

These are among the most controversial disorders, not least because it is not at all clear where these end and schizophrenia begins. The ICD-10 recommends restricting the use of this category to disorders that have an abrupt onset (within 2 weeks) and where there is a typical syndrome and an associated acute stress. There are said to be two typical syndromes. In the first, hallucinations, delusions and perceptual disturbances are marked but highly changeable from day to day and even hour to hour. Emotional turmoil with intense but transient feelings of elation, irritability and anxiety is common. Complete recovery usually occurs within a couple of months. In the second syndrome, the picture is that of schizophrenia, with relatively stable symptoms, but with an explosive onset and a very short course with recovery occurring within a month of onset. The validity of these syndromes as separate diagnoses is hotly disputed. It is likely, for example, that they represent one end of the spectrum of schizophrenic disorder or some variant of an affective psychosis.

Schizoaffective disorder

The co-occurrence of typical schizophrenic and affective symptoms is well recognised and presents a challenge to all diagnostic systems. In ICD-10, this is classified in the same broad group as schizophrenia. The affective symptoms can be either depressive or manic in nature. The diagnosis should be made only when the schizophrenic and affective symptoms are prominent within the same episode of illness, either simultaneously or within a few days of each other, and not in cases where the client has experienced schizophrenic symptoms and mood symptoms in quite separate episodes of illness. Other systems, such as the American DSM-IV (1994), categorise these disorders separately from both schizophrenia and mood disorders

2. Mood (affective) disorders: mania, depression and bipolar disorders

The ICD-10 approach to the classification of mood disorders is shown in Figure 4.1. The fundamental disturbance for all these disorders is a change in

Manic episode

	Lower	Hypomania
Severity	⇩	Mania
	Higher	Mania with psychotic symptoms

Bipolar affective disorder – at least two episodes

	Lower	Currently hypomania
Severity	⇩	Currently mania
	Higher	Currently mania with psychotic symptoms

Depressive episode

	Lower	Currently mild/moderate depression
Severity		Currently mild/moderate depression with somatic symptoms
	⇩	Currently severe depression
	Higher	Currently severe depression with psychotic symptoms

Recurrent depressive disorder

Mild (± somatic symptoms)
Moderate (± somatic symptoms)
Severe (± psychotic symptoms)

Persistent mood disorder

Cyclothymia
Dysthymia
Other

Figure 4.1 ICD-10 classification of mood (affective) disorders.

mood, which may be in the direction of depression or elation. The mood change is accompanied by changes in level of activity and interests, most other symptoms being secondary to these. The disorders tend to be recurrent, the onset of individual episodes typically being triggered by stressful circumstances.

Manic episodes

In a manic episode the client is euphoric with grandiose ideas and excitement. The elation is accompanied by increased energy, overactivity, pressure of speech and a decreased need for sleep. Self-esteem is inflated, with feelings of improved mental and physical well-being. Normal social inhibitions are lost so that the sufferer may be overfamiliar, intrusive and boorish. The sufferer may embark on extravagant schemes, spend money unwisely, or display other immoderate behaviour. Perceptual disorders are common (heightened perceptions such as seeing colours more vividly or being unduly sensitive to sounds). In some episodes the mood is irritable and suspicious rather than euphoric and elated.

When psychotic symptoms occur, these are typically congruent with the mood disorder. So, for example, the sufferer may claim to have special powers, to be related to royalty or to be God. The pressure of speech may be so great as to make speech unintelligible. Motor excitement may result in profound self-neglect and dangerous states of dehydration and self-neglect.

Mania with psychotic symptoms can be very difficult to distinguish from schizophrenia, the delusions, hallucinations and apparent thought disorder obscuring the underlying change in mood. The distinguishing feature is most often the history of the illness, whether previous episodes of mood disorder have occurred and how the current episode began. The difficulty in diagnosis largely explained the large differences in the 1960s in the observed rates of schizophrenia between the USA and the UK. It has been suggested that the failure to recognise core symptoms of mania and to attribute these wrongly to schizophrenia is still a problem where ethnic minority groups are concerned.

Bipolar affective disorder

This term is applied to those who have experienced at least two episodes of mood disturbance, at least one of which was mania. The ICD-10 subclassifies each episode according to whether the current episode involves mania, depression or both together, the severity of the mood disorder and whether psychotic symptoms are present. Recovery is usually complete between episodes. The frequency of episodes and remissions is variable between sufferers though there is a tendency for the remissions to get shorter as time passes. Psychotic symptoms may be present and will tend to be congruous with the predominant mood change.

Depressive episode

The sufferer experiences low mood, a loss of energy and a reduction in the capacity to enjoy their usual pursuits and activities. There seems to be little point in the future and the sufferer may express the desire to die or be contemplating suicide. The low mood tends to persist with little change from day to day and is unresponsive to circumstances. Concentration is impaired and marked tiredness may be common even after slight effort. Appetite is usually disturbed (typically a loss of appetite), as is sleep. The sufferer often feels a sense of failure, worthlessness or guilt.

The ICD-10 takes a rather complex approach to the classification of depression based on symptom patterns and the longitudinal course of the disorder (Box 4.3). Depressive episodes are classified as mild, moderate or severe depending on the number of symptoms and their intensity. Episodes may be further subclassified according to the presence of one or more 'somatic symptoms' and according to whether psychotic symptoms are also present. Single episodes are distinguished from recurrent depression (where there are two or more episodes not involving mania).

Severe depressive episodes are characterised by marked distress and agitation, feelings of guilt and hopelessness. Somatic symptoms are always present. Some will experience delusions of guilt, catastrophe or nihilism (see above) and auditory or visual hallucinations. The sufferer may be retarded to the point of stupor, at which point there may be difficulties differentiating this from catatonic schizophrenia and organic brain diseases that also give rise to stupor. The diagnosis in such instances may depend on obtaining a good description of the evolution of the condition and investigations to exclude organic disease.

Recurrent depressive disorder

The client reports repeated episodes of depression without any history of mania. As with other episodes of depression, the current episode is coded as mild, moderate and severe, with/without somatic and psychotic symptoms.

Persistent mood disorders

Two disorders are recognised. First is *cyclothymia*, in which the sufferer reports a protracted period of unstable mood, lasting at least 2 years and involving multiple periods of both depression and hypomania that were not sufficiently severe to meet criteria for a manic or a depressive episode alone.

Box 4.3 ICD-10 and depressive episodes

Core symptoms

a. Depressed mood

b. Loss of interest and enjoyment

c. Decreased energy or increased fatigability

d. Reduced concentration and attention

e. Reduced self-esteem and self-confidence

f. Ideas of guilt and unworthiness (even in a mild type of episode)

g. Bleak and pessimistic view of the future

h. Ideas or acts of self-harm or suicide

i. Sleep disturbance

j. Change in appetite and corresponding weight change

Severity classification

◆ Duration must persist for at least 2 weeks

◆ Core symptoms

— mild   at least two of a–c plus at least one from d to j

— moderate   at least two of a–c plus at least three from d to j

— severe   all three from a–c plus at least four from d to j

◆ Somatic syndrome: at least four of:

— marked loss of interest/pleasure

— lack of emotional reactions to events

— waking in the morning 2 or more hours before usual time

— depression worse in the morning

— marked psychomotor retardation or agitation

— weight loss of 5% or more body weight in previous month

— marked loss of libido

◆ Psychotic symptoms – mood congruent delusions and hallucinations

The disorder is frequently found in relatives of those who have a bipolar affective disorder and some go on to develop this condition eventually. In *dysthymia* the sufferer reports a chronic low grade depression that does not currently meet criteria for a depressive episode. It is not unusual for this to appear as a prolonged 'tail end' of an earlier depressive episode. To meet ICD-10 criteria, the disorder must have lasted for 2 years with no periods of hypomania and no recoveries longer than a week or two. In earlier classifications, this disorder was commonly referred to as 'neurotic depression' or as a depressive personality disorder.

CONCLUSIONS

The diagnostic categories outlined in the last section represent the current consensus of how abnormal mental experiences should be grouped together. These will certainly be modified and eventually abandoned as the biological and social processes that underpin mental illness are elucidated. In fact, none of the psychoses have ever clearly been demonstrated to be a disease entity in the sense that all sufferers with the particular condition share all the features. But, by these criteria, few conditions in medicine qualify. For example, even simple infectious diseases fail in the sense that not everyone who is infected with the same bacillus experiences the same symptoms, course or outcome, while many different infections share common symptoms. For much of medicine the resolution of this conundrum has only followed greater understanding of the basic biological processes that are disturbed by disease and how a particular disturbance leads to specific symptoms. For mental disorders, the equivalent step is now under way with increasingly successful efforts to link symptoms to neuropsychological processes and brain structures. New classifications will eventually emerge from this research but in the meantime, the simple descriptive approach continues to be an essential underpinning of everyday clinical practice.

Cross references

Chapter 3 – should be read prior to exploring diagnosis as stress vulnerability complements this chapter.

All of Section 2 assumes diagnosis. Therefore, this chapter should be read prior to exploring the interventions mentioned.

References

Bleuler E 1911 Dementia praecox or the group of schizophrenias. International Universities Press, New York

Diagnostic and statistical manual of mental disorders, 4th edn (DSM-IV) 1994. American Psychiatric Association, Washington DC

References (cont'd)

Foulds G A 1965 Personality and personal illness. Tavistock, London
ICD-10 1992 Classification of mental and behavioural disorders. World
  Health Organization, Geneva
Kopelman M D 1994 Structured psychiatric interview: assessment of the
  cognitive state. British Journal of Hospital Medicine 52:277–281
Kraepelin E 1896 Dementia praecox. In: Cutting J, Shepherd M (eds) The
  clinical roots of the schizophrenia concept. Cambridge University Press,
  Cambridge, pp 15–24
Schneider K 1959 Clinical psychopathology (transl Hamilton M W). Grune
  & Stratton, New York
Sturt E 1981 Hierarchical patterns in the distribution of psychiatric
  symptoms. Psychological Medicine 11:783–794

Annotated further reading

Diagnostic and statistical manual of mental disorders, 4th edn (DSM-IV) 1994.
American Psychiatric Association, Washington DC

*A comprehensive description of all mental illness from the perspective of American
psychiatrists.*

Gelder M, Gath D, Mayou R 1989 Oxford textbook of psychiatry, 2nd edn.
Oxford University Press, Oxford

*One of the leading textbooks of psychiatry. Useful as a reference source to current
thinking about mental illness and disorder.*

ICD-10 1992 Classification of mental and behavioural disorders. World Health
Organization, Geneva

*The internationally agreed definitions of mental illness and disorder. Similar to DSM-
IV in approach. Contains helpful descriptions of all the common disorders and should
be widely available in most clinical settings.*

Kopelman M D 1994 Structured psychiatric interview: assessment of the
cognitive state. British Journal of Hospital Medicine, 52:277–281

*An introduction to clinical tests for the cognitive and memory impairments that
accompany organic brain disease. Describes how to carry out both the common tests
of memory and concentration as well as some more specialised tests of parietal and
frontal lobe disorder.*

Mueser K T, Tarrier N 1998 Handbook of social functioning in schizophrenia.
Allyn & Bacon, Boston

*Multiauthor textbook that includes descriptions and examples of the assessment of
social function and disability.*

Section 2

Assessments: choosing and using

5

Assessments: a rationale and glossary of tools

Catherine Gamble   Geoff Brennan

KEY ISSUES

- ◆ Systematic assessment: a rationale for.
- ◆ Core elements of information gathering.
- ◆ Standardised tools glossary.
- ◆ Implementation of assessment data: practical guide.

INTRODUCTION

A recent survey identified that standards of care and provision of service for people who experience serious mental health problems were inadequate (Department of Health 1995). Quality assessment is the cornerstone of effective interventions, indicating directions for treatment at point of contact and a baseline to judge the effects of these interventions. The philosophy of measuring health and social functioning is set to become a major aspect of clinical practice following the 'Health of the Nation' recommendations and implementation of the care programme approach (Department of Health 1992). Therefore, assessment of an individual with a serious mental health problem presents a huge challenge (Gournay 1996). Mental health practitioners need to be familiar with global needs assessments and more symptom or need specific assessments in order to plan their own individual treatment strategies and provide evidence of need to influence multidisciplinary decision making.

Nevertheless, despite the demand to measure clinical outcomes of persons with serious mental illness, there is no consensus about how to do this task (Dickerson 1997). This chapter seeks to address this issue by:

1. presenting a rationale for undertaking a systematic assessment
2. outlining the core elements of the information-gathering process
3. providing a practical guide to choosing and using assessments and outlining standardised tools via a glossary
4. considering practical strategies to aid interpretation and effective implementation of assessment data.

A RATIONALE FOR UNDERTAKING A SYSTEMATIC ASSESSMENT

Hall (1981) outlines the purposes of assessment to include:

◆ judging the individual's level of disability
◆ planning a programme of care and observing progress over time
◆ planning of service provision and conducting research.

While each of the above are interconnected, their focus and use are different. The expansion of each item below highlights this:

Judging the individual's level of disability

Ascertaining the individual level of disability helps to fulfil the following:

1. to reach a diagnosis of the main problems (see Ch. 4)
2. to determine the most appropriate interventions.

This is the most recognised focus for practitioners, yet it is often carried out with little or no scientific rigour. Assessment of disability relies on accurate observation and on the use of sound, practical interviewing and rating procedures. It is no longer acceptable to 'think' an intervention is appropriate – we should know and be able to provide evidence to this effect.

Planning a programme of care and observing progress over time

This aspect of care delivery is particularly important as it helps practitioners demonstrate whether or not their interventions are effective. Indeed the process can be likened to pre- and postresearch studies. Here a baseline is taken prior to intervention and subsequently reassessed to measure any changes that have taken place. We need to be careful in these situations that change does not equate with improvement and that prescribed interventions are not seen to occur within a vacuum. The individual will experience and be subject to many other variables that affect health outcomes, such as: life effects, family environments, drug use, etc. (Repper & Brooker 1998). Nevertheless, a systematic assessment procedure does help to construct a tentative prognostic statement regarding the probability of the success of interventions. The process of setting a baseline and then evaluating change can be carried out by utilising either standard assessment tools or clients' own assessment of their problems and progress (for further discussion on clients' own assessment see Ch. 6). The common feature of both standard tools and clients' own assessment is that they encourage a formalised measure of problems or needs. Such measures will facilitate a more robust, scientific method of setting baselines and evaluating change.

Planning of service provision and conducting research

The above have focused on the rationale for undertaking assessments with individuals. However, the process can also help practitioners and their organisations to audit need within whole populations. Reliable, valid instruments help to ascertain need and the subsequent allocation of resources. Indeed they can also help to highlight and plan for any shortfall in service provision. For example, when making the transition from hospital- to community-based care there is a need to collect some basic but extremely important data, such as: the length of time people have been in.hospital, the levels of dependency, mental and physical disabilities, community provision, etc. Again, as with individual assessment, population need should be continually evaluated to ensure that service provision adapts to any change in need.

Research is an integral part of clinical work, although the majority do not recognise it. This is possibly because 'research' is perceived to be in the domain of academics who arrive in the clinical area asking to interview staff or clients. Not all practitioners will carry out formal research work, so it is seen as elusive, exclusive and outside of normal everyday practice. In this instance, however, 'research' should be reframed as a process of 'gathering evidence to facilitate understanding and enhance decision making'. Within this reframe, it is possible to deduce that all the aforementioned is, in fact, 'research'.

OUTLINING THE CORE ELEMENTS OF THE INFORMATION-GATHERING PROCESS

The gathering of information should be conducted in a systematic way and is comprised of a number of core elements. The first step is to gather information from all reliable sources. The procedure should elicit the following:

1. **History of psychiatric disorder and past physical history:**
   ◆ family and social background

◆ relevant chronological details of the individual's past treatment, contact with services and risk levels
◆ current medication and its side-effects.

2. Current financial, social functioning and environmental factors: particular attention should be paid to the duration and stability of personal relationships and employment since they have prognostic implications.

3. The psychiatric diagnosis and current symptoms: these should be noted and more importantly, the degree to which these may influence behaviour. This is of particular relevance because behaviour rather than symptoms is a decisive factor in community survival.

4. Personal insights: information should be sought that may help to estimate persons' insight into their difficulties.

Rather than merely reading old medical notes, it is highly advisable that much, if not all, of the aforementioned process is conducted with clients and their 'significant others'. Indeed, Nelson (1998) recommends meeting before reading the medical notes for the following reasons:

◆ rather than gaining one narrow professional view this allows you to get a clearer three-dimensional picture of how things seem to clients and their carers
◆ it prevents you from prejudging the issues
◆ it will help you to be more empathetic and ask the appropriate questions naturally
◆ if clients cannot recall some of their experiences and symptoms you can genuinely offer to look in the notes and find out for them.

Box 5.1 covers the core elements that should be considered prior to formulating any treatment plan.

A PRACTICAL GUIDE TO CHOOSING AND USING STANDARDISED ASSESSMENT TOOLS

Assessment is a complex process, especially when one considers the amount of conflicting interests of various stakeholders involved in care. Therefore we need to be clear about why a particular tool is chosen and be able to present a rationale as to who it is for and what purpose it serves.

The general principles surrounding this issue are:

1. Practitioners should be wary of choosing and using only one type of assessment method. Indeed, one alone is not sufficiently sensitive enough to assess all aspects of a client's needs. An example of this is: during the process of preparing for a care programme meeting a practitioner, filling in a care

Box 5.1 Summary of areas to be assessed prior to developing a treatment plan:

- risk
- physical and mental health status
- social needs and functioning
- symptomatology and coping skills
- quality of life and its effects on others
- housing and money
- social support
- medicine and its effects
- work skills and meaningful daily activity

programme assessment (CPA) form, asks clients if they have any unmet needs. When a client replies 'everything is OK' it is reported that all needs have been met. In this instance, a formalised, thorough needs assessment would have to be completed for this statement to be correct.

2. Only valid and reliable methods that are sensitive to change should be used. However, it should not be assumed that, because a scale is used or frequently referred to in professional journals, that it is reliable or indeed valid (Pilling 1991). When choosing a particular tool, practitioners should ascertain whether it is pertinent, and easy to follow and use. When a tool does not appear applicable or relevant to the practice setting, some practitioners have a tendency to cut corners and make modifications. A possible example of this is when an acute ward team tries to adapt a tool designed for use in community settings. Modifying tools can bring the validity and reliability of the instrument and the results the practitioner identifies into question. Any modifications should be made on the basis of careful rationale and in consultation with recognised experts in the area. When doubting whether the aforementioned has occurred it is highly advisable to visit the library, read the literature and examine the original evidence.

As mentioned previously, we need to be able to clarify why we are assessing someone and to what purpose the process serves. This is particularly relevant if the assessor is not in a position to act on information gathered. An example would be when a practitioner is assessing side-effects of medication but is not able to adapt the medication regimen. In this situation we should ask ourselves: do all relevant parties know the assessment procedure is taking place? To carry out a side-effects assessment without informing medical staff

---

Box 5.2 Questions to ask before commencing an assessment procedure

◆ Am I the best person to carry this out – if so, why?

◆ Do I have an ulterior motive? – is this assessment in the client's and/or their carers' best interest or has the need been identified by someone else?

◆ Has the assessment been carried out already – if so, what is the benefit for a new or different assessment and who is it for?

◆ Have I chosen the correct battery of tools or am I making presumptions?

◆ Will the results have implications for another practitioner?

◆ Who else will be informed of the assessment process and the results?

◆ How can I translate what I have learnt to the wider care team and in which format or forum should this occur?

◆ What immediate feedback should I give and how do I summarise this for clients and their carers?

◆ Are there any subsequent assessments I may need to undertake as a consequence of this initial process – if so when should I do it and how do I inform the client that this may happen?

---

of the concerns that lead to this is not good practice. They may feel coerced into making treatment changes before they feel it is appropriate, or they may have wished to carry out the assessment themselves.

When you can answer the questions in Box 5.2 to your own satisfaction you are ready to formulate a rationale for your client and the care team. The flowcharts in Figures 5.1–5.3 are intended to guide practitioners through an assessment process.

Use of flowcharts and assessment scales glossary

The flowcharts in Figures 5.1–5.3 give a rough guide to processing assessment in three areas:

◆ needs
◆ symptomatology
◆ informal carers.

The flowcharts break the possible assessment tools into two categories:

1. **global**: these are assessments that give an overall view of the area being assessed

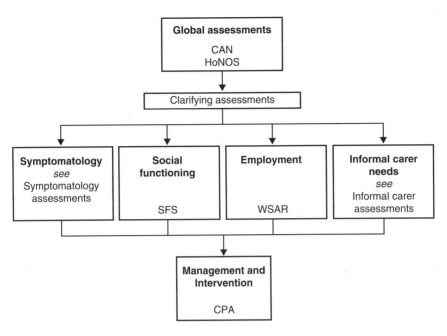

Figure 5.1 Needs assessments (for explanation of abbreviations see Table 5.1).

2. **clarifying**: these are assessments that focus on more specific aspects of the area to be assessed.

Table 5.1 gives a brief glossary of assessment tools and where they can be obtained. For tools that are listed as unpublished manuscripts, it is advisable to write directly to the author or organisation indicated. The glossary contains additional tools to the flowcharts that may be useful to practitioners and clients. Neither the flowcharts nor the glossary should be thought of as definitive, however. They are simply a guide to thinking and processing.

There is, at present, some debate as to the assumptions underpinning carer assessment. Early assessment concerned itself with the concept of 'carer burden'. Carer burden assumes that the experience of caregiving is a negative one and, therefore, the assessments looked for areas of difficulty in the caregiving relationship, carer coping and carer health.

Professionals working in the field have since realised that the assumption of caregiving as being exclusively negative needs to be challenged. This is not to say that an individual informal carer may not find the experience a negative one, but rather that professionals should not automatically assume that all carers will find caregiving a burden. The danger here is that, if we assume that carers are burdened and ask only about negative aspects, we will invariably create a bias. An assumption that closely follows the burden assumption is

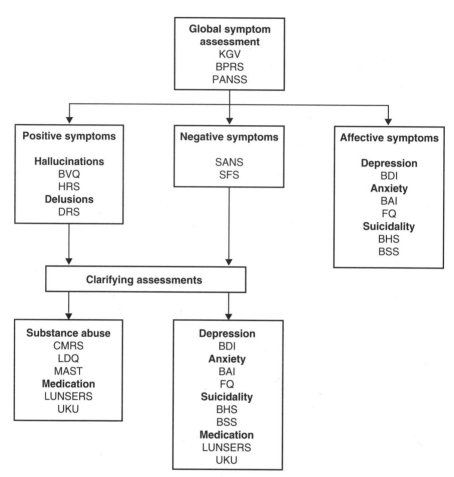

Figure 5.2 Symptomatology assessments (for explanation of abbreviations see Table 5.1).

that carers are unable to cope. Many carers cope well and create environments in which the client is not only valued and respected, but carers themselves are able to maintain their health and be in control of very difficult situations. Newer assessment tools have attempted to address some of these issues by assessing positive attributes within the caregiving relationship. The introduction of the positive aspects tend to be called 'coping' rather than 'burden'. Any assessors undertaking informal carer assessment need to be aware of their own assumptions as to the caregiving role and not dismiss, reduce or ignore any positive coping or attitude expressed by informal carers as these aspects are crucial in getting the balance between understanding the burden that informal carers face and the personal strengths they can marshal to help them cope. In many ways, this topic mirrors the strengths versus deficit debate within client assessments, where some assessments assume a

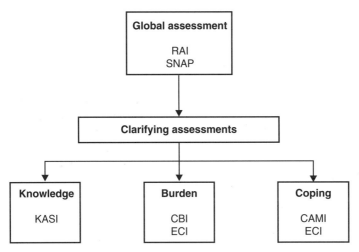

Figure 5.3 Informal carer assessments (for explanation of abbreviations see Table 5.1).

person will be disabled and handicapped by illness and therefore finds this to be the case, whereas other assessments assume that clients will have a range of strengths they can utilise to control the illness. In this case also, assessors need to be cautious that the tool they use and the assumptions they have do not introduce a bias.

PRACTICAL STRATEGIES TO AID INTERPRETATION AND EFFECTIVE IMPLEMENTATION OF ASSESSMENT DATA

One of the main issues for practitioners is what to do with the information once it has been obtained. All too often, practitioners encourage relatives and clients to undertake and complete assessments. However, once this procedure has occurred, the majority of the information gets filed into medical notes and is rarely referred to or looked at again. This can be very frustrating and can lead to the perception that a rigorous assessment process is a waste of time for all concerned. Therefore, practitioners need to present a clear rationale and be able to demonstrate that assessments are not paperwork exercises and just about statistics. Indeed, they can in fact play a useful part in care, as results from well-constructed scales can be discussed with clients and carers and incorporated into empowering, needs-led treatment plans.

To achieve this successfully it is important to become familiar with the tools and manuals (e.g. administration and scoring); in this way you will be in a better position to value the assessment procedure and understand the reasons for conducting it. A thorough assessment process can be a rewarding

Table 5.1 A glossary of standardised assessment scales

Assessing	Abbreviation	Suggested scales/tools
Anxiety	*BAI	*Beck Anxiety Inventory.* Beck A T, Steer R A 1990 Manual for Beck Anxiety Inventory. Psychological Corporation, San Antonio, TX
	FQ	*Fear Questionnaire.* 16 item scale that rates on a Likert scale, 0 (would not avoid it) to 8 (always avoid it), how much a person avoids certain situations. Can be used as a self-report instrument or when practitioners wish to assess clients' fears re travelling alone or going into crowded shops. Marks I M 1997 Living with fear: understanding and coping with anxiety. McGraw-Hill, Cambridge
Carers	CSI	*Caregiver Strain Index.* Assesses strain using a simple questionnaire. Comprises 13 pre-determined questions answered as yes or no by interviewee. Has the benefit of being simple and quick, although crude. Robinson B C 1983 Validation of a caregiver strain index. Journal of Gerontology 38:344–348
	CAMI	*Carers' Assessment of Managing Index.* Assesses coping styles and management of stress by questionnaire. Carers are given examples of coping strategies, asked if they use these and if they are effective. Important in that it assumes carers have coping strategies that can be enhanced. Nolan M, Keady J, Grant G 1995 CAMI: a basis for assessment and support with family carers. British Journal of Nursing Quarterly 4(14):822–826
	ECI	*Experience of Caregiving Inventory.* Assessment of both burden and coping. Comprises 66 questions that cover ten areas; eight areas described as 'negative'; two described as 'positive': negative – difficult behaviours, negative symptoms, stigma, problems with services, effects on family, need to back up, dependency and loss; positive – positive personal experiences, good relationships with patients. Note that areas such as stigma and relationship with care team are covered. Szmukler G I, Burgess P, Hermann H, Benson A, Colusa S, Bioch S 1996 Caring for relatives with serious mental illness: the development of the Experience of Caregiving Inventory. Society for Psychiatry and Psychiatric Epidemiology 31:137–148
	KASI	*Knowledge About Schizophrenia Interview.* Assesses and evaluates relatives' knowledge, beliefs and attitudes about six broad aspects of schizophrenia: diagnosis,

Table 5.1 (cont'd)

Assessing	Abbreviation	Suggested scales/tools
		symptomatology, aetiology, medication, prognosis, management. Barrowclough C, Tarrier N 1995 Families of schizophrenic patients: cognitive behavioural intervention. Chapham & Hall, London (see Ch. 11)
	RAI	*Relatives' Assessment Interview.* Based on the Camberwell Family Interview, but modified for clinical use. Aims to obtain essential information that helps to direct family intervention work. Covers seven main areas summarised as: client's family background and contact time, chronological history of the illness, current problems/symptoms, irritability, relatives' relationship with client, effects of the illness on relatives. Barrowclough C, Tarrier N 1995 Families of schizophrenic patients: cognitive behavioural intervention. Chapham & Hall, London (see Ch. 11)
	RAISSE	*Relatives' Assessment Interview for Schizophrenia in a Secure Environment.* Adaptation of RAI for secure environment. Assessment based on a semistructured interview, three areas covered: schizophrenia, admission, visits. Whole not as robustly researched for validity as other assessments, has been constructed by experts in this area who have tested it in the field. McKeown M, McCann G A 1995 A schedule for assessing relatives. The relatives' assessment interview for schizophrenia in a secure environment (RAISSE). Psychiatric Care 2(3): 84–88
	SNAP	*Schizophrenia Nursing Assessment Protocol.* Assesses all family members, including the client. Covers four main areas in a semistructured interview format: clients' relationships with people with whom they live, clients' psychiatric and personal history, nature of present episode, families' understanding/knowledge of the illness. Particularly useful for quick assessment of main problem areas. Brooker C, Bagley I 1990 'SNAP Decisions'. Nursing Times 86(41):56–58
Depression	*BDI	*Beck Depression Inventory.* Beck A T, Greer R 1987 Beck Depression Inventory Scoring Manual. Psychological Corporation, New York
	CDS	*Calgary Depression Scale.* A nine-item structured interview scale developed to assess depression in schizophrenia sufferers. Addington D, Addington J M, Maticka M N, Dale E 1993 Assessing depression in schizophrenia: the Calgary Depression Scale. The

Table 5.1 *(cont'd)*

Assessing	Abbreviation	Suggested scales/tools
		Calgary Depression Scale for Schizophrenia (CDSS). British Journal of Psychiatry (suppl): 22 Dec, 39–44
Delusions	DRS	*Delusions Rating Scale* (Haddock G 1994). Structured interview designed to elicit details regarding different delusional beliefs. Consists of six items that range from the amount of preoccupation to intensity of distress and disruption. The Delusions Rating Scale. Unpublished scale, University of Manchester
	IS	*Insight Scale.* Self-report instrument. Consists of eight statements (four negative and four positive). Clients can agree, disagree or be unsure. Statements include the need for: medication, to see a doctor, illness recognition and relabelling of psychotic experiences. Birchwood M, Smith J, Davry V, Healy J, Macmillan F, Slade M 1994 A self-report insight scale for psychosis: reliability, validity and sensitivity to change. Acta Psychiatrica Scandinavica 89:62–67
Early signs of relapse	ESS	*Early Signs Scale.* Describes problems and complaints people sometimes have prior to relapse. It contains 34 items that describe feelings and behaviours that can occur prior to relapse. Each item is rated on a 0 (not a problem) to 3 (marked problem) scale. Birchwood M, Smith J, Macmillan F et al 1989 Predicting relapse in schizophrenia: the development and implementation of an early signs monitoring system using patients and families as observers. Psychological Medicine 19:649–656
Global need	CPA	*The Care Programme Approach.* Provides for the continuity of care and accountability for clients and the managing agency. Department of Health (1990) The Care Programme Approach for people with a mental illness referred to specialist psychiatric services. Joint health/social services circular HC (90) 23/LASSL (90) 11. HMSO, London
	CAN	*Camberwell Assessment of Need.* Rates met and unmet service needs. Phelan M, Slade M, Thornicroft G et al 1995 The Camberwell Assessment of Need: the validity and reliability of an instrument to assess the needs of people with severe mental illness. British Journal of Psychiatry 167:589–595
	GHQ	*General Health Questionnaire.* Measures neurotic symptoms. To ensure that this instrument is not used inappropriately it is not in the public domain. Goldberg D, Williams P 1988 A user's guide to the General Health Questionnaire. NFER-Nelson, Windsor

Table 5.1 (cont'd)

Assessing	Abbreviation	Suggested scales/tools
	HoNOS	*Health of the Nation Outcome Scale.* A 12 item health and social functioning scale. Measures risk behaviours, physical problems, deterioration and/or improvement in symptoms and social functioning. Can be completed by the care team and/or the individual practitioner. Wing J, Curtis R, Beevor A 1995 Measurement for mental health: Health of the Nation Outcome Scales. Royal College of Psychiatrists' Research Unit, London, pp 33–46
	SFS	*Social Functioning Scale.* Assesses aspects of day to day social functioning that are adversely affected by client's mental health difficulties. It covers seven main areas of social functioning, e.g. social engagement, interpersonal behaviour, independence in living skills (competence and performance). It can provide a guide to goals and interventions, as well as measure progress and outcome. Birchwood M, Smith J, Cochrane R 1990 The Social Functioning Scale: the development and validation of a new scale of social adjustment for use in family interventions programmes with schizophrenic patients. British Journal of Psychiatry 157:853–859
	WSAR	*Work and Social Adjustment Ratings.* Marks I M, Bird J, Brown M, Ghosh A 1986 Behavioural psychotherapy: Maudsley pocket book of clinical management. Wright, Bristol
Hallucinations	BVQ	*Beliefs About Voices Questionnaire.* Chadwick P, Birchwood M 1995 The omnipotence of voices II: The Beliefs About Voices Questionnaire (BAVQ). British Journal of Psychiatry 166:733–776
	HRS	*Auditory Hallucinations Rating Scale* (Haddock G 1994). An 11 item checklist for auditory hallucinations. Assesses distress control and belief re origin of voices in addition to how client experiences voices. The Hallucinations Rating Scale. Unpublished scale, University of Manchester
Medication: side-effects	LUNSERS	*Liverpool University Neuroleptic Side-Effect Rating Scale.* Enables clients to rate their own side-effects. A simple measure that covers 51 side-effects, ten of which are red herrings, such as hair loss. Day J C 1995 A self rating scale for measuring neuroleptic side effects: validation in a group of schizophrenic patients. British Journal of Psychiatry 166: 650–653
	UKU	*UKU Side Effect Rating Scale.* Breaks side-effects into distinct groupings: psychic, neurological, autonomic,

Table 5.1 (cont'd)		
Assessing	**Abbreviation**	**Suggested scales/tools**
		other. Also assesses global interference of side-effects on daily performance and includes action planning section. Lingjaerde O, Ahlfors U G, Beck P, Dencker S J, Elsen K 1987 The UKU side effect rating scale. A new comprehensive scale for psychotropic drugs and a cross-sectional study of side effects in neuroleptic-treated patients. Acta Psychiatrica Scandinavica (suppl) 334:1–100
Substance abuse	CMRS	*Case Managers' Rating Scale* (Drake R, Noordsy F 1994 Case management for people with coexisting severe mental disorder and substance use disorder. Psychiatric Annals 24:427–431). Contains a five point scale with each point operationally defined in terms of levels of substance abuse and their biopsychosocial consequences (see Ch. 12)
	LDQ	*Leeds Dependence Questionnaire* (Raistrick D, Bradshaw J, Tober G, Weiner J, Allison J, Healey C 1994 Development of the Leeds Dependence Questionnaire (LDQ): a questionnaire to measure alcohol and opiate dependence in the context of a treatment evaluation package. Addiction 89:563–572). Designed to detect and rate the severity of illicit substance abuse. Contains ten items that are rated on a four point scale (see Ch. 12)
	MAST	*Michigan Alcoholism Screening Test* (Selzer M 1971 The Michigan Alcoholism Screening Test: the quest for a new diagnostic instrument. American Journal of Psychiatry 127:1653–1658). Designed to detect problematic alcohol use by rating its effect on an individual's psychical and social circumstances (see Ch. 12)
Suicidality/ risk	*BHS	*Beck Hopelessness Scale.* Beck A T, Steer R A 1988 Manual for Beck Hopelessness Scale. Psychological Corporation, San Antonio, TX
	*BSS	*Beck Scale for Suicide Ideation.* Beck A T, Steer R A 1993 The Beck Scale for Suicide Ideation. Psychological Corporation, San Antonio, TX
Symptoms	BPRS	*Brief Psychiatric Rating Scale.* A well-validated measure of general psychiatric symptoms. Originally contained 16 items; nine of these are scored on verbal responses (somatic concerns, anxiety, guilt, grandiosity, depressive mood, hostility, suspiciousness, hallucinatory behaviour and unusual thoughts), the other seven are scored on observation at time of interview. Scoring is on a Likert scale from 1 (not present) to 7 (extremely severe). Developed by

Table 5.1 (cont'd)		
Assessing	**Abbreviation**	**Suggested scales/tools**
	KGV	Overall J E, Gorham D R 1962 The Brief Psychiatric Rating Scale. Psychological Reports 10:799–812 *Manchester Symptom Severity Scale.* A simplified version of the BPRS. It identifies the type and severity of psychiatric symptoms and contains 12 items. The first five are rated on verbal responses; the remainder are rated on observation at interview. Krawiecka M, Goldberg D, Vaughn M 1977 A standardised psychiatric assessment scale for rating chronic psychotic patients. Acta Psychiatrica Scandinavica 55:299–308
	PANSS	*Positive and Negative Syndrome Scale.* Thirty item scale for practitioners: seven items address negative symptoms and seven positive symptoms; the remaining 16 focus on general psychopathology. Some items are based on interview; others on observation. Each item rated using Likert scale (0–6 with 6 most severe). Kay S R, Fiszebein A, Opler L A 1987 Positive and Negative Syndrome Scale. Schizophrenia Bulletin 13:261–276
	SANS	*Schedule for the Assessment of Negative Symptoms.* Assesses 20 of the negative symptoms: affective flattening, alogia, avolition/apathy, anhedonia/asociality and attention. Symptoms are rated on a 0–5 scale of increasing severity. Andreasen N 1982 Negative symptoms in schizophrenia: definition and reliability. Archives of General Psychiatry 39:784–788

*These instruments are not in the public domain. Some organisations and institutions have licence to use these for clinical practice and research purposes. This should be clarified prior to use. If not, they can be purchased from the Psychological Corporation, USA.

experience for clients, their carers and the professionals involved. It can empower all concerned. In many instances, clinicians who do not routinely complete formalised assessments have reported being amazed and slightly ashamed about how little they knew and how much clients have been willing to tell them. Such positive experiences have been achieved because the aforementioned practitioners have 'owned' and familiarised themselves with a battery of assessment tools and have been able to interpret wisely the data they have obtained. For example:

> *We have recently completed a number of assessments; one helped us to identify what needs you have generally (HoNoS), and some of the symptoms*

you are currently experiencing (KGV). The third one gave me an idea of how you and your family are coping at the moment (RAI). I know this seemed like a long process, but I was keen to obtain as clear a picture as possible. The overall process has helped us identify that you have numerous coping strategies and strengths. For example, if we look at the SFS, it shows us that you score highly in independent living skills – you cook, clean, take care of your home and personal appearance and you have a large, supportive social network. Your sister and dad also reported that they feel you are coping very well. However, would I be right in saying that we have deduced that you wish to be slightly more independent? Should we therefore think about how to address the difficulty you identified about using public transport and going out alone?

It is important to know how to feed back information to the client and informal carer and not overload them. Indeed, the example above illustrates that it is not necessary to flood clients. Information obtained from baseline assessments can be gradually fed back and used on other occasions as and when the need arises.

Not being overzealous is something that is learnt over time. What may be tolerable for one client will not be for another and all practitioners should strive to ensure that the assessment process is flexible and tailormade to suit individuals. There will be cases when clients do not wish to participate; there are numerous reasons for taking this stance, such as lack of rapport, communication and language, literary skills, past experiences and/or practitioners making assumptions or jumping to the intervention stage before properly identifying what the real need is for the client. Having said this, clients come to services for specific interventions (e.g. help with completing DLA forms and housing). In this situation it is advised to assist clients to achieve these aims. This engages them and shows them that their needs will be addressed. Further assessment can then take place naturally, for example, in the above situation, saying to the client 'now we have done this – should we check if you have any other unmet needs?'

CONCLUSIONS

Assessments are an integral part of any practitioner's work. In practice, clients and their carers complain that they repeat the same information over and over again. This indicates that practitioners do not follow a structured process that leads naturally on to intervention. This chapter should guide and clarify the process. The overall aim of assessment is as much to engage clients in the process of treatment as it is to identify their needs and problems. It cannot be emphasised enough that old-fashioned qualities, such as respect, empathy, politeness, punctuality and genuine concern, can help to create collaboration and understanding.

Other chapters in this book identify how the assessment process leads to intervention and change. Whilst reading these it should be noted that using and choosing appropriate assessments is the foundation on which successful, collaborative intervention is built.

Summary of practical strategies identified

- ◆ Always endeavour to match need with appropriate assessment tools.
- ◆ Ask 'Am I the best person to carry out this assessment?'
- ◆ Use Table 5.1 as a guide to choosing assessment tools.
- ◆ Give preference to validated tools.
- ◆ Provide a rationale for and inform client of process and outcome.
- ◆ Be respectful, empathetic, polite and punctual.
- ◆ Attempt to obtain a culturally sensitive, collaborative history from clients and their 'significant others'.

References

Birchwood M, Tarrier N 1995 Innovations in the psychological management of schizophrenia. Wiley & Sons, Chichester

Day J C 1995 A self rating scale for measuring neuroleptic side effects: validation in a group of schizophrenic patients. British Journal of Psychiatry 166:650–653

Department of Health 1990 The Care Programme Approach for people with a mental illness referred to specialist psychiatric services. Joint health/social services circular HC (90) 23/LASSL (90) 11. HMSO, London

Department of Health 1991 Care management and assessment. HMSO, London

Department of Health 1992 Health of the Nation. HMSO, London

Department of Health 1995 Report of a clinical standards advisory group on schizophrenia, vol 1. HMSO, London

Dickerson F B 1997 Assessing clinical outcomes: the community functioning of persons with serious mental illness. Psychiatric Service July 48(7):897–902

Gourney K 1996 Schizophrenia: a review of the contemporary literature and implications for mental health nursing theory, practice and education. Journal of Psychiatric and Mental Health Nursing 3:7–12

Hall N 1981 Psychological assessment. In: Wing J K, Morris B (eds) Handbook of psychiatric rehabilitation practice. Oxford University Press, Oxford

Nelson H 1998 Cognitive behavioural therapy with schizophrenia: a practical manual. Stanley Thornes, Cornwall

References (cont'd)

Pilling S 1991 Rehabilitation and community care. Routledge, London
Repper J, Brooker C 1998 Difficulties in the measurement of outcome in people who have serious mental health problems. Journal of Advanced Nursing 27:75–82

Annotated further reading

Kavanagh D J 1992 Schizophrenia: an overview and practical handbook. Chapman & Hall, London

Contains an entire section on the assessment process that is comprehensive and accessible. Covers life skills assessment; social skills assessment; family assessment; predicting relapse and dangerousness.

Fowler D, Garety P, Kuipers E 1995 Cognitive behaviour therapy for psychosis. Wiley, Chichester

Contains an informative chapter entitled 'Getting started: engagement and assessment'. This provides an overview of rationale for assessment and some practical ways to carefully examine clients' current behaviour and psychotic experiences.

6

Assessing clients' needs: the semistructured interview

Jayne Fox   Paddy Conroy

KEY ISSUES

◆ Introduction to the concept of structured assessment for people with SMI.
◆ Overview of the assessment procedure including:
— clinical case example
— tips for smooth running assessment.
◆ How to formulate assessment information using problems and goals methodology.
◆ How to clinically measure baseline assessment information.

INTRODUCTION

An accurate assessment of the client's main problems is an essential requirement prior to the application of any intervention. Richards & McDonald (1990) argue that 'any treatment plan is only as good as the information it is based upon'. Whilst meaningful and accurate assessment is essential for all disorders, it is particularly important if the individual's problems are long term and have a high degree of complexity associated with them. This is often the case with those who suffer from a serious mental illness, for example schizophrenia or bipolar disorders. That is not to say that other mental health problems are less severe but the authors believe that, in some instances, they present with greater and more long term impact on lifestyle. This often requires individuals to make permanent changes to large aspects of their day to day lives; and engage in treatments that they often find unpleasant (e.g. medication). This is not always the case, and to the same degree, with other illnesses. In almost all cases a large part of any therapeutic intervention requires the health professional to help the individual to make the required lifestyle adjustments and this process should begin at assessment.

Almost all interventions or approaches begin with assessment and there are, of course, many different ways of assessing. The authors do not intend in this chapter to review the many differing approaches or to suggest that one is superior to another. Whilst we will be describing and advocating the use of one particular model this is intended mainly to demonstrate for the reader the importance of clear and meaningful assessment as a beginning to any intervention. It is important, and often the case, that health professionals develop their own style of assessment, based upon the needs of the individual at the time, using assessment formats merely as a guide. This chapter will describe our preferred style and format for assessment, which has been successfully applied to individuals with a range of mental health problems in a range of settings.

THE SEMISTRUCTURED ASSESSMENT INTERVIEW

This type of assessment is commonly associated with cognitive–behavioural approaches. Its simple principles, format and aims make it relatively easy to apply. In addition it provides the structure and logic required to complete a useful assessment (Hawton et al 1989). According to Clinton & Nelson (1996) 'assessing the problems of a client typically involves a semistructured interview that deals with the client's thoughts, feelings and behaviours at any one time'. In addition, McFarland & Thomas (1990) argue that the semi-structured assessment interview provides a framework for the total assessment – 'it functions to establish rapport and gain knowledge of characteristic patterns of living and coping behaviours'. When considering semistructured assessment for problems associated with serious mental illness, Birchwood & Tarrier (1992) postulate that 'a thorough assessment of the patient's symptomatology and coping skills should be covered through a semistructured interview'. It is important that the assessor appreciates clients' understanding of their problems or difficulties. Whilst it may be more straightforward to plan interventions according to 'textbook' procedures, this does not necessarily lead to a successful outcome. Anecdotal evidence suggests that, far too often, clients with serious mental illness feel uninvolved in their care, which does not reflect their personal needs or aspirations.

In light of this, the authors believe that the semistructured interview is a sensible choice to begin the assessment process. However, the reader must understand that, whilst this assessment gives a clear overall picture of the individual's main problems or difficulties, the assessor may need to complement this assessment with other tools designed to clinch specific information.

Beginning the process

Prior to outlining the structure of this assessment it is important for the reader to understand some of the underlying principles associated with this approach.

1. Be pragmatic

The assessor should approach the interview with a clear outcome in mind. The intention is to establish what problems currently cause this individual difficulty in day to day life and what are the implications or consequences of this. In short, emphasis is placed on practical consequences of problems rather than why they exist or how they began.

2. Expectation

Richards & McDonald (1990) argue that 'clients will have expectations of us, but they will also be influenced by what we expect from them'. In light of this it is important early on in the assessment to demonstrate positive assumptions about clients. They propose these to be:

◆ Clients will be responsive to the help that is offered and that they will be working with you in a partnership that allows them to have control and take responsibility.
◆ Clients try to cope with the problems they have and that they are real problems that do not exist merely because the individuals are not trying to help themselves.
◆ Clients are honest and telling the truth about their problems. Spending time trying to prove that clients are not being honest about their problems is pointless and potentially damaging to the therapeutic relationship and contradicts the underlying principles of this assessment.

Note: Refer to Chapter 8 for more details.

Questioning style

The main aim of this assessment is to allow clients an opportunity to describe their problems as they experience them. This information is then formulated into a short sentence, known as a 'problem statement'. Once this is completed clients are able to identify their own goals describing what they wish to achieve or work towards. (Examples of these will be described later in this chapter.)

The primary role of the assessor in this process is to enable individuals to 'tell their story' by asking a series of questions, beginning with simple open-ended questions and then clinching specific details by asking closed questions. This is known as the 'funnelling technique'. (See Fig. 6.1 for details.)

By applying this approach to questioning throughout the assessment interview the assessor establishes a clear and accurate definition of the main problem. Note how in the above example the questions are begun openly; then, based upon information the client gives in responses, they become more specific and details are gathered. An outline of the assessment format containing information from a client assessed by one of the authors is described below. In addition, examples of how questions could be formulated are also described. To help enhance the assessment process the reader should be mindful of the tips given at the end of the chapter under 'Summary of practical strategies identified'.

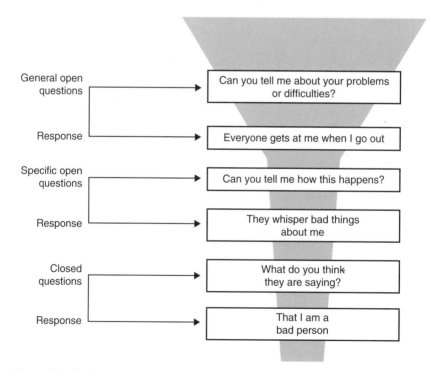

Figure 6.1 The funnelling technique.

Assessment format

1. The five 'Ws'

This part of the assessment allows clients to begin describing their problem in their own words. In addition, any patterns or predictors of the problem can also be established (Table 6.1). Once this is completed you should have a fairly detailed description of the main problem, as the client perceives it.

2. FIND

Once the initial details of the problem have been described it is now time to funnel down and gather some more specific information (Table 6.2). This helps build a clearer picture of the problem and how it impacts upon the client's day to day life.

3. A behavioural analysis

Arguably the most central and perhaps important part of this assessment, a behavioural analysis allows individuals to describe their problem in three parts. If this part of the assessment is fully completed it will prove to be useful when planning interventions as it draws out strategies that are used to help cope with the impact of the problem (see Table 6.4). In addition the individual's

Table 6.1 The five 'Ws'	
Questions	**Responses**
What: what do you see as being your main problem?	Every time I go out people talk about me. They make fun and try to stop me from doing things.
When: when is the problem worse?	It's bad at night-time, when it starts to get dark.
When is the problem better/improves?	In the mornings it's better, because I can see better.
Where: in what situations is the problem most difficult?	At the day centre they talk about me and I don't like it there.
Are there any places/situations where the problem is better?	At home my brother talks to me and this helps.
With: are there any people who help you with the problem?	My brother helps and so does my mum; they try to understand.
Are there any people who hinder you or make things worse?	The day centre people upset me – they make things worse for me.
Why/consequences: what do you think causes/maintains your problems?	People don't like me – the world is a bad place sometimes and is full of bad people.

Table 6.2 Funnelling down

Questions	Responses
Frequency: how often does the problem you have described occur?	Every day, except Sunday. On Sundays I can stay at home and read my magazines.
Intensity: how intense do you feel as a result (on a scale of 0–100)?	At the day centre it's really bad, about 100% bad I would say.
Number: are there any patterns or particular times it occurs?	On Tuesdays, the manager is always there and it happens a lot but I can't remember exactly.
Duration: how long does it last?	Ages – a long time. About 2 hours.

emotional experience of the problem can be captured during this part of the assessment by applying a three systems analysis (Richards & McDonald 1990).

An example of a behavioural analysis is as follows:

Antecedent: 'What happens before or what triggers the problem?'
Response: 'When I am getting ready to go to the day centre. I begin to feel scared.'

4. The impact of the problem

The next part of the assessment involves questions designed to elicit the impact and consequences of the problem (Table 6.3). Although some of this information may have already been gathered, it is important to clarify it, as this will form part of the overall problem definition and will also act as a springboard into meaningful goals.

PROBLEMS AND GOALS

Capturing the assessment information

Once the assessment information has been gathered, it is then summarised into a short structured sentence known as a 'problem statement'. In addition, clients are asked to describe the things they wish to work towards that, when achieved, would indicate that the impact or severity of the problem had reduced. These are known as 'goal statements'. This is an important process as the semi-structured interview provides a wealth of information that, whilst useful, can be hard to evaluate. Summarising the assessment information in this way allows the health professional and the client to evaluate objectively both the ongoing severity of the problem and how close they are to achieving the agreed goals.

Table 6.3 Impact and consequence

Questions	Responses
Behavioural excesses: what things do you do more of because of the problem?	I stay at home more often. I sleep a lot and watch TV.
Deficits: what things do you do less of because of the problem?	I don't see my friends or go out with my brother any more.
Modifiers: is there anything that you do to help?	I get my mum to come out with me. Sometimes I walk around with my hands over my face or close my eyes.
Onset: when did it begin? Did anything significant happen?	When I was at school, the others in my class used to say things about me.
Fluctuations: has it got better at all?	At Christmas, after I came home from hospital it was OK. They stopped talking about me.
Has it got worse at all?	It gets worse every day.
Past treatment: describe any past treatment you have had. Did it help?	Tablets, which I hate. They make my mouth dry. Mum says they help and so does the doctor but I hate them.
Impact: how would you sum up the impact this problem has on your lifestyle?	It makes me scared all of the time. Because I am scared I don't see my friends. I am lonely.
Motivation: are there any things you would like to do that this problem currently prevents?	Go to the pub with my friends. Try and get back to college.

The following guide can be used to establish meaningful problem and goal statements.

Problem statements

Problem statements should focus directly on difficulties that:

◆ have been identified by the client during the semistructured assessment interview
◆ have been written, whenever possible, in the client's own words; this helps to reduce the use of jargon and provides meaning to the client
◆ describe the problem in observable behaviours – for example, Michael described feeling afraid and was encouraged to say how this affected the way he behaved, thus transferring 'feeling afraid' into avoiding going to the day centre
◆ indicate the impact and consequences the problem has on the client's lifestyle.

As described above, each problem statement should include an accurate description of the current presenting problem, its immediate impact and the subsequent consequences.

Goal statements

Goal statements should:

◆ describe what the client would like to achieve in relation to the identified problem
◆ describe a behaviour that, when consistently implemented, would indicate a reduction in problem severity
◆ where possible, describe a positive change to be worked towards as opposed to simply stopping certain behaviours; for example, during assessment Michael described using alcohol as a way of blocking out his voices, although this led to additional problems; it was important when formulating goals with Michael that they were aimed at achieving alternative coping strategies, such as listening to music as opposed to solely refraining from alcohol consumption
◆ be reflective of something that the client wishes to and can be realistically expected to achieve
◆ indicate how frequently and for how long the behaviour would be sustained for. This helps to ensure some permanency as opposed to 'one-off' goal achievement.

Table 6.4 demonstrates a guide that can be used to help with formulating problem and goal statements.

Table 6.4a Problem statement guide

Problem definition	Impact	Consequences
Avoids going out. Believes others say bad things.	Stays at home in bedroom.	Feels lonely and isolated.

Table 6.4b Goals statement guide

The behaviour	Conditions	Frequency	Duration
Attend day centre	Go to groups	Three times per week	12 hours

A good start when writing problem statements with clients is to ask them to try and sum up in one sentence what they believe their problem is. As they talk through it, you could fill in the above boxes and pull together a statement. This should then be read back to the client to ensure that it fulfils the above check list. The same can be applied to goals, except you could ask clients to think of something they would like to work towards that the current problem prevents.

Measuring problems and goals

Increasingly, health professionals are being asked to demonstrate the effectiveness of their interventions; subsequently the use of clinical measures to evaluate practice is becoming routine. This is reflected in many training programmes, including the Thorn Initiative (Gamble 1997), which encourages the use of validated questionnaires and other measures to evaluate practice. Marks (1986) argues that the evaluation of any treatment requires some predetermined criteria for outcome and suggests that problems and goals can be measured using a 0–8 point scale. Boxes 6.1 and 6.2 show examples of a problem statement and goal statement respectively, along with the rating scale. Problems and goals should be rated at assessment to give a baseline rating and then at subsequently prearranged (by the client and assessor) intervals thereafter. It is important that clients understand what and why they are rating; this is best achieved by either asking them to read, or reading to them, the sentence directly above the rating scale shown in Box 6.2. Both clients and

---

Box 6.1 Problem statement

Avoidance of going out because I believe others say bad things about me, leading to me staying at home resulting in my being lonely.

Rating scale
This problem interferes with my daily activities:

```
       0-------1-------2-------3-------4-------5-------6-------7-------8
  Does not          Slight        Definite      Often         Severe
```

	Assess						
Date							
Client							
Assessor							

Box 6.2 Goal statement

To attend the day centre, and to go to the groups, remaining 2 hours three times weekly.

Rating scale

My progress towards achieving this goal:

```
0-------1-------2-------3-------4-------5-------6-------7-------8
```
Complete success   75%   50%   25%   No success

	Assess					
Date						
Client						
Assessor						

assessors should rate the problem and goals as this helps demonstrate mutual and equal commitment. In addition it gives a focus to feedback at subsequent sessions.

Acknowledgement

The authors would like to acknowledge the work of Dave Richards and Bob McDonald in their book *Behavioural psychotherapy: a handbook for nurses,* and in particular their description of the Problems and Goals Rating Scale used in this chapter.

Summary of practical strategies identified

Assessment interview

- ◆ Establish mutually agreed assessment boundaries at the beginning – for example, the agenda and time frames.
- ◆ Encourage the client to expand on information by asking the question: 'Is there anything you would like to add?'
- ◆ Keep questions simple, avoid asking double-barrelled questions and allow the client time to answer.
- ◆ Avoid using jargon. If possible, try and use similar language to that of the client.

Summary of practical strategies identified (*cont'd*)

◆ Recap information to gain clarity and more detail. (This is also a good strategy to use when the interview loses its flow.)

◆ Take written notes. It is hard to remember information unless you write it down. Most clients will not object but remember to ask permission and keep note taking discreet.

Problems and goals

◆ Do not write problem and goal statements for clients; this defeats the object and contradicts the philosophy of this assessment. It is more appropriate to work with clients to help them achieve this.

◆ Be flexible; although it is desirable that the statements follow the suggested format, adherence to this should not take precedence over a statement that has meaning to the client.

◆ Be prepared to compromise; remember these are the client's goals, not yours.

References

Birchwood M, Tarrier N 1992 Psychological management of schizophrenia. Wiley, Chichester

Clinton M, Nelson S 1996 Mental health and nursing practice, Prentice Hall, Sydney

Gamble C 1997 The Thorn nursing programme: its past, present and future. Mental Health Care 1(3):95–97

Hawton K, Salkoskis P, Kirk J, Clark D 1989 Cognitive behavioural therapy for psychiatric problems: a practical guide. Oxford Medical Publications, Oxford, p 13

McFarland G K, Thomas M D 1990 Psychiatric Mental Health Nursing: application of the nursing process. Lippincott, London

Marks I M 1986 The Maudsley handbook of behavioural psychotherapy. Croom Helm, London

Richards D, McDonald B 1990 Behavioural psychotherapy: a pocket book for nurses. Heinemann, Oxford

Annotated further reading

Fowler D, Garety P, Kuipers L 1995 Cognitive–behavioural interventions for psychosis: a practical guide. Wiley, Chichester

Annotated further reading (cont'd)

A simple structured format that gives the reader a step by step guide through some strategies to help with psychotic symptoms. It also uses excellent clinical examples to demonstrate this, which bring the interventions to life.

Birchwood M, Tarrier N 1992 Psychological interventions for schizophrenia. Wiley, Chichester

Although this book is a few years old, it still has one of the best chapters on assessment, providing a logical and straightforward approach. In addition, it has some chapters that look more broadly at service provision for this client group and it includes an introductory chapter on family interventions and assessment.

Haddock G, Slade P D (eds) 1996 Cognitive–behavioural interventions for psychosis. Routledge, London

This is more of a reference book and includes a good review of literature. In addition, the chapter by Jenny Day related to medication is an essential read as it includes some useful ways of helping clients assess and measure side-effects.

7

Assessing risk

Iain Ryrie

KEY ISSUES

- ◆ The meaning of risk.
- ◆ Principles of risk assessment.
- ◆ The process of risk assessment.
- ◆ Assessments of suicide risk.
- ◆ Assessment for risk of violence.
- ◆ Assessing the care environment.
- ◆ The process of risk management.

INTRODUCTION

Clinical risk assessment is an established tenet of psychiatric treatment. In varying degrees it forms an integral part of any decision concerning the provision of care. Recent additions to legislation (Mental Health [Patients in the Community] Act 1995), as well as the publication of national frameworks and guidelines (Department of Health 1990, NHS Executive 1994), have refocused practitioners' attention on its importance. Additionally, concerned members of the public, following publicised tragedies involving psychiatric patients and the subsequent formation of lobbying groups, are more able to articulate their expectations of the health care professions. This chapter offers the reader a conceptual framework for the comprehensive assessment of clinical risk. It deals with the nature of risk and the types of harm that might occur. The basic principles of risk assessment are then presented. In turn, these are used to guide the reader through the systematic assessment of risk to others and to oneself.

THE NATURE OF RISK

Before describing any methods for assessment it is necessary to understand what constitutes risk and how it may manifest itself. In our personal lives we are all familiar with notions of risk: 'if I make this luxury purchase today will I manage financially until pay day?' or, perhaps of a more serious nature, 'I've tried to stop, but not recently, because my work and social life revolves around other smokers'. In the latter example, risk is equated with danger, in so far as the individual may suffer debilitating or life-threatening consequences. Clinical risk is also concerned with danger, in terms of that which an individual might pose to themselves or others. However, recent literature conveys dissatisfaction with the term 'dangerousness'. Some commentators deem it to be pejorative (Snowden 1997), whilst others believe it implies an inflexible and static personality state that leads to clinical assessments as one-off yes/no predictions (Blom-Cooper, Hally & Murphy 1995).

Consideration of risk, rather than dangerousness, provides a more comprehensive basis for clinical decisions. It is concerned not simply with the individual, but also with the circumstances they are in and their perception of those circumstances. Since circumstances are subject to change, levels of risk will equally fluctuate. Clinical risk assessment therefore deals with the probability of an event occurring and needs to address the types of harm that might occur as well as the likelihood of their occurrence.

Self-harm, suicide and homicide are the types of harm that threaten the lives of individuals. Other types of harm also constitute risk even if a life is not immediately threatened. On a daily basis clinical staff make decisions concerning the relative merits of different treatment interventions. Their selection will involve consideration of the possible harms and benefits each option has for their client's health. Clinical risk assessment is therefore concerned with threats to health as well as life. This concern extends beyond the individual client to their family and friends, and others who they will encounter in their communities. These elements delineate the scope of clinical risk assessment, and can be understood by viewing them as two continua crossed as axes (Fig. 7.1). This framework provides a conceptually coherent resource that is also fundamentally practical. Additionally, it draws attention to those areas of risk assessment which healthcare staff regularly undertake, thereby aligning their existing skills with the more onerous task of determining levels of risk in life-threatening situations.

PRINCIPLES OF RISK ASSESSMENT

Whether assessing risk of harm to others, or to self, the process is similar but

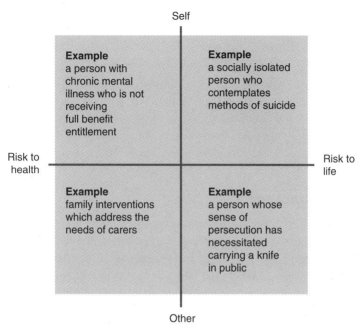

Figure 7.1 The scope of clinical risk assessment.

with a slightly different emphasis (Gunn 1994). A number of principles underpin the approach; they are listed in Box 7.1 and then briefly elaborated.

Instrumentation

It is appealing to envisage a quantitative fixed response instrument that enables clinicians to accurately predict who will be violent or self harming. However, no such instrument exists. Whilst certain objective individual

Box 7.1 Principles of risk assessment

◆ Do not rely on clinical instruments to determine risk
◆ Risk assessment is an interpersonal process
◆ Focus on probability rather than certainty
◆ Ground assessments in history
◆ Utilise collateral data sources
◆ Focus on 'at risk' situations rather than 'at risk' people
◆ Risk management is an ongoing process

attributes do correlate with risk, of greater importance are the subjective or phenomenological perspectives that individuals bring to bear on their circumstances (Keirle 1997). Risk assessment does not rely on a 'tick box' type of clinical instrument but requires a collaborative and sensitive exploration of a client's circumstances. Whilst some quantitative instruments are available in the literature, such as Pierce's (1981) 'Suicide Intent Scale', it is advisable to use these as global assessments of need, before undertaking a more detailed and discursive assessment, rather than as ends in themselves.

Interpersonal processes

If risk assessment involves collaborative exploration of a client's circumstances then it is predicated on an interpersonal process. The utility of assessment data will therefore reflect the quality of the interpersonal relationship. Since the subject matter to be explored may be upsetting or provocative to the client, staff will need to employ appropriate strategies to minimise distress and client resistance. Staff should appraise their communication style and endeavour to generate accurate empathy with the client through the use of open-ended questions and reflective listening skills. They should also assess their own stressors and personal concerns, which might affect their interaction with clients. Although still poorly understood, the literature increasingly reports associations between staff behaviour and client violence (Maier et al 1987, Whittington & Wykes 1994). Morgan & Priest (1991) also report that over 50% of a sample of psychiatric patients who committed suicide had been viewed by staff as complaining and manipulative, had become the focus of critical comments and negative judgement, and were alienated within the care environment.

Probability

Risk assessment is an inexact science based ultimately on clinical judgement. Its purpose is to minimise risk rather than eliminate it. The accuracy with which clinicians are able to predict risk is a contentious issue and estimates of this vary in the literature. Traditionally it was reported that one in three predictions of violent behaviour would be accurate (Monahan 1988). Recent investigations, utilising more rigorous methodologies, have found that approximately two-thirds of predictions are accurate (Lidz, Mulvey & Gardner 1993, McNeil & Binder 1995). Despite inaccuracies, Lidz, Mulvey & Gardner (1993) conclude that clinicians are able to predict violent behaviour more accurately through comprehensive risk assessment than by chance alone.

History

An old adage recurs in the literature that 'nothing predicts future behaviour better than past behaviour'. Health care staff employ this principle on a daily basis. It is central, for example, to decisions concerning the suitability of a client for atypical antipsychotic medication. Staff will draw on their knowledge of clients' previous management of medication to determine their ability to adhere to a more onerous regimen involving regular blood cell monitoring. Equally, a previous history of violence or self harm is one of the most useful indicators of risk available to clinicians. It has been estimated, for example, that parasuicide increases the risk of suicide tenfold (Rorsmann 1973). Similarly, in a study of psychiatric patients discharged from hospital, nearly two-thirds of those with a history of violence were violent again within a year of discharge (Klassen & O'Connor 1989). Whenever possible therefore, risk assessments should be grounded in history, not simply because of the correlation between past and future behaviour, but because the circumstances surrounding past behaviour will provide useful insights to reduce the likelihood of its reoccurrence.

Collateral sources

To ensure comprehensive assessment of risk clinicians need to seek information from all possible sources and create opportunities to share this information with others. CPA meetings provide one such opportunity. Information will be gathered from multidisciplinary team members, but also from others involved in the client's care, including the general practitioner, relatives, social workers, housing officers, the probation service and the police (Snowden 1997). The acquisition and sharing of information between parties raises concern over a patient's right to confidentiality. However, the common law duty of confidence should not be applied so rigidly as to jeopardise the well-being of an individual or the public at large. The Department of Health (1996) have issued useful guidance on these matters.

Risk situations

Of paramount importance in clinical risk assessment are situational determinants. The assessor should be concerned with those factors that, from past experience, have been associated with poor health or relapse and the occurrence of violence or self harm. It is therefore more appropriate to think in terms of 'at risk' situations rather than 'at risk' people.

Ongoing risk management

If the nature of risk is variable, dependent as it is upon any one set of circumstances, then it follows that risk assessments should form part of an ongoing process of risk management rather than being one-off decisions (Keirle 1997). This is particularly true when an individual's circumstances change, such as during admission or discharge from hospital, or following changes in housing or support networks. Chadwick (1997) also draws attention to anniversaries, such as that of a relapse or suicide attempt, which can engender fear in patients and increase current levels of risk. At such times staff need to be flexible in their convening of meetings to share information and reassess risk, rather than adhering to a preset CPA review date.

THE PROCESS OF RISK ASSESSMENT

Various methods are reported in the literature to guide clinicians through the risk assessment process. Common to most is a staged approach involving a global assessment of risk followed by a specific assessment of the likelihood of its occurrence. This approach is now considered in relation to the assessment of suicide risk and risk of violence to others.

Suicide

In some situations evidence of risk is immediate, as in the case of a patient admitted to a psychiatric unit from an accident and emergency department following a suicide attempt. In other cases evidence is less tangible and clinicians will require a template against which they can gauge the overall, or global, risk that their client might face. Table 7.1 presents a number of individual attributes that have been shown to correlate with suicide. These factors have an accumulative effect and their presence should raise the index of concern among staff. Data are also available for the lifetime prevalence of suicide among certain psychiatric diagnostic groups (Department of Health 1993):

◆ schizophrenia 10%
◆ affective disorders 15%
◆ personality disorders 15%
◆ alcohol dependence 15%.

Less attention has been paid in the literature to those personal factors that might protect individuals from taking their own life in the face of unbearable circumstances. However, this type of information can counterbalance an otherwise high risk situation (Appleby 1992). In a study by Linehan et al (1983) the most frequently cited reasons for not attempting suicide were concern for children, religious beliefs and fear of pain.

Table 7.1 Suicide risk factors

Variable	Risk categories
Age	Generally increases with age but also: ◆ young men ◆ young Asian females
Gender	More common in men than women
Physical health	Chronic life-threatening illness Chronic pain
Psychological health	Low self-esteem Depression Feelings of hopelessness Experience of significant loss Unrelenting and distressing delusions/hallucinations Command hallucinations Impulsiveness
Social health	Social isolation with poor social supports Conflict with supportive others Social upheaval, e.g. divorce, accommodation changes
History	Suicide attempt in previous 12 months

Assessment of suicide intent

When global assessments indicate a risk of serious self harm or suicide a more detailed assessment of the individual's intent in relation to any action is required. Before embarking on such an exploration it is important to remember the potentially distressing nature of the subject matter and create an environment that is conducive to sensitive discussion. The process follows a funnelling of questions, which begin with open-ended, indirect enquiries and lead on to more specific, direct questioning.

Areas for indirect enquiry:

◆ explore what hopes or plans your client has for the future
◆ ascertain whether they are able to see any way out of their current difficulties
◆ explore whether they have ever felt overwhelmed or have wanted to escape because of their difficulties.

If responses to these enquiries continue to suggest that the client is at risk then it becomes necessary to ask specific questions about the client's intent. This requires a much more direct approach that might typically involve asking clients whether they have ever considered harming themselves or ending it all, or whether they have ever felt suicidal.

When clients confirm suicidal intent then further assessment of risk can be made. Ratna (unpublished study 1990) identifies three indices that warrant attention. First, there is an index of seriousness, which requires assessors to ask whether clients have considered how they will harm themselves and whether any plans have been made. Secondly, there is an index of management, which requires assessors to ascertain what has led clients to this conclusion and whether they have considered any alternatives to suicide. Thirdly, there is an index of urgency, which involves assessors asking when clients think this might happen and whether there is any deciding factor or event that might influence them. These indices provide valuable information for the management of clients.

The collation and synthesis of this information will provide an indication of the likelihood that individuals will act upon their feelings. It was also suggested earlier that previous attempts at suicide can provide valuable information concerning current intent. These events should also be assessed by means of a functional analysis that retrospectively looks at the antecedents and behaviours involved, as well as the consequences. Table 7.2 presents areas for enquiry in a functional analysis.

Violence

Research has a identified a number of individual attributes that correlate with violent behaviour (Table 7.3). Their presence does not necessarily indicate the inevitable occurrence of violence, since this will depend on additional situational factors. However, their accumulation should draw attention to an increased risk of violence and the need for further assessment.

Table 7.2 Assessment of intent following a suicide attempt

Antecedents	Was the act prepared for in advance? Were steps taken to deal with the aftermath such as a will or suicide note?
Behaviour	Was the person alone when suicide was attempted? Were any steps taken to avoid the person's discovery by others? What is the person's perception of the lethality of the method they used?
Consequences	Was any assistance sought after the event? Did the person resist assistance from others? Does the person express any regret at the failure of the attempt?

Table 7.3 Risk factors for violence

Variable	Risk categories
Age	Generally decreases with age
Gender	More common in men than women
Physical	Drug or alcohol intoxication Medication side effects, e.g. disinhibition, disorientation
Psychological	Fears for personal safety Feelings of anger Delusional beliefs of persecution Command hallucinations Low intelligence
Social	Unstable living arrangements Poor educational attainment Exposure to violence in social milieu, e.g. home, environment
History	Previous history of violent behaviour

When determining whether an individual has a history of violence, several points need to be considered. Documentary evidence may not be immediately available. In such circumstances, if a possible risk of violence has been identified, clinicians may deem it appropriate to seek historical information directly from clients. This reflects a shift in focus from global to specific assessment data. It should not be conducted through the delivery of a series of closed-ended questions concerning the clients' past behaviour. For some, this will be provocative and for most, demeaning. Staff must judge their enquiry according to the clients' verbal and non-verbal communication patterns and the level of rapport that has been established. Clients may be encouraged to share information related to the areas of enquiry listed below. During this process staff need to demonstrate empathy through the use of reflective listening and convey a personal interest in the clients' histories:

◆ experiences of anger and frustration, and methods of coping
◆ juvenile involvement in fighting or other violence
◆ episodes of verbal or physical hostility to partners or family members
◆ episodes of verbal or physical hostility to offspring or other children
◆ episodes of indiscriminate verbal or physical hostility
◆ criminal records
◆ use of weapons or implements.

Previous incidents of violent behaviour provide important information concerning the circumstances in which its reoccurrence is more likely as well

Table 7.4 Assessment of intent following violent behaviour

Antecedents	Circumstantial factors that motivated client Provocation Drug or alcohol intoxication Treatment status
Behaviour	Was behaviour planned or impulsive? Was behaviour directed at a specific individual? Were weapons used? How was the behaviour stopped, and by whom?
Consequences	Degree of resultant harm or damage Victim empathy Positive reinforcers for past behaviour Current perception of past behaviour

as indicators for how that risk might be minimised. A functional analysis, similar to that outlined for the assessment of acts of self harm, can be conducted to elicit this information (Table 7.4).

Assessment of intent to harm

When serious risk of harm is identified, a more detailed assessment of an individual's intent in relation to any action is required. Communication strategies similar to those used when eliciting a client's history of violent behaviour should be employed. The client's current thoughts and feelings are explored in relation to the following areas:

◆ experiences of hopelessness, frustration or anger in relation to circumstances
◆ focus of anger and any thoughts of revenge
◆ frequency, intensity and perception of thoughts
◆ current and intended methods of coping.

This information provides insight into a client's current thinking and as such is an indicator for short term risk. Generally, the greater a client's preoccupation and willing indulgence in thoughts of violence, the higher is the risk.

Assessment of the care environment

The environment influences, and is influenced by, human behaviour. This reciprocity illuminates the potential impact of service provision upon an individual's behaviour. In relation to both self harm and harm to others, studies demonstrate a positive association with certain types of care environment. For example, Crammer (1984) in the United Kingdom and

Coser (1976) in the USA have both studied inpatient settings following sharp increases in suicide rates. Both studies identified similar characteristics of the care environment, which were thought to contribute to the elevated rates. These included: inadequate plans for the rehabilitation process prior to an individual's discharge; poor communication among staff; inconsistent observation of patients by staff; low staff numbers, morale and training opportunities; and poor supervision of junior staff.

The Royal College of Psychiatrists (1998) have recently published clinical practice guidelines for the management of violence that address the clinical environment. The following areas are highlighted for attention and each is broken down in greater detail with a comprehensive list of implementation points:

◆ calming features and ensuring a safe environment
◆ activities
◆ day accommodation
◆ protocols for effective care environments
◆ policies for effective care environments.

Readers are encouraged to refer to this work and to employ the implementation points in an assessment of the care environments they create or contribute to. This can form part of an ongoing process of multidisciplinary audit. At the very least it requires staff to recognise their own influence upon patient behaviour and incorporate such considerations into any clinical risk assessment process.

RISK MANAGEMENT

Clinical risk management is the intended purpose of the assessment process. It involves the development of treatment strategies to reduce both the severity and frequency of identified risks (Snowden 1997). A client's key worker, case manager or other main service provider has responsibility for formulating the risk management plan and securing consensus, regarding its content, from other disciplines, agencies and individuals involved in the client's care. Listed below are the necessary contents of a risk management plan:

◆ the circumstances associated with previous risk behaviours
◆ any early warning signs that immediately precede risk behaviours
◆ a description of what must change to reduce risk
◆ the presentation of possible strategies to enable change to occur
◆ an assessment of the client's likely collaboration with each strategy
◆ the roles and responsibilities of those involved in the client's care
◆ responsibilities for responding to emergency situations
◆ dates for routine review and circumstances that would necessitate an immediate review.

The plan does not signify an end point in the risk assessment process. Risks will vary over time and in relation to different circumstances. Failure to share information and take a long term view of risk are significant factors for the occurrence of dangerous incidents and tragedies in mental health services (Lipsedge 1995). The risk management plan is therefore only a short term strategy and should be subject to constant review. It follows that all individuals involved in a client's care have a responsibility to fulfil their specific role but also to communicate progress, and any perceived changes in the client, to the coordinator of the plan. Similarly, this coordinator may have specific treatment responsibilities but will also have a duty to maintain effective lines of communication with other treatment and care providers.

CONCLUSIONS

This chapter has presented a framework to understand the scope of risk assessment and a series of principles that should underpin its process. The assessment of risk to self and others has been presented as a staged approach to aid clarity although, in practice, the sequence and inclusion of elements will vary considerably. It should not be viewed as a stand-alone process but one that permeates all aspects of the treatment culture. This will include multidisciplinary decisions concerning the relative merits of routine treatment options, multidisciplinary and interagency collaborations to minimise the risk of serious harm, and the integration of risk management principles in a rolling programme of clinical audit. It is inevitable that incidents involving violence or suicide will occur from time to time since risk assessment is ultimately based upon clinical judgement. However, providing a comprehensive assessment has been undertaken, a coherent rationale documented for any intervention offered, and an ongoing process of review operationalised, then healthcare staff will have fulfilled their responsibilities.

Summary of practical strategies identified

- ◆ All clients attending should receive a risk assessment not simply to determine possible violence or self-harm but also to identify any factors that may compromise their health or the health of their 'significant others'.
- ◆ The validity of clinical risk assessments will depend on the quality of the therapeutic relationship and the application by staff of various principles that underpin the process (see Box 7.1).

Summary of practical strategies identified (cont'd)

◆ Whether assessing risk to others or to self, the process is similar and involves an initial global assessment of risk followed by a specific assessment of the likelihood of its occurrence.

◆ Risk factors for self harm and violence are presented in Tables 7.1 and 7.3 and can be used to undertake initial global assessments.

◆ Any history of previous risk behaviours should be sought and these events can be assessed in greater detail to determine the likelihood of their reoccurrence (Tables 7.2 and 7.4).

◆ When potential risk is identified a more detailed assessment of current intent is undertaken; this follows a funnelling process beginning with open-ended, indirect enquiries and leading to more specific, direct questioning.

◆ Clinical risk management is the intended purpose of the assessment process and involves the development of a risk management plan, which identifies strategies to reduce both the severity and frequency of risk behaviours.

◆ Risk will vary over time in relation to different circumstances and should be subject to regular review.

References

Appleby L 1992 Suicide in psychiatric patients: risk and prevention. British Journal of Psychiatry 161:749–758

Blom-Cooper L, Hally H, Murphy E 1995 The falling shadow – one patient's mental health care 1978–1993. Duckworth, London

Chadwick P 1997 Recovery from psychosis: Learning more from patients. Journal of Mental Health 6:577–588

Coser R 1976 Suicide and the relational system: a case study in a mental hospital. Journal of Health and Social Behaviour 17:318–327

Crammer J 1984 The special characteristics of suicide in hospital in-patients. British Journal of Psychiatry 145:460–476

Department of Health 1990 The care programme approach for people with a mental illness referred to the special psychiatric services (HC(90)23, LASSL (90) 11). Department of Health, London

Department of Health 1993 The Health of the Nation: key area handbook, mental illness. Department of Health, London

Department of Health 1996 The protection and use of patient information. Department of Health, London

References (*cont'd*)

Gunn J 1994 Dangerousness. In: Gunn J, Taylor P (eds) Forensic psychiatry: clinical, legal and ethical issues. Butterworth-Heinemann, Oxford, pp 624–625

Keirle P 1997 Psychiatric patient violence: assessment and management of risk. British Journal of Community Health Nursing 2:191–194

Klassen D, O'Connor W 1989 Assessing the risk of violence in released mental patients: a cross-validation study. Psychological Assessment 1:75–81

Lidz C, Mulvey P, Gardner W 1993 The accuracy of predictions of violence to others. Journal of the American Medical Association 269:1007–1011

Linehan M, Goodstein J, Nielsen S, Chiles J 1983 Reasons for staying alive when you are thinking of killing yourself: The Reason for Living inventory. Journal of Consulting and Clinical Psychology 51:276–286

Lipsedge M 1995 Psychiatry: reducing risk in clinical practice. In: Vincent C (ed) Clinical risk management. British Medical Journal Publishing Group, London, pp 18–29

McNeil D, Binder R 1995 Correlates of accuracy in the assessment of psychiatric inpatients' risk of violence. American Journal of Psychiatry 152:901–906

Maier G, Stava L, Morrow B, Van Rybroek G, Bauman K 1987 A model for understanding and managing cycles of aggression among psychiatric inpatients. Hospital and Community Psychiatry 38:520–524

Monahan J 1988 Risk assessment of violence among the mentally disordered: generalising useful knowledge. International Journal of Law and Psychiatry 11:249–257

Morgan H, Priest P 1991 Suicide and other unexpected deaths among psychiatric inpatients: the Bristol Confidential Inquiry. British Journal of Psychiatry 158:368–374

NHS Executive 1994 Guidance on the discharge of mentally disordered people and their continuing care in the community (HSG994)27. Department of Health, London

Pierce D 1981 The predictive validation of a suicide intent scale: a five year follow up. British Journal of Psychiatry 139:391–396

Rorsmann B 1973 Suicide in psychiatric patients: a comparative study. Social Psychiatry 8:55–66

Royal College of Psychiatrists 1998 Management of imminent violence: clinical practice guidelines: quick reference guide. Royal College of Psychiatrists, London

Snowden P 1997 Practical aspects of clinical risk assessment and management. British Journal of Psychiatry 170 (suppl 32):32–34

Whittington R, Wykes T 1994 An observational study of associations between nurse behaviour and violence in psychiatric hospitals. Journal of Psychiatric and Mental Health Nursing 1:85–92

Annotated further reading

Duggan C (ed) 1997 Assessing risk. British Journal of Psychiatry 170: suppl 32

This comprehensive account of contemporary knowledge concerning risk assessment has been collated into a single British Journal of Psychiatry supplement by Conor

Annotated Further Reading (*cont'd*)

Duggan. The contributors are eminent clinicians and academics who deal with a diverse range of issues from sexual offending to the rights of the person who is being assessed for levels of risk. Overall the text is rather more analytical than practical but nevertheless equips the reader with a sound grasp of relevant issues.

Royal College of Psychiatrists 1998 Management of imminent violence: clinical practice guidelines to support mental health services. RCP, London

These guidelines were developed to reflect the current levels of knowledge concerning the effective and appropriate treatment of potentially violent persons. They are based upon a rigorous and systematic review of research evidence as well as the views of practitioners, service users and their carers. They are fundamentally predicated upon the provision of an environment that reduces the likelihood of violence but deal also with the management of actual violence.

Gunn J, Taylor P 1994 Forensic psychiatry: clinical, legal and ethical issues. Butterworth-Heinemann, Oxford

A comprehensive textbook that integrates forensic treatment with its wider legal and moral ramifications. The book is written in an easily accessible format and provides practice-orientated recommendations for this field of care.

Section 3

Interventions

8

Using a low Expressed Emotion approach to develop positive therapeutic alliances

Catherine Gamble

KEY ISSUES

◆ Addressing beliefs, assumptions and stigma.
◆ Therapeutic qualities and characteristics of high and low Expressed Emotion.
◆ Using such approaches in clinical practice.

INTRODUCTION

With the changing context of mental health care delivery and the development of the user movement, clinicians, researchers and clients themselves have begun to place greater emphasis upon learning how to develop positive working alliances with each other. From the literature it is clear that, in order for any intervention to be successful, clients need to feel safe to disclose important and often distressing information (Hawton et al 1989). Therefore the relationship between themselves and the practitioner has to be based upon non-judgemental support, honesty, warmth and concern. In this way, clients will be more likely to achieve their personal goals and learn how to manage their symptoms as they will feel reassured that their experiences and needs will be taken seriously (Sainsbury Centre 1998). These concepts are not new and this chapter does not intend to reinvent the wheel. Instead, its aims are to examine the qualities and characteristics required, challenge some of the beliefs and attitudes that some practitioners hold and provide practical advice and strategies to aid the development of positive therapeutic alliances.

QUALITIES REQUIRED BY PRACTITIONERS

Throughout any mental health practitioner's training and working life, constant reference is made to the sort of personal qualities that are required to develop relationships with clients, their families and carers, but it is only recently that correlations between the importance of therapeutic relationships and the effect of therapy outcome has been recognised (Blaauw & Emmelkamp 1994). These qualities range from having a considerable degree of sensitivity, knowledge and expertise (Perkins & Repper 1996) to being self-aware, approachable, purposeful, flexible and ordinary. Having the ability to be a companion with a sense of fair play and humanity is what matters, as these qualities can be extraordinarily effective in helping clients find a sense of affinity with professionals (Taylor 1994). The effectiveness of such characteristics in helping clients learn and achieve their personal goals remains difficult to define (Burnard 1988); nevertheless, specific and sometimes counterintuitive skills are needed to work successfully with this client group (May 1976, Tuma et al 1978).

Overall such characteristics are compatible with Rogers' (1983) view of a facilitator. These are based on the value of individual freedom and responsibility, which are vital in order for meaningful learning to occur. Rogers (1983) believes the therapist–client relationship to be as important to learning as the teacher–student relationship and finds similarities between them, seeing the qualities that facilitate learning to be: realness, prizing, acceptance, trust and empathetic understanding. Indeed, when participants attending the recent Mind Annual Conference were asked to brainstorm what qualities and characteristics they thought practitioners required (Gamble 1998) they were readily able to identify similar, if not identical, characteristics (Box 8.1).

Such qualities can be inherent and/or developed over time, using communication and observation, and throughout a mental health practitioner's training there are numerous opportunities to reflect on the acquisition of these skills. However, after qualifying, some practitioners appear to have difficulty remembering to use these skills in everyday clinical practice. Indeed, all too frequently in the clinical area, professionals can be heard to make sweeping generalisations and judgements about clients and their needs, such as:

1. 'Oh yes, him again. Send him straight to the ward, we know all about him – we've treated him before.'

> **Box 8.1** Qualities and characteristics required in mental health professionals: a brainstorm
>
> Empathy. Sympathy. Non-judgemental. A friend. Being there when needed. Knowing when to back off. Being trustworthy. Believing in the person, letting me live my own life – not imposing own opinions and ideas upon me. Having the ability to listen. Providing supportive practical advice and help. Respectful of culture and beliefs. Perseverance, tolerance and acceptance. Flexible. Resourceful. Knowledgeable. Committed. Having a sense of humour.

2. 'The fact is that, despite every effort being made, he refuses to take medication, so what do you expect?'

3. 'This is the third time she's been in this year and its only July! What she really needs to do is leave her boyfriend – he's a nightmare and makes her condition worse, but there's no telling her.'

4. 'No, there is no point organising that for him, we tried it before and he said he couldn't be bothered – don't you remember?'

5. 'We've dealt with cases like this on numerous occasions – what we need to do is review the treatment again. Get him back on depot medication and then get the social worker involved to sort out his housing.'

6. 'Don't you realise how difficult it is for your family to cope with your behaviour?'

If the above statements were attributed to relatives their ability to provide a caring environment would be questioned, as clients exposed to emotionally critical, hostile or overinvolved environments have a greater tendency to relapse. To reduce this risk, the research and surrounding work on EE (see Ch. 2) highlights the importance of being warm, empathetic, objective, non-confrontational and adaptive (Leff & Vaughn 1985). Yet, despite this efficacious research, some professionals continue to be punitive, confrontational and authoritarian and as a direct consequence clients and relatives can become ostracised. This increases the likelihood of frustration, anger and incidence of relapse.

When one considers how difficult it is to cope with a serious mental illness such as schizophrenia and its consequences in today's under-resourced, stressful clinical environments, these reactions are *sometimes* understandable. However, such responses should be avoided. It is no longer acceptable to tell someone to stop doing something or behaving in a certain way, as this does not take into consideration the caring emotion behind the perceived behaviour or comment. Being critical or hostile is sometimes the only way that some people can relay how frightened and concerned they feel.

Therefore, professionals should challenge their own and each other's assumptions and strive towards using the aforementioned positive attributes, because until a sound, collaborative rapport is formed it is not possible to facilitate a psychoeducation approach and teach clients about their illness or the effects of medication (Weiden & Havens 1994). Indeed, none of the interventions described in this book will ever be truly effective if practitioners are not prepared to foster such an approach.

So how can this change be brought about?

REVIEW OF PERSONAL ATTITUDES, KNOWLEDGE AND BELIEFS

First, the most important step practitioners can make is to review their own response characteristics, attitudes, beliefs and knowledge base. A useful exercise is to examine Table 8.1, then observe your colleagues and your own interactions with clients and note which characteristics you exhibit.

During this process you may notice that you respond differently towards some clients than you do with others; this is not uncommon and such observations confirm the findings of Moore, Ball & Kuipers (1992) and Finnema et al (1996). Nevertheless, you and your colleagues should be striving towards responding in a low EE manner with all clients, as these positive attributes have been found, with the help of medication, to reduce relapse

Table 8.1 Response characteristics of low and high EE

	Low EE	High EE
Cognitive	Recognise illness as genuine	Legitimacy of the illness in doubt
	Lower expectations of the individual	Expectations unchanged
Emotional	Other-focused	Self-focused – 'my goals and needs are more important'
	Empathetic	
	Calm	Intense anger and/or distress
	Objective	
Behavioural	Adaptive	Inflexible
	Problem-solving approach	
	Non-intrusive	Intrusive
	Non-confrontational	Confrontational

Source: Adapted from Leff & Vaughn (1985)

rates (see Lam 1991 for a review). Although it is acknowledged that this is sometimes easier said than done, the first step to changing interaction patterns is to challenge assumptions, understand the reason for their occurrence and consider why practitioners make them in the first place. For example, in statement 1 (see p. 116) in the earlier list, there is an assumption that a person never changes and that they should always be treated the same way despite what may have happened between admissions. Statements 2, 3 and 4 (see p. 117) give the impression that clients wilfully contribute to their condition. Indeed, these examples present clients as being part of the problem itself and therefore they are not perceived as having the ability or desire to contribute to possible solutions. In none of these cases are the professionals questioning their own attitudes. In statement 5 the client is removed from the decision-making process altogether and the issues are reduced to practical problems, with treatment being decided *for* rather than *with* the patient. The practitioner is also making assumptions about another professional's role and this further reduces the possibilities of collaboration. Statement 6 is a direct criticism and also patronising. It induces guilt and makes the assumption that the remark will stop the behaviour. This is never the case.

If, at this point you are thinking 'I've made those type of statements' – good, we all have. Irrespective of whether we are practitioners, carers or clients, we all make such comments without thinking of their consequences. No one is perfect. It is a fact of life that we will not always get on with everybody we come in contact with. But we should try to avoid writing off individuals for this reason alone. If a relationship has been established for some time, it may be initially difficult to change entrenched interaction patterns. Nevertheless, it is important to realise the need for change, and as professionals share similar attitudes to those of relatives (Oliver & Kuipers 1996) it is worth assessing and continually re-evaluating your own EE characteristics.

To enhance this process, begin by asking yourself: 'When was the last time I thought or said something positive about the clients I am working with?' An important technique is to reframe client behaviour and interactions positively. In other words, we need to have the ability to redirect or change the perception of a situation and place it in another more appropriate context. Begin then by thinking about your clients, how you perceive them and the work you are doing together; that is, try to stop viewing clients as a problem and start seeing them as people facing problems. To achieve this successfully, remember that no one knows more about their illness than clients themselves and a diagnosis of schizophrenia or other SMI does not indicate complete mental incapacity.

Ultimately, an individual's choice is of paramount importance. Therefore, the second part of the aforementioned process is to make time to listen to clients. As mentioned earlier, clients, not professionals, are the experts in serious mental illness, and the majority (if they are provided with the appropriate opportunity) are quite able to tell about their experiences (see Ch. 1). Indeed, when asked, users appreciate having someone to talk to and perceive this to be a 'safety net' (Hannigan, Bartlett & Clilverd 1997). Listening, however, is an art. If you are prepared to concentrate 100%, hear what is said and not contaminate what you heard with your own thoughts and ideas, your attitude towards the client will undoubtedly change for the better.

Another way to change attitude in a positive direction is through education. Professionals need to keep abreast with current thinking and, rather than solely relying on medication, they should learn how to use problem-orientated, efficacious interventions (Kuipers 1996). By doing so many of the myths and misunderstandings about how to treat and deal with serious mental illness will be defused, because these approaches focus upon the here and now rather than personality and therefore can help to dissipate negative emotions, which, in turn, will provide another step towards reducing levels of EE (Leff & Vaughn 1985).

In this context 'strength through knowledge' has significance for both the client and the practitioner, as without the appropriate knowledge neither can help each other to make informed health choices. When clients are deprived of adequate information about their illness and feel lost and alone, it is very reassuring to meet a competent and knowledgeable practitioner. They do not wish to be bombarded with facts and figures and there is nothing worse than being attended to by someone who perceives themselves to be an enlightened sage, when all they really do is pass on partisan pearls of wisdom. Nevertheless, clients do appreciate being treated by someone who is well informed and has the ability to: (1) overcome the fear of losing authority if information is shared and (2) provide practical help through a needs-led assessment and empowering treatment plan.

Finally, to promote and develop positive relationships there is a need to examine beliefs and prejudices about serious mental illness. The intolerance to mental illness is overwhelming in current society and clients have to live and cope with these negative perceptions every day of their lives. Haywood & Bright (1997) identify four possible explanations for the root cause of these unfavourable views, they are: (1) dangerousness: people fear the mentally ill because they believe they are prone to violence, (2) attribution of responsibility: there is a belief that the mentally ill 'choose' to behave as they do, (3) poor prognosis: they are chronic and difficult to treat, and (4) disruption of social interaction: the mentally ill are unpredictable and don't behave 'normally', so people feel uneasy interacting with them in social situations.

If mental health professionals are honest they have at some time or other shared a number or all of these views. Indeed, before entering into any relationship with a client, it is essential that you take time to review your own belief systems. For example, consider your 'off duty' reaction when you encounter someone exhibiting bizarre behaviour on the bus or in the street and/or how you would respond if you found out that the house next door was to be converted into a large rehabilitation hostel for the seriously mentally ill?

A number of the negative reactions you identify may be addressed if the following adapted model is utilised (Haywood & Bright 1997):

◆ **Assess specific beliefs:** challenge maladaptive views of the causes of serious mental illness, in regards to dangerousness and prognosis. Consider the degree to which your efforts can ameliorate the effects of the illness and the stigma it causes.

◆ **Challenge others' views on a wider social level:** take time to educate the lay person and those in your social network and do not shy away from this responsibility when such opportunities arise.

◆ **Question what are 'normal' beliefs and what are not:** consider any 'strange' experiences or ideas you have: for example: déjà vu, a belief in ghosts, reincarnation, aliens, astrology and tarot, etc.

◆ **Attack the view that the mentally ill are different:** try to portray clients with serious mental illness as rounded individuals; they are not 'nutters', they are human beings and this diagnosis is not self-inflicted.

◆ **Promote and encourage positive interactions and discussion with service users.**

◆ **We all have had periods when we have been 'ill', i.e. unable to function as we would normally expect:** consider how you would cope with such a situation if it went on for more than a few weeks.

Lastly, develop a holistic conception of mental illness that incorporates cultural, psychological and biological models of health care. In doing so, you will have a greater sense that there are self-management steps that can be used to enhance relationships, reduce the effects of stigma (Kingdon & Turkington 1994) and also help to ensure that a low EE approach is routinely practised.

CONCLUSIONS

Throughout this manual, numerous practical strategies will be described to help practitioners engage and work with service users who experience serious mental health problems. Although acknowledging that the development of alliances with clients can sometimes be a difficult task and may take a considerable amount of time (Frank & Gunderson 1990), this chapter has argued that the identified methods will be effective only if practitioners are prepared from the onset to keep abreast and continue to reassess their own assumptions, attitudes and beliefs. All too often professionals make sweeping generalisations about clients and have inappropriate expectations of what can and cannot be achieved. Putting these ideas into practice will be an ongoing challenge, especially if the practitioner is working in isolation, does not have access to an appropriate clinical supervisor, or is surrounded by team members who are unwilling to change or reflect upon their behaviours or assumptions. Nevertheless, whatever the circumstances, we have a professional responsibility to ensure that everyone who uses mental health services is treated fairly by objective, flexible, knowledgeable mental health professionals.

Summary of practical strategies identified

- ◆ Have the ability to reframe client behaviour and interactions positively.
- ◆ Avoid viewing clients as a problem and start seeing them as people facing problems.
- ◆ View clients as experts – a diagnosis of schizophrenia or other serious mental illness does not indicate complete mental incapacity.
- ◆ Actively listen – concentrate 100%, hear what is said, don't contaminate what you hear with your own thoughts and ideas.
- ◆ Keep abreast with up to date knowledge and thinking.
- ◆ Examine own beliefs and prejudices about serious mental illness.
- ◆ Avoid working from the standpoint of 'I am the only one who understands this client' – regularly evaluate your work and role, and use peer and individual supervision.

References

Blaauw E, Emmelkamp P M G 1994 The therapeutic relationship: a study on the value of the therapist client rating scale. Behavioural and Cognitive Psychotherapy 22:25–35

Burnard P 1988 Equality and meaning: issues in the interpersonal relationship. Community Psychiatric Nursing Journal Dec:17–21

Finnema E J, Louwerens J W, Slooff C J, Van den Bosch R J 1996 Expressed emotion on long stay wards. Journal of Advanced Nursing 24:473–478

Frank A F, Gunderson J G 1990 The role of the therapeutic alliance in the treatment of schizophrenia. Relationship to course and outcome. Archives of General Psychiatry 47:228–236

Gamble C 1998 Using a low expressed emotion approach in clinical practice: a challenge for professionals? Mind Annual Conference, Brighton

Hannigan B, Bartlett H, Clilverd A 1997 Improving health and social functioning: perspectives of mental health service users. Journal of Mental Health 6:613–619

References

Hawton K, Salkovskis P M, Kirk J, Clark D M 1989 Cognitive behaviour therapy for psychiatric problems. Oxford University Press, Oxford

Haywood P, Bright J A 1997 Stigma and mental illness: a review and critique. Journal of Mental Health 6(4):345–354

Kingdon D G, Turkington D 1994 Cognitive behavioural therapy of schizophrenia. Lawrence Erlbaum Associates, Hove, UK

Kuipers E 1996 The management of difficult to treat patients with schizophrenia, using non drug therapies. British Journal of Psychiatry 169 (suppl 31):41–51

Lam D 1991 Psychosocial family intervention in schizophrenia: a review of empirical studies. Psychological Medicine 21:433–441

Leff J, Vaughn C 1985 Expressed emotion in families. Guilford, New York

May P R A 1976 Rational treatment for an irrational disorder: what does the schizophrenic patient need? American Journal of Psychiatry 133:1008–1012

Moore E, Ball R A, Kuipers L 1992 Expressed emotion in staff working with the long term mentally ill. British Journal of Psychiatry 161:802–808

Oliver N, Kuipers E 1996 Stress and its relationship to expressed emotion in community mental health workers. International Journal of Social Psychiatry 42(2):150–159

Perkins R, Repper J 1996 Working alongside people with long term mental health problems. Chapman & Hall, London

Rogers C 1983 Freedom to learn for the 80's. Merrill, Columbus

Sainsbury Centre 1998 Keys to engagement. Sainsbury Centre, London

Taylor B 1994 Being human: ordinariness in nursing. Churchill Livingstone, New York

Tuma A H, May P R A, Yale C, Forsythe A B 1978 Therapists characteristics and the outcome of treatment in schizophrenia. Archives of General Psychiatry 35:81–85

Weiden P, Havens L 1994 Psychotherapeutic management techniques in the treatment of outpatients with schizophrenia. Hospital and Community Psychiatry 45(6):549–555

Annotated further reading

Perkins R, Repper J 1996 Working alongside people with long term mental health problems. Chapman & Hall, London

The title of this book clearly reflects its content. It provides an informative, thought-provoking explanation about how to work positively with people who experience long term mental health problems. The authors address how to enhance collaborative working relationships, so that a greater understanding of clients' personal needs can be achieved. In doing so, the text is refreshingly controversial. It explores the attitudes and assumptions professionals often make about people who have a serious mental health problem, by challenging the notion that clients are unable to control their own lives, or take an active role in treatment and service provision.

9

Dealing with voices and strange thoughts

Jem Mills

KEY ISSUES

◆ Voices and strange thoughts as part of the normal range of human experience.

◆ Adjusting the helping process to suit individuals.

◆ Encouraging service users and professionals to work alongside each other.

◆ Using specific assessments to develop a shared understanding of the problem, based on psychological models.

◆ Developing useful ways of coping with voices and strange, worrying beliefs.

◆ Exploring and testing out the specific beliefs about symptoms that are associated with a person's distress.

INTRODUCTION

For nearly half a century the most effective treatment for people with psychosis has been, and still is, to take powerful antipsychotic drugs. Despite the effectiveness of these substances, the majority of people taking them continue to experience some level of distressing symptoms. Other difficulties that people have with the chemical approach include the burden of unwanted effects and forgetting or deciding not to take the advised course. It is then a great advantage that this approach can now be complemented by other, more palliatable interventions.

Psychological approaches to the symptoms of psychosis have, in recent years, shown some remarkable developments. The application of cognitive behavioural therapy to these problems is a predominantly British endeavour and one that is proving to be quite successful (Kuipers et al 1997). Whilst we pride ourselves in these innovations we also need to take up the complex question of how to make the approaches more readily available to the people that need them.

This chapter deals with that challenge. I have attempted to identify important elements of the approach that might be useful to those mental health professionals seeking to help people with psychosis. I have avoided producing a 'cook book' of techniques in the hope that the reader will realise the importance of the process of helping someone with voices or delusions. In the spirit of collaborative working I have tried to present some ideas about dealing with these problems in a way that might be accessed by anyone. With this in mind I have also taken up the challenge of avoiding technical language, hence the use of the terms 'voices' and 'strange, worrying beliefs' rather than 'hallucinations' and 'delusions'. This use of language reflects another emergent principle of the work, namely that people with psychosis experience something that is quite naturally human. The tragic predicament in psychosis is the disabling regularity of intense psychotic experiences rather than the phenomena themselves.

Intervening too soon is often the cause of common problems encountered by mental health professionals learning to help people with psychosis. The iceberg model (Fig. 9.1) shows that there are a number of things to consider before crossing the water line into practical interventions. Sometimes the steps below this line are overlooked because they have a low visibility and there is currency in being seen to be doing something. Sometimes the professional assumes that enough information has been gathered to suggest a solution to the problem. Whatever the reason it is important to develop conceptual ways rather than intervention-led ways of understanding psychotic symptoms. It is also important to pay attention to the process of helping. The practical interventions shown in the figure (in the shaded area) are often the icing on a cake that has taken a long time to cook. Essential to the recipe is attention to those processes that underpin the interventions.

ADJUSTING THE THERAPEUTIC APPROACH TO SUIT PEOPLE WHO EXPERIENCE PSYCHOSIS

Naïveté

It is very hard to understand what it must be like to have psychosis and this can often make empathising with the sufferer difficult. Adopting a naïve approach is helpful in a number of ways. It gives a clear message that you are interested in finding out about a person's problems and that you are not setting

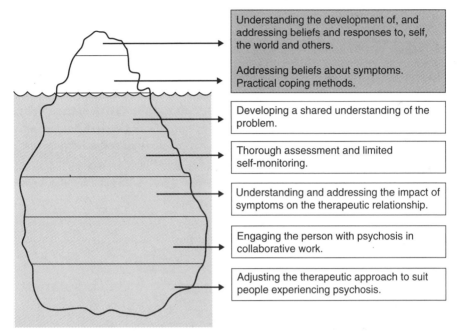

Understanding the development of, and addressing beliefs and responses to, self, the world and others.

Addressing beliefs about symptoms. Practical coping methods.

Developing a shared understanding of the problem.

Thorough assessment and limited self-monitoring.

Understanding and addressing the impact of symptoms on the therapeutic relationship.

Engaging the person with psychosis in collaborative work.

Adjusting the therapeutic approach to suit people experiencing psychosis.

Figure 9.1 Iceberg model showing the importance of low visibility work in psychosis.

yourself up as an expert. It also allows you to explore people's thinking on their terms. The approach involves an open questioning style. You should try to put your own expectations out of mind and explore people's own understanding of their problems. Adopting the principle that you might think the same way given similar circumstances is helpful. If the story seems difficult to understand at first do not assume that this is the storyteller's fault. Allow the confusion to wash over you and ask for clarification as you go. Many times adopting this approach has led to new insights into problems that were already considered well understood.

It will probably be necessary to adjust your therapeutic approach when beginning to help people with psychosis. Usual ways of working such as hour long, weekly sessions, setting tasks to be completed between sessions and having an active and lively pace may well be appropriate for some people. However, it might be that some people have never been asked to participate actively in their care. It is also possible for people to be hampered by difficulties with concentration and motivation. Consideration should be given to how individuals' particular problems might affect the therapeutic process. This often means:

◆ being flexible about the timing and frequency of sessions
◆ negotiating regular breaks

◆ regularly checking out how the person is finding the experience
◆ agreeing to stop the session if necessary
◆ being creative about the setting for the session.

In practice this means having an open discussion about expectations for the work ahead. It is important to set out the options and to explore any likely obstacles at an early stage. When in doubt, start slowly and build the pace after reflecting on the process together. Another difficulty with this approach can be that people are not used to the increased sense of responsibility that often comes with collaboration. Again, adjusting the pace of work helps this. The guiding principle should be one of moulding the process to suit individuals, rather than the other way around. This was helpful in Nigel's case:

Case study – Nigel

Nigel had been referred by his occupational therapist for some specific help in coping with voices. He found discussing them very upsetting and was understandably wary. He also had problems at home with his heating breaking down and had to visit the local inpatient unit to use its bath. It was suggested that working on his voices would be hard with so many practical problems taking up his time. He agreed that he was distracted by these difficulties and that he did not want to add to his stress. This approach acknowledged his difficult circumstances and made his well-being a clear priority. It also gave the message that learning to deal with his voices would involve some effort on his part, requiring him to devote time and motivation to the process. However, he was keen to start something and so a suitable compromise was negotiated. After some discussion he decided that he would call in over the following month when attending appointments with his occupational therapist. He wanted us to get to know each other and as the visits progressed he started asking questions about the ways we would be working together. After a month his home life was more stable and he felt able to begin. It was quickly established that even thinking about his voices was distressing. To lessen this distress it was agreed that appointments should last no more than 20 minutes. As the work progressed Nigel felt confident about trying more frequent and longer sessions.

This tailoring of the approach was begun to sow the seeds of some important principles that would guide the process of helping him to deal with his voices. These principles apply generally to helping people with psychotic symptoms:

◆ Alleviating distress is the prime focus of the work.
◆ Staying engaged with the process is more important than pushing ahead for results.

◆ The way to tackle big problems is to break them down into manageable steps.
◆ Each step of the process is openly negotiated.

Engaging the person with psychosis in collaborative work

Collaboration in this sense involves the person with psychotic symptoms working alongside the professional. The term implies that both parties have a role to play in the development of new understandings and coping methods. The venture is characteristically open and honest within the confines of a professional relationship. The professional needs to be clear about the boundaries of the therapeutic relationship including rules of confidentiality and duty of care. Because of this, collaboration can also be threatening to both parties. People with psychosis have often had little active involvement in their own care. For some the idea of participation is a welcome and refreshing change. For others the increased responsibility can be quite daunting and unwelcome. Some can feel quite hopeless about the prospect of change whilst others might be weighed down with low motivation. An individual's ability to participate will guide the pace of the process. If the person with psychosis is not able to take part in decision making it will be very difficult to proceed. With this in mind it is often useful to discuss how the referral came about. Useful questions will include:

◆ Was the referral made collaboratively?
◆ What are the person's expectations?
◆ What has been said about the service on offer?
◆ How does it feel to consider new ways of dealing with psychotic symptoms?

As with the previous section the guiding principle here is that large obstacles are tackled in small steps. Any difficulties with collaboration should be identified and the problem solved. For instance the person may have worries about medication being increased or reduced as a result of disclosing information about symptoms. A common worry is that full and open discussion of symptoms will lead to admissions or labelling of the person as mad.

Open discussion about the limitations of medication is often useful. Curson et al (1988) show that the majority of people taking neuroleptic medication continue to have residual symptoms. It is commonly thought that, when leaving hospital, rather than having had a complete recovery, people with psychosis have improved to a degree whereby they are able to disguise symptoms and avoid talking about them. Acknowledging that residual symptoms are sometimes to be expected rather than seen as a sign of relapse can relieve fears about disclosure. Often the early practical stages of helping a person with psychosis can be beneficial in demonstrating the value of collaborative work. It is important to foster this approach rather than press ahead with interventions that might be passively received by the unmotivated person. Many things can derail the process; working collaboratively at least ensures that if something goes wrong it will not be due to factors that one party has obscured from the view of another.

UNDERSTANDING AND ADDRESSING THE IMPACT OF SYMPTOMS ON THE THERAPEUTIC RELATIONSHIP

As described in Chapter 8, the therapeutic relationship is vital to this kind of work. Psychotic symptoms can have a profound effect on a person's ability to maintain a relationship of this nature. A popular training exercise for mental health professionals involves a role-played interview between two people whilst a third person whispers into the interviewee's ear. The result is meant to approximate what it might be like to hear voices and answer questions at the same time. People find themselves losing concentration, feeling wary of the interviewer and having seemingly inappropriate emotional responses. This simple exercise can be a useful and powerful learning tool.

Chadwick, Birchwood & Trower (1996) suggest that the professional should assume that a person's symptoms will be active in a new and potentially threatening situation like an assessment interview. For instance it is expected that voices will comment on the interview and that people prone to feeling paranoid will often have misgivings about the interviewer.

It is useful to bring this subject up early on by asking whether the voices are speaking during the interview and whether they are commenting on the process. It can be useful to state that other people often find symptoms disruptive. Stating that it is common for people's voices to make comments, especially negative ones, about the interviewer is often useful. Once this is out in the open then difficulties arising from the predicament can be solved. Sometimes voices warn against disclosure of information to the interviewer. This can lead to the person feeling unsafe and can disrupt the development of trust. Interestingly some people find that voices are not present during conversations with others. As will be mentioned later, talking aloud often forms part of the person's repertoire of coping skills. However, this was not the case with Lucy, who found her voices warning her that her problems would not be taken seriously.

The process above includes:

◆ assuming that voices will comment on the interview
◆ being willing to address openly any warnings the voices are giving about the interviewer

Case study – Lucy

Lucy, whilst living in a local authority group home, was referred to the local mental health centre asking for help with voices. She had four voices that she recognised as deceased family members. She had a lot of difficulty concentrating during the assessment interviews owing to them saying that she was evil and worthless and that no one would believe her story. She believed that they had power over her and that they could harm her by urging her to take an overdose. We noted that it was very difficult for her to discuss her voices during our sessions together. After a while she was able to say that they were commenting on the interviewer. However, she felt very uncomfortable talking about the content of their comments. We discussed the reactions of people that I had seen before and I told her that one man had found his voices saying that I would not be interested in his story and that I would laugh at him if he told me. She was able to say that, although she did not think that I would laugh at her, something similar worried her. I asked her if the voices had ever told her something that later turned out to be false and she replied that it happened all the time. She realised that there was a possibility that they were wrong on this occasion but said that the thought of being mocked was too much to bear. On further questioning it became clear that being mocked would mean having everyone she knew knowing about her voices and laughing at her because of them. Once this was clear we were able to discuss the boundaries of confidentiality. She was surprised at how little information would have to be passed around the professionals at the mental health centre, and her fears that someone at her home might find out about her through their own community nurse were alleviated. Despite feeling nervous about trying, Lucy agreed to disclose a little of the voices' content and then see if the information got back to her friends. She returned the next week more confident that the process was safe despite what the voices told her. We acknowledged that it had been good to discuss this and Lucy agreed to bring up similar worries if they occurred again.

◆ showing that voices commenting in this way is a usual occurrence
◆ acknowledging that disclosing details of the voice content can be very distressing
◆ moving the discussion away from the specific to more general aspects of the voices – such as whether they always tell the truth
◆ trying to identify information that might reassure the person hearing voices
◆ negotiating a small test of whether the voices will react in the predicted way
◆ discussing the results of the test and making plans for the future.

THOROUGH ASSESSMENT AND LIMITED SELF-MONITORING

Assessment methods are discussed in detail in Chapter 5. The purpose of addressing the subject here is twofold. First, this is to highlight specific information that is useful to helping people with voices or strange, worrying thoughts. Secondly, it enables the process to be followed with some basic principles in mind to serve several purposes.

The process of assessing psychosis is vital for a number of reasons. First, a comprehensive understanding of the problem is essential in the search for new ways of dealing with the problem. Secondly, the process itself can be useful in helping the person experiencing symptoms to gain a better understanding of them. It can also be a time when principles that underlie the work ahead are first established.

Activities that promote this opportunity include:

◆ working collaboratively to collect information on the symptoms
◆ examining the way that stress precipitates the symptoms
◆ looking at the way vulnerability factors like poor social support affect the problem
◆ promoting the idea that symptoms are on a continuum with normal psychological processes.

The assessment process often blends well with the relationship-forming process. The endeavour should be collaborative – that is, done *with* rather than *to* the person experiencing symptoms. (Follow Ch. 6 for guidelines of the assessment interview.)

Specific questionnaires that are useful in assessing the nature of and fluctuations in a person's experience of voices or strange, worrying thoughts are given in Box 9.1.

Specific information relevant to the assessment of voices will include:

◆ the characteristics of the voice (e.g. identity, age, loudness, how threatening it is)
◆ what the voice says exactly; this often relates to other problems that the person has such as low self-esteem
◆ the person's explanation of how the voice is heard (e.g. telepathy, radio waves)
◆ what it means to the person to hear voices (e.g. madness, specially gifted)
◆ whether the voice makes commands and if so how easy it is to resist these at different times.

Specific information relevant to the assessment of strange, worrying thoughts includes:

Box 9.1 Questionnaires that assess experiences of voices or worrying thoughts

◆ The Topography of Voices Scale (Hustig & Hafner 1990)
◆ The Cognitive Assessment of Voices Schedule (Chadwick & Birchwood 1994)
◆ The Hallucinations Rating Scale (Haddock, unpublished scale, 1994)
◆ The Delusions Rating Scale (Haddock, unpublished scale, 1994)
◆ The Beliefs about Voices Scale (Chadwick & Birchwood 1995)

◆ what the central belief is about (e.g. 'there is a plot against me' or 'I am being experimented on by aliens')
◆ what general rules and assumptions the person has developed in response to this belief (e.g. 'never trust new people', 'do not talk to the neighbours' or 'do not go out at night')
◆ what specific situations this leads to difficulties with (e.g. not being able to reply to the lady at the paper shop when she says good morning or avoiding catching the bus)
◆ how much conviction the person has in these beliefs (e.g. 0–100%)
◆ how much distress the beliefs cause
◆ how much time is spent thinking about the beliefs.

Information that is useful to collect on both voices and strange, worrying thoughts includes:

◆ how easily ignored the problem is
◆ triggers that start the problem off
◆ things that make it better or worse
◆ ways of coping with the problem.

Much of this type of information will be collected with the questionnaires mentioned above and the interview methods described in Chapter 6.

It can be helpful to include self-monitoring in the assessment process (e.g. asking the person to keep a record of the voices including the content). Monitoring a problem can help with:

◆ identifying patterns in the experience (e.g. the voice changing from comments to threats in response to feelings of sadness)
◆ identifying things that help (e.g. being with a trusted person reducing the distress experienced when leaving the house)
◆ generally providing more detailed information around that discussed

during assessment; this often leads to new ideas about dealing with the problem.

However, this needs careful consideration. Some people find this quite threatening or at least very difficult to remember. If a person is unable to keep a simple tick-box record it may be possible to enlist the help of a relative or another carer. Experiences of failure should be avoided particularly in the early stages of the process as this can disrupt enthusiasm and hope. Therefore if there is any doubt over the person's ability or motivation to keep diaries they should not be used, but these methods may be considered later if levels of concentration and motivation improve. Once it is collected the assessment information will help with the development of a conceptualisation of the person's problems, i.e. a way of understanding how it all links together. This is one of the most important aspects of this type of work. Without a shared understanding of the problem the process of learning to deal with symptoms can become overprescriptive, unstructured, disorganised or even demoralising.

DEVELOPING A SHARED UNDERSTANDING OF THE PROBLEM

There are a variety of psychological theories or models of psychotic symptoms. These are helpful in piecing together the information gained during the assessment phase. The application of these ways of understanding symptoms to the actual experience of the person who has them forms the basis of a shared understanding of the problem. The professional's skill and experience in this part of the helping process will show in how well the person with psychosis accepts the explanation. It takes practice to present theoretical models in lay terms and to work on them with people experiencing symptoms. The result should be an individualised picture based on an understanding of the theory. In practice the shared understanding is constantly developing as new information arises. It is also guided by the following principles:

◆ Psychotic symptoms become largely understandable once enough information about the person's experience of them has been gathered.
◆ Many of the characteristics of psychotic symptoms fluctuate as if on a continuum so that, for instance, levels of conviction in strange, worrying thoughts vary and voices change in volume.
◆ All psychotic experience is on a continuum with normal psychological functioning so that symptoms represent an extreme of normality rather than something that is categorically different.
◆ Developing a shared understanding of psychosis is underpinned by a knowledge of theoretical models.

Only three models will be presented here for simplicity. The Further reading section at the end of this chapter lists a number of practice manuals, each of which will contain a review of theoretical models.

Stress and vulnerability

There are a number of theories relating stress and vulnerability factors to psychosis. A classic one is Zubin & Spring's (1977) stress vulnerability model. It proposes that psychosis is an episodic problem and that episodes are precipitated by a variety of factors. Stressful life events are said to interact with vulnerability factors determining whether someone is pushed over a psychosis threshold. Vulnerability factors include family history of psychosis, birth complications, poor social support, poor self-care, lack of sleep, etc. The model in Figure 9.2 shows that if several of these factors are present then just a small amount of stress may tip the balance into psychotic experience.

The model allows for conversations about the nature of psychotic symptoms such as:

◆ symptoms appear to be an extreme form of normal experiences
◆ all people have a degree of susceptibility to psychosis
◆ symptoms are precipitated by stress
◆ looking after physical and social needs can protect against psychosis.

Kingdon & Turkington (1994) review the literature that supports these ideas. It is suggested that results from sleep deprivation and sensory deprivation experiments, along with studies of people's reactions to extreme stress, show that in these circumstances psychotic experience is the most common

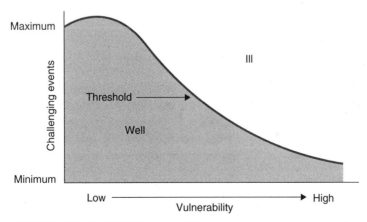

Figure 9.2 Zubin & Spring's (1977) model of the interplay between stress and vulnerability in episodes of schizophrenia.

reaction. Indeed, when asking groups of mental health professionals whether they have ever had an auditory hallucination, I have found the majority report that they have, at least once. Feeling paranoid or thinking someone is watching you is, of course, commonly seen as being within usual human experience. Although not the same as having continuing problems with psychosis, they surely point towards a continuum between the two. This kind of information can be reassuring to people with psychotic symptoms. Another useful discussion to have that is advocated by Kingdon & Turkington (1994) is about the cultural differences in the way people who have these problems are received. In much of Western culture, people who hear voices for instance are feared, whereas in Native American culture hearers of voices are often revered as being in contact with spirits. This can be especially helpful to people whose self-esteem is badly affected by hearing voices.

A powerful message from the stress vulnerability model is that there are things the person with psychosis can do to help towards reducing vulnerability to symptoms. These include:

◆ trying to maintain a regular sleep pattern
◆ reducing alcohol and drug intake
◆ maintaining self-care (e.g. in diet and hygiene)
◆ keeping in touch with supportive friends and family
◆ keeping active (e.g. keeping up exercise or some form of employment)
◆ taking regular medication.

A review of the person's previous experiences of relapse or recent history of symptoms will often show changes in many of these areas. It can be encouraging to know that there is more to managing psychotic symptoms than being a passive recipient of medication. Helping somebody to deal with voices and strange, worrying thoughts begins with reviewing these ideas in relation to the person's own experiences. The stress vulnerability model is used in this initial collaborative search for understanding of the person's distressing experiences.

The ABC model – the relationship between symptoms and a person's responses to them

The ways of dealing with symptoms addressed in this chapter have an underlying assumption that a person's responses to a problem are central to how it is experienced. One of the central messages of cognitive therapy of psychosis, for instance, is that a person's beliefs about symptoms are strongly associated with the way that person reacts, both emotionally and practically. How people actively respond to their symptoms can play a large part in whether or not the problems escalate.

> **Box 9.2** The ABC model
>
> ◆ **Activating events:** with *strange, worrying thoughts* these will be trigger situations such as a stranger making eye contact in the case of paranoia, with *voices* the voice itself is classed as the activating event, in other cases such as *physical symptoms* of anxiety the symptom itself can be classed as the initial event
> ◆ **Beliefs** about the event or symptom
> ◆ **Consequences** of the problem including emotional responses such as depression or anxiety or actions like hiding in a bedroom or shouting at neighbours

The ABC model shown in Box 9.2 is central to this way of working and helps to unravel the various facets of a problem. This is of course a grossly simplified description but it is where most conversations with people experiencing symptoms will start. The important points are, first, to establish what factors precipitate the problem or, as is the case with voices and physical concerns, the exact nature of the voice or feeling. Secondly, it is important to ascertain what interpretation is being made of the event – that is, exactly what the person thinks about the event, voice or feeling. Lastly, it is vital to note all the ways in which the person responds to the problem – that is, what emotions, thoughts, actions, or physical feelings occur.

These responses are often helpful, such as removing oneself from a threatening situation, but they can also have unhelpful consequences, as in the case of Ken (mentioned later) who threatened his neighbours with a bat. Many of the responses that people have to symptoms are understandable but in the end feed back into the problem. These may include responses such as those given in Box 9.3.

It is important to use the thorough assessment methods mentioned earlier to ascertain as many of these responses as possible and to think about what effect they in turn might have on the problem.

Different levels of belief

When trying to understand strange, worrying thoughts it can be helpful to think in terms of three levels. These correspond to the types of beliefs described by Beck (1979) in his seminal cognitive model of depression, which has underpinned many consequent developments. At the centre of a person's problem with strange, worrying thoughts there will be a core belief. This is

Box 9.3 Some responses to problems

Emotions:
◆ Becoming depressed and hopeless
◆ Feeling stressed and anxious
◆ Feeling angry towards people

Thoughts:
◆ Spending time worrying about the problem
◆ Generally spending a lot of time thinking about the problem
◆ Thinking of the worst possible scenario

Actions:
◆ Keeping a special lookout for the problem
◆ Spending time alone
◆ Complying with demands that voices make
◆ Being aggressive to others

Physical feelings:
◆ Tense muscles
◆ Headaches
◆ Any physical sign of stress that could be mistaken for something else such as: thinking that dizziness has been caused by being poisoned

often related to self-esteem and contains meaning about relationships with other people and the world in general.

The next level corresponds to general rules or assumptions by which the person acts. Much of the time we are unaware that we are living by these rules, sometimes recognising only that we end up responding to events in similar ways.

The third level concerns specific situations – for instance, the specific judgements or predictions we make about particular events. If these three levels are pictured as a target with the core belief at the centre (Fig. 9.3) then what emerges is a model that is helpful in directing which beliefs to address at what times.

The first step in helping someone to cope with strange, worrying thoughts is to start with situation specific beliefs – that is, at the outer ring of the target. Moving inwards towards the assumptions and core beliefs requires a degree of specialist skill and good supervision. It is therefore inadvisable to tackle beliefs at this level without appropriate training. Core beliefs are by nature firmly held in place and premature intervention can strengthen them.

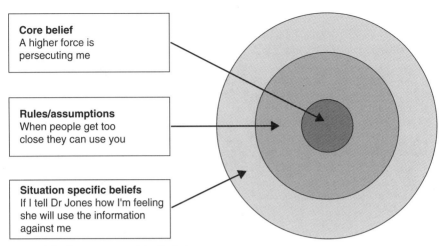

Figure 9.3 The target model of beliefs.

When summarising a person's problem using this model it is helpful to acknowledge emergent themes from the rules or assumptions level – that is, the second level of the target. This is done to support the rationale for addressing the situation specific beliefs that cause distress in the person's everyday life. This will often mean inquiring about general attitudes towards other people and will lead to a wider picture that includes the person's world view. Pointing out the link between assumptions and beliefs about specific events will begin to reveal the person's tendency towards jumping to conclusions. Developing a shared understanding of the person's expectations about others will open up discussions about events that the person has had mixed feelings about. People that operate on fixed generalisations often jump to conclusions about others. Consequently they find themselves in situations that are expected to turn out badly only to find that the opposite is true. Acknowledging this jumping to conclusions style of summing up situations is often the first step towards acting differently in them and will be discussed later in relation to helping people respond differently to their beliefs.

The following case studies illustrate the usefulness of different models.

Box 9.4 shows the ABC model for David.

Box 9.5 shows the ABC model for Lorna.

Box 9.6 shows the ABC model for Carol.

Checking for shared understanding

The collaborative effort in developing shared understanding involves the mental health professional in presenting an appropriate model from the ones mentioned above. The skill in this lies in one's ability to describe the model in

Case study – ABC model, David

David had a single female voice that sounded like one of his primary school teachers, Miss Imelda. The voice would tell him that he was useless and stupid. He found attempting anything new very distressing and would feel hopeless after making even the slightest mistake. He found that situations like these would start the voice off and would consequently avoid them as much as possible. Using the ABC model above we were able to discuss a specific recent example and identify what was particularly distressing for him. David had been advised by his key worker to try and get to know people at the local day hospital but was very worried about what to say. When thinking about approaching someone his voice started.

Box 9.4 ABC model – David

Activating event: In this case the voice of Miss Imelda was saying 'You'll never be able to talk properly; they'll all find out you're stupid'.

Belief: David was convinced that he would be unable to start a conversation and that he would look foolish; he also predicted that this would lead to everyone at the day hospital thinking he was stupid and that, as a result of this, nobody would want to know him.

Consequence: He started to feel very tense and anxious. He found himself shaking and feeling quite flushed. This convinced him even more that he would mess up any attempt at a conversation. As a result he avoided talking to anyone that day and went home feeling dejected and worried that he had let his key worker down.

Case study – ABC model, Lorna

Lorna also found herself worrying that people would reject her, but for different reasons. Lorna heard the voice of a famous dead writer urging her to commit suicide and join him. She found talking about the voice very upsetting and had until recently denied hearing voices at all. She found that having a normal conversation with people helped to distract her from the voice. Unfortunately the voice would often start taunting her when she woke up in the middle of the night. Although there was a member of staff awake during the night at her home she would not seek help and had on occasion overdosed on her medication. Weeks after the following event she was able to describe it in some detail.

Box 9.5 ABC model – Lorna

Activating event: Voice repeatedly saying 'Go on do it, come to me'.

Belief: 'If I tell the night staff about this they'll think that I'm mad they'll tell everyone else in the house and no one will want to know me. If people find out I'm hearing voices I'll be put in hospital and be given electrical treatment like my mum. The voice will make me kill myself.'

Consequence: Lorna buried her head under her pillow and screamed for the voice to leave her alone. This woke up the person in the next room who complained the next morning. Lorna denied that anything was wrong and started spending more and more time alone in her room. She began to feel quite depressed as a result.

Stress and vulnerability model – Lorna

One thing that Lorna found helpful was discussing the relationship between stress, vulnerability and hearing voices. She was also particularly taken with the idea that, in some cultures, voice hearers are respected. She was able to identify aspects of her lifestyle that might make her vulnerable to hearing voices. These included:

◆ *spending too much time alone*
◆ *not sleeping very well*
◆ *acting on her low opinion of herself (e.g. never putting her own needs first)*
◆ *always turning down offers of support.*

We talked about studies that showed that people's thinking changes when they are deprived of sleep (see Kingdon & Turkington 1994 for a review). She could relate this to her own experiences over the previous month that had seen her becoming increasingly worried about not sleeping. She found herself in a vicious cycle where sleep was prevented by worrying that the voice would start as a consequence of not sleeping. These night-time experiences had provided a hotbed for worry about what the other people in her house thought about her. One of the first steps towards reducing the distress caused by her voice was to make changes in these areas. She decided to visit her family more. As well as feeling more comfortable with talking about her voice with them, she also found that the long walk to her mother's house was good exercise and this helped her to sleep at night.

lay terms using individualised information. Wherever possible use the person's own language to describe symptoms and difficult situations. The general principle is to develop the information in small steps. This can involve

Case study – target model of beliefs, Carol

Carol was troubled by a belief that other people could hear her thoughts. Her mother had been a strong believer in psychic powers and had often talked of receiving telepathic messages. Carol's worries led her to trying very hard to avoid having critical thoughts about other people in case they heard them telepathically. At its worst Carol could not face people and worried that they would reject her if they knew she was having bad thoughts about them. After a number of assessment sessions we were able to start thinking about her beliefs using the target model. She had a core belief that she was guilty and evil and this seemed related to her worries about people finding out what she was really like. She was often anxious in the television room of her shared house.

The target model for Carol is shown in Figure 9.4.

Using this model we were able to make a list of specific situations that caused Carol distress. She could not recall whether she had ever later discovered her first impressions of a situation to be wrong. She started to look out for these situations and talked with a few people that she trusted. She eventually decided that she did sometimes jump to the wrong conclusions, but not always. Carol was later able to find ways of entering situations that she had avoided for a long time. Whilst she still had the belief that people could read her thoughts, she found that focusing on specific beliefs about here and now situations helped her to find ways of coping. We were also able to use the ABC model in trying to understand more about the specific situations that caused her distress. One that regularly upset her was meeting with her psychiatrist. Although she got on very well with him she found herself trying to control her thoughts so much that it interfered with her concentration.

pausing after each idea or small set of ideas. Connections between concepts can be highlighted so that the whole picture builds up slowly. Each pause should be accented with a check for understanding and an invitation to elaborate further if the person feels that important points have been missed. Finally, it is useful to check for understanding by asking the person to repeat an impression of what has been discussed. In Carol's case above, a conversation similar to the one below was helpful in establishing a shared understanding.

JM: Carol I'd like to spend some time making sure that we understand this problem in the same way, how would that be?

Carol: How?

JM: Well, how about if I tell you what my understanding is and you can tell me if that's right?

Carol: OK.

JM: Well, from what you've said it seems that a lot of your distress

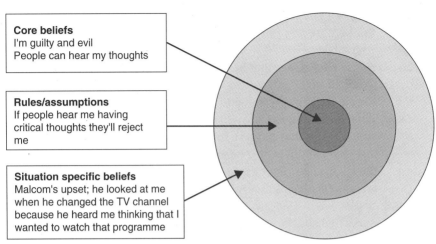

Core beliefs
I'm guilty and evil
People can hear my thoughts

Rules/assumptions
If people hear me having
critical thoughts they'll reject
me

Situation specific beliefs
Malcom's upset; he looked at me
when he changed the TV channel
because he heard me thinking that I
wanted to watch that programme

Figure 9.4 The target model of beliefs – Carol.

comes from worrying about people hearing your thoughts. Is that right?

Carol: Yes, people do hear my thoughts.

JM: And you find that very upsetting.

Carol: (Nods.)

JM: And you were saying that, because of this, you spend a lot of time checking people's expressions to see if they have picked up on what you're thinking.

Carol: Yes, I have to watch people all the time.

JM: And that this is because you worry that people won't want to know you if they find out you've had bad thoughts about them.

Carol: That's why I have to stop myself thinking bad thoughts.

JM: Yes, and you were telling me earlier that that's what was happening when the doctor said you looked distracted.

Box 9.6 ABC model – Carol

Activating event: Carol had a thought about not taking her new medication.

Belief: 'He can hear me thinking this. He will think that I am going to stop taking my tablets and put me on a section because of it.'

Consequence: Purposely repeating the thought: 'I will take my tablets'. Feeling afraid and not paying attention to the meeting.

Carol: I worried that he'd have me taken in.

JM:　Yes, because you worried that he could hear you thinking about your tablets.

Carol: But he always says that he can't hear me thinking. Sometimes I worry for nothing.

JM:　How about if we try and pull all of this together?

Carol: What do you mean?

JM:　Well it seems that all these things go together somehow. You have this worry about people hearing your thoughts because you think they won't like you if they hear them. This leads you to look out for it happening. Is that right?

Carol: Yes.

JM:　And when you are looking out for signs of this you often find this makes life quite difficult around other people because you're watching them carefully and trying not to have bad thoughts. Have I got that right?

Carol: Yes, I have to watch myself and everyone else.

JM:　But sometimes you get it wrong and find out that even though you really believed that someone could hear you thinking they couldn't all along. It's like if you really expect them to hear you hard enough you convince yourself that they can.

Carol: It's so hard.

JM:　You must work very hard at keeping all this under control.

Carol: (Nods.)

JM:　So let's see if we can sum this up. Stop me if I get this wrong. You really worry that people can hear your thoughts and that if they do they won't like you. (Pause.) This means that you try to control your thoughts and look out for signs that people can hear them. (Pause.) The problem makes life very upsetting sometimes. (Pause.) And we know that, at least sometimes, people can't really hear your thoughts even though you really believed they did. How was that Carol, does it sound like I've got it right?

Carol: I think so.

JM:　Did I miss anything out?

Carol: Well, only that my Mum always said that I was telepathic as a child.

JM:　OK, so that might explain where the worry came from. I need to see if I've explained myself properly, Carol. Can you say something about how you understand this problem?

Carol: What like you just did?

JM:　Yes, but from your point of view.

Carol: Well it's the same. I get upset because people can hear me thinking bad things about them.

JM: And what do you do about that?

Carol: I stop myself having bad thoughts and watch out for them getting upset. But sometimes people just get upset and it's nothing to do with my thoughts, but I can't tell the difference.

JM: How about if we try and find some things that might help with this problem?

Carol: Like what?

JM: Well you said that when you told your friend that you have this worry you felt better about it and stopped watching her for a while. Maybe we could look at why that was helpful.

Carol: All right.

Small summaries and reflective statements along with regular requests for feedback were helpful in breaking down the information. This helped Carol to piece it together with me and in the end we had some common ground to start from. This enabled us to move on to discussing ways of coping with the problem.

COPING WITH VOICES AND STRANGE, WORRYING THOUGHTS

The way people respond to symptoms of psychosis can be compared to the way people respond to headaches. Headaches are a common experience but everyone has different ways of dealing with them. Some people reach for tablets immediately whilst others try to get on with whatever they are doing. Others would never or only rarely take medication. A similar picture emerges from talking to people with voices or strange, worrying thoughts, especially if the person has been experiencing the problem for a long time.

Coping methods are not always helpful in the long term and some only partially reduce the distress associated with the problem. With this in mind it is useful to spend time developing three aspects of coping:

1. increasing the effectiveness of current coping methods
2. reducing the use of harmful ways of coping
3. introducing previously untried methods.

The first step is to examine current ways of coping. These might fall into one of the following categories (Table 9.1).

Building on coping methods

The person may have a variety of ways of coping with symptoms. It will be helpful to discuss how effective each one is. Some people use their coping

Table 9.1 Ways of coping

Distraction	Interacting
Voices and strange, worrying thoughts: ◆ Listening to music ◆ Reading aloud ◆ Counting backwards from 100 ◆ Describing an object in detail ◆ Watching TV	**Voices:** ◆ Telling the voices to go away ◆ Talking to the voices whilst pretending to use a mobile phone ◆ Agreeing to listen to the voices at particular times **Strange, worrying thoughts:** ◆ Testing out beliefs (see next section)

Activity	Social	Physical
Voices and strange, worrying thoughts: ◆ Walking ◆ Tidying the house ◆ Having a relaxing bath ◆ Playing the guitar ◆ Singing ◆ Going to the gym	**Voices and strange, worrying thoughts:** ◆ Talking to a trusted friend or member of the family ◆ Phoning a helpline ◆ Avoiding people ◆ Going to a drop-in centre ◆ Visiting a favourite place	**Voices and strange, worrying thoughts:** ◆ Taking extra medication ◆ Using ear plugs (voices) ◆ Breathing exercises ◆ Relaxation methods

methods only when the symptoms are very bad, whilst others get through most days using them. As before, thinking about recent examples often helps, especially when detail is needed. When trying to develop the coping method's effectiveness consider the following:

◆ What type of coping method is it (distraction, activity, interacting, social or physical)?
◆ How could it be made more absorbing or intense?
◆ Are there any similar ones that might be more helpful?

Spending time thinking about what the essential qualities of a coping activity are (Table 9.2) can help in the process of making it even more effective.

The next step will be to practise the new or improved way of coping repeatedly. This is started during a session and practised in between. When the person feels confident other methods can be added to the repertoire.

Table 9.2 Essential qualities of coping activities

Problem and coping method	Possible effective ingredients	Intensified version
Marie believes that the Masons are plotting to kidnap her sons. She finds that when she is anxious it can help to lie on the sofa and watch TV	Relaxation Distraction	Lying in a hot bath with aromatherapy oils Listening to soft music and reading magazine
Jonathon finds that having to talk to his friend on the phone sends his voices into the background	Speaking aloud Distraction Social contact	Visiting parents or friends and talking about things other than his voices

Tarrier's (1990) Coping Strategy Enhancement is a well structured, researched and clearly outlined method for developing coping.

Coping methods with harmful effects

Methods of coping often emerge that are effective but costly in the long term. However, the person may feel reluctant to give them up if they are seen as the only means of control. The use of these should also be explored in detail. These ways of coping can themselves become uncontrolled, causing problems of their own. This can be especially true for the use of alcohol and drugs. Serious problems of this nature will need to be dealt with separately (see Ch. 12).

A balanced view of the short and long term effects of coping methods will inform any discussion of this nature. The short term usefulness should be acknowledged but offset against the damage likely to occur in the medium and long term. Harmful ways of coping include ones that:

◆ eventually cause more emotional distress
◆ are detrimental to physical health
◆ actually involve physical harm
◆ lower confidence and self-esteem
◆ cause other people to react badly.

Examples are included in Table 9.3.

Considering what the effective part of the coping method is can lead to more suitable alternatives. This often means undertaking a collaborative period of trial and error where the person with psychosis agrees to try out

Table 9.3 Harmful ways of coping

Problem	Coping method	Short term effect	Medium/long term effect
Ken hears voices that sound like his neighbours planning to break into his flat	Threaten them with a bat	Voices stop, leaving Ken feeling safer	The police are called and they take the neighbours' side. People in the area avoid Ken. He begins to feel that everyone is against him
Carrie hears voices saying that she is a prostitute	Shouts at the voices during meal times	Feels that she has made her point and that the voices will stop for a while	Staff ask her to leave and eat in her room. Carrie begins to feel depressed about having no one to talk to
Mark believes that he has defrauded the benefits agency and that he will be prosecuted	Visits the benefits office daily to confess	Feels reassured when he is told that there is no problem	Has little time in the day to do things he enjoys. Later thinks that it is too serious for the desk clerk to know about and feels even worse

new ideas that have been discussed and practised in session. Examples are included in Table 9.4.

If a less harmful version of the same coping method cannot be identified then the person may agree to using it less often if other alternatives are suggested. Again, every effort should be made to maximise the beneficial effects of the coping method. This will include thinking of ways to make distraction methods more absorbing or social methods more engaging.

The coping plan

Once information about all types of coping has been collected and new and improved versions have been identified, then a summary can be made possibly using a 'coping grid'. This is a plan that is individualised using the person's own language. It can be kept in a prominent position at home, and some

Table 9.4 Alternative coping methods

Problem and coping method	Possible effective ingredients	Alternative coping method
Ken threatens his neighbours with a bat because of the voices he hears	Activity Exercise Adrenaline	Kicking a football very hard and chasing it in the field behind his house
Barbara feels embarrassed when she is compelled to shout at her voices whilst walking down the street	Answering the voices Talking aloud	Pretends to use a replica mobile phone and answers the voices in a normal voice
Cyril feels upset when his neighbours get angry about him playing his music very loud to drown out the voices	Distraction	Listening to the same music on a personal stereo

people find it helpful to identify a trusted family member or friend to help them put the plan into action. Ken's plan looked like Table 9.5.

DEALING WITH STRANGE, WORRYING BELIEFS

Any attempt to deal with this problem should take into account the effects of:

◆ the distress associated with the belief
◆ the preoccupation with the belief
◆ the strength of belief (conviction)
◆ the person's responses:
  — acting as if it were true
  — looking out for things associated with the belief
◆ the increased tendency to jump to conclusions in people with psychosis.

As seen earlier, people respond to problems in ways that are designed to keep themselves safe. However, these responses can in fact make the problem worse and this process is just as evident with strange, worrying beliefs (Fig. 9.5). To emphasise that this way of responding to beliefs is part of human nature rather than being unique to those experiencing psychosis we can use the example of superstitious beliefs.

It is part of being human that people often have strong beliefs despite having little or no real evidence to support them. Superstitious beliefs are like this. For instance, there is no conclusive evidence of unfortunate events being

Table 9.5 A coping plan

Things I do to get rid of the voices of my neighbours	Inside the house	Outside the house
Helpful ways of coping to use more	◆ Listening to my personal stereo (but not the really heavy music) ◆ Reminding myself that the police said they would watch my flat ◆ Reading the paper aloud ◆ Phoning my brother to talk about the football	◆ Having a hard run in the field with the football ◆ Visiting mum and dad ◆ Phoning my keyworker ◆ Get out and do the shopping ◆ Talking to the doctor about having a little more medication to calm me down
Bad ways to use less	◆ Turning the TV up very loud ◆ Shouting to the neighbours through the window ◆ Drinking a bottle of cider	◆ Threatening the neighbours with violence ◆ Complaining at the police station ◆ Shouting in the street

precipitated by ignoring magpies, walking under ladders or putting new shoes on a table. It is, however, common for people to believe these things. These examples can serve to highlight two of the processes that affect people with psychosis when they have strange, worrying beliefs:

◆ acting as if the belief were true
◆ looking out for signs that support the belief as well as ignoring evidence against it (consciously and unconsciously).

Keeping a lookout

Consider people who worry about not saying hello to every magpie that they come across. When confronted with a situation that makes this inevitable, such as seeing seven all together whilst driving along a fast road, such a person would naturally feel quite distressed. Once the worrying belief is activated, in this case 'that unfortunate events come after ignoring magpies', the person will be on the lookout for bad luck. This happens purposefully as well as automatically. The automatic process is the same one that causes us to

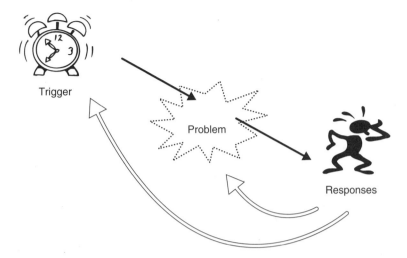

Figure 9.5 A generic view of how responses can feed back into a problem.

notice more Volkswagen camper vans if we are thinking about buying one. Of course, if something is being looked out for more then it is much more likely to be noticed. In this way people concerned with magpies increase the number of unfortunate events that they notice. Strong beliefs also cause us to ignore evidence against them. Strong prejudicial beliefs, for instance, survive this way. Hence the person who worries about having ignored a magpie is also more likely to discount automatically any good events that happen that day.

The same process applies to all strange and worrying beliefs. The more time a person spends dwelling on a belief the stronger it gets as more supportive evidence is collected and refuting evidence is ignored. Therefore one of the first steps in coping with strange and worrying beliefs is to find ways of being less preoccupied by them (Box 9.7).

Box 9.7 Tips for dealing with strange, worrying beliefs

◆ Preoccupation leads to greater conviction
◆ Greater conviction leads to more distress
◆ Distress is what we work with
◆ Helping someone to be less preoccupied with their distressing beliefs will help to prevent increasing conviction; commonly helpful coping strategies include absorbing and distracting activities such as structured time with trusted friends (e.g. playing a game or going shopping)

Acting as if the belief were true

A second process that leads to the maintenance of strange, worrying beliefs is that of responding to them as if they were true. This is understandable given that we all have a powerful need to protect ourselves from harm. Unfortunately, the avoidance of predicted harm strengthens the notion that it would have happened if action had not been taken. Take, for example, somebody who avoids putting new shoes on the table owing to a belief that this will lead to unspeakable tragedy. If no such tragedy occurs the person will explain this in terms of the safe handling of shoes rather than attributing it to sensible precautions, the happily infrequent nature of disasters or even, for that matter, not walking under ladders. Following this pattern can intrude more and more on a person's quality of life. People with distressing beliefs often find themselves so convinced of them that they adapt their lives around the belief to a disabling extent. In this way people can often end up housebound and extremely socially isolated.

Jumping to conclusions

When we are tired or experiencing distress we tend to leap to conclusions that are not always accurate. A classic analogy used to illustrate this is that of waking up in the middle of the night to the sound of breaking glass. Imagine that this happened to you and that you were alone in the house. Would you feel anxious? What would be the first conclusion to enter your mind? Most people answer that they would feel distressed, thinking that an intruder had entered the house. The story continues that on bravely venturing downstairs you discover that your cat has woken up and broken a vase whilst exploring the mantelpiece. The jumping to conclusions style of thinking would in this case have been helpful in preparing to deal with an intruder. However, the resolution of the story points to the frequent false alarms set off by this quick but often inaccurate automatic thinking process.

Jumping to conclusions is something that people with psychosis are particularly prone to. Garety & Hemsley (1994) describe some research that involved asking people to guess the proportions of coloured beads in a hidden jar. For instance, it might contain 70 black beads and 30 yellow beads. Beads were taken out, one at a time, and displayed so that the participants could hazard a guess as to whether there were more yellow or black beads in the jar. It was discovered that people with psychosis were more likely to come to a firm conclusion after fewer beads had been drawn. So, although it is naturally human to jump to conclusions on the basis of small amounts of information, it seems that this is more pronounced for people experiencing psychosis.

Jumping to conclusions too quickly can lead to regular misunderstanding of events. Thus people with psychosis can often find themselves making mistaken assumptions about people and situations. Unfortunately, if this is followed by the types of responses mentioned above, the mistaken assumption can become increasingly believable as it is bolstered with more supportive evidence and the seemingly protective effects of evasive action.

Exploring the effects of jumping to conclusions – testing beliefs

As mentioned earlier, this phase is impossible to engage in successfully without the thorough groundwork described in the first part of the chapter. A shared rationale for exploring the effects that jumping to conclusions has on a person's lifestyle will emerge from assessment and the development of coping techniques. As the work continues, opportunities should arise to discuss recent examples of how the tendency to view the world in a certain way leads to mistaken assumptions. This happened in Neil's case.

Case study – Neil

Neil had been seen on six occasions for help with his voices and paranoia. He found it particularly difficult to trust people and this was exacerbated by the voices, which would tell him that people were collecting information about him so that he could be banned from the ward. At the beginning of the session Neil was asked how the previous few days had been and he described an upsetting event that had taken place the day before. It transpired that he had gone to attend a discussion group facilitated by his primary nurse Sue (whom he was just beginning to trust). When he entered the group room Sue was sat with her back towards the door. The voices told him that she did not want him there and for a while he was convinced that she would turn around and ask him to leave. Neil bravely stayed and was eventually greeted by Sue as she turned around. Neil was quite shaken by the experience but remained in the group despite not contributing a great deal. This became an ideal opportunity to discuss Neil's tendency towards jumping to conclusions that did not always turn out right. The discussion ended with the following summary:

JM: Neil, this event seems quite important. I think it tells us a lot about the kinds of situations that you find difficult.

Neil: How do you mean?

JM: Well, it seems to me that this tendency you have to think of the worst in certain situations causes you a lot of grief. Let's imagine that you had left the group room when you felt sure that Sue was against you. How would you have felt?

Neil: Well I probably would have gone back to my room and wound myself up about it.

JM: Right, but you didn't, you took the plunge and stayed.

Neil: Yeah, sometimes it's easier than others.

JM: OK, I wonder if there might have been other occasions when you jumped to a conclusion that someone was against you and later found out that they were OK?

Neil: It does happen sometimes but, most of the time, I avoid people that I'm not sure about.

JM: I wonder if sometimes you avoid people that are actually OK but you don't get to find out?

Neil: I suppose that could happen, but its better to be safe than sorry!

JM: That's true, it is good to be safe, but I wonder if there's such a thing as being too safe. I mean what kind of effect does this strategy have on your life?

Neil: Well, you know that it makes me very edgy around people and that I sometimes upset them because I have a go. But I'm not about to start running up to people with open arms just because I sometimes make mistakes.

JM: I don't think that's what I'm going to suggest.

Neil: What then?

JM: Well, how about looking at the people that you think might be OK? Is there any way we could check out to see if you're jumping to conclusions with them?

Neil: You mean like Sally? I suppose I could stop and say hello to her rather than keep walking by.

JM: That sounds like the kind of thing. Let's see if we can work this out as something for you to try in the week.

A specific test was then negotiated with Neil. He was encouraged to work out the details following the guidelines given in Box 9.8.

A test is, generally, more effective the simpler it is. In the case above, for instance, Neil decided that he would spend 5 minutes talking to Sally to see if she would (as he predicted) turn nasty towards him. The specific signs of nastiness that he expected to see were written down, as well as his own evidence for and against the prediction. One strong piece of evidence was his 'gut feeling' about the situation. After he discovered that Sally was in fact very pleasant towards him, we discussed the results and Neil decided that it might be worth exploring other areas where his strong intuitive sense might lead him to jump to incorrect conclusions.

Pitfalls to avoid include:

◆ imposing your own ideas for a test

Box 9.8 Guiding principles for tests of strange, worrying beliefs

◆ Start with beliefs about specific events so that the knowledge that beliefs are sometimes wrong can be used as a method of coping with future events.

◆ Ask whether the person has ever jumped to a conclusion that was later found to be wrong.

◆ Explain common effects of factors such as stress and lack of sleep on thinking (e.g. selective attention and jumping to conclusions) – ask if anything like this could be happening.

◆ Clarify a particular belief about a particular situation that the person feels able to tackle.

◆ Discuss the evidence for and against the belief using a naïve approach that allows a development of the person's own perspective with as few suggestions from you as possible.

◆ Discuss the quality of the evidence for the worrying belief. People often base important predictions and conclusions on intuition or insufficient information.

◆ Work together to devise a way of safely testing the belief.

◆ Take time to prepare the test including recording predictions about what might happen and what this might mean.

◆ After carrying out the test, spend time discussing the meaning of what happened; ask how the client might use the information gained.

◆ any approach that involves you trying to prove something to the client
◆ lack of preparation and preliminary discussion.

ADDRESSING BELIEFS ABOUT VOICES – EXPLORING CONTROL OVER VOICES

Most people, when asked about how much control they have over their voices, will report having very little or none at all. Voices can make people feel weak, hopeless and powerless. With this is mind, a significant step towards dealing with voices can be discovering just how much control can be gained over them. This is a sensitive area to work with, requiring good supervision for the mental health professional and much preparation for the person with voices.

Previous discussions about the nature of psychosis will be essential to this work. If a person is to give up an idea that voices are uncontrollable because they come from an outside source then consideration must be given to the alternative explanations. Without the underpinning work described earlier, people can be faced with frightening misconceptions about voices and what it means to have them. As discussed previously, accounts of psychosis that emphasise the role of stress and vulnerability will be crucial to this foundational work.

Helping a person to develop a greater sense of control over a voice involves identifying, clarifying and testing out the specific beliefs that are held about the power of the voice. In essence the method is similar to the guidelines for testing out beliefs set out in Box 9.9. It is worth reviewing how this process relates specifically to beliefs about the power of voices.

The case study of Anne-Marie is an example of exploring control over voices.

Box 9.9 Guiding principles for testing beliefs about voices

◆ Discuss the person's current beliefs about how controllable the voice is.

◆ Discuss the link between lack of power over the voice and the distress it causes.

◆ Review the person's evidence for having no control over the voice. This usually amounts to 'not being able to switch it off'.

◆ Discuss how having more control over the voice would affect the person's level of distress.

◆ Discuss actions that demonstrate a person's control over things such as a radio, car or heater. This discussion explores the idea that turning things up and down is as good a demonstration of control as switching them on and off.

◆ Propose that being able to make the voice louder then quieter, at will, would demonstrate a high degree of control over it.

◆ Collaboratively plan a test of whether the person can develop this kind of control. This involves:

Picking a useful coping method developed during previous work

Making the voice louder by listening to it intently (this may have to involve bringing the voice on by thinking about it)

Using the coping method to reduce the volume of the voice

Repeating this process until the person can call up the voice, make it louder and then reduce the volume at will.

◆ Review the person's previous ideas about control over the voice in relation to this process and develop ideas for further coping.

Case study – Anne-Marie, turning the voices up and down

Anne-Marie was very distressed by a voice that sounded like her late grandfather's. The voice would comment on her actions and say very upsetting things about her. At its worst the voice shouted that she was evil and demanded that she hurt herself. Earlier work with Anne-Marie had concentrated on understanding the experience of hearing voices. She developed ideas around stress and vulnerability and was able to identify a number of factors that would make her particularly vulnerable to hearing voices. For instance she had a poor view of herself having been regularly beaten by her grandfather when she was a child. She had experienced bouts of depression on and off for most of her life. Two family members on her mother's side experienced emotional problems requiring long term medication. Her sleep was regularly disturbed and she frequently forgot to take her tablets owing to waking up late. Anne-Marie was very worried about upsetting people and consequently found spending time in new social situations very difficult. She had recently been introduced to a new keyworker and two new residents at the group house where she lived. This stress, coupled with her particular vulnerability, had, she thought, led to her problem with the voice becoming worse.

Practical ideas developed from this understanding included working to improve sleep, asking a friend who called by her room every morning to remind her to take medication and talking to her new keyworker about her shyness with a trusted person present. Anne-Marie later found that talking aloud was helpful in reducing the volume of her voice. She would sing along to her stereo in her room, talk to her friend or read the newspaper to a fellow resident whose sight was bad. She found all these things to be helpful to a greater or lesser degree. Anne-Marie's voice had reduced in intensity and frequency but it was still very distressing to her, especially as she believed that it might make her harm herself and that she had no power over it whatsoever. She looked to the times that she had very nearly followed its instructions to hurt herself and thought that without the reassurance and help of either her best friend or her sister she would not have been able to resist. She saw these near misses as proof that she could succumb if the voice pushed too hard when she was alone.

Exploring control *Anne-Marie agreed that worrying about the power of the voice was one of the worst aspects of the problem. She was also intrigued about my suggestion that her seeking help from her sister and friend was a successful coping method rather than a failure to cope. We used her demonstrating control over her stereo as an analogy. She identified that she could show that she was in control of her stereo by turning it on and off, changing the tape in it or by turning the volume up and down. I suggested that the last method might be useful for our purposes and began:*

JM: So, Anne-Marie, are you saying that if you were able to change the volume on the stereo, turning it up and down when you decided, that you would be showing you were in control of it?

Case study – Anne-Marie, turning the voices up and down

AM: Of course I can control the volume, I have to in case the others complain about the noise.

JM: Yes. How about thinking about the voice in the same way?

AM: What, turning it up and down?

JM: Yes. If you could turn the volume of the voice up and down just like that, how would that be?

AM: That would be great but I can't see it happening.

We discussed the arrangements for trying this out, including the art of bringing the voice on. Anne-Marie was very unsure of this and wanted to try it out with her friend first rather than with me. We set this up and agreed that she should have something to do shortly afterwards in case the voice became very distressing; she also informed her keyworker what she was going to do. We spent the next session discussing her success in bringing the voice on and planning the test. Anne-Marie brought a newspaper to the session and spent 15 minutes thinking about and listening to the voice for 1 minute followed by reading aloud for 2 or 3 minutes. After 15 minutes she was happy that she could bring the voice on, make it louder and then reduce the volume at will. We discussed what this meant to her. She was excited about the finding but remained a little cautious.

Over the coming weeks she tried the technique regularly and eventually decided that she did indeed have more power than the voice. This helped to decrease her fear of hurting herself and we discussed the implications that this might have for her. Anne-Marie began to be a little more adventurous socially, chancing that the voice would increase with stress. It did worsen on a few occasions but she was happy to just ignore it or to continue a conversation rather than leave, which is how she would have responded previously.

Useful ideas from Anne-Marie's experience of exploring control include:

◆ use an effective coping method that is already well practised
◆ use analogies relevant to the person's lifestyle (e.g. in Anne-Marie's case the stereo volume)
◆ move forward at the person's own pace
◆ practise turning the volume of the voice up and down until it becomes easy.

CONCLUSIONS

I am always humbled by people's ability to bear the adversity associated with psychotic symptoms. Often people have adapted their lifestyle so much that the small sense of well-being they do have feels precariously balanced. It is enthusing to be able to offer some degree of help to a group of people who have historically had limited access to anything other than drug treatments. However, learning to deal with psychosis can in itself be worrying and so I have tried to emphasise the sensitive nature of this approach. There is a fine balance in the therapeutic stance between caution and confidence. For instance, offering suggestions tentatively and carefully negotiating the pace of the process, whilst maintaining a quiet confidence that small things can helpfully change, is a useful position to adopt.

There are many ways that the ideas presented in this chapter can be taken forward practically. Putting the ideas into practice and discussing them with people who experience symptoms is by far the most effective method. However, launching into new ways of working without guidance is unwise. Meeting with an experienced professional for regular supervision sessions is vital in the development of any new skills and for many professionals it is necessary for continued registration. Further reading from the list at the end of the chapter will be essential for the person looking to develop skills beyond those covered here. Workshops and conferences around the subject are frequent in the UK and can provide a useful as well as cost effective further introduction. There are a number of courses that prepare professionals to work in this way; a few of which are listed at the end of the chapter. In my experience, courses that can demonstrate a high level of skills-focused training are most useful. This can be verified if the course includes high levels of practice scrutiny through the mediums of role play, feedback on taped clinical work, and supervision.

Dealing with psychosis is a challenge to those who experience it as well as to those from whom help is sought. With the right support, however, the process can be both fruitful and rewarding.

Summary of practical strategies identified

- ◆ Sharing worrying experiences with a trusted person.
- ◆ Having that person, or someone else, to help work out practical strategies.
- ◆ Trying to maintain a regular sleep pattern.
- ◆ Reducing alcohol and drug intake.
- ◆ Maintaining self-care (e.g. diet and hygiene).

Summary of practical strategies identified (*cont'd*)

◆ Keeping in touch with supportive friends and family.

◆ Keeping active (e.g. exercise, some form of daily activity or employment).

◆ Taking regular medication.

◆ Reducing potentially harmful ways of coping.

◆ Building up useful coping methods and learning new ways of coping from other people. These might include:
— telling the voices to go away
— agreeing to listen to the voices at a particular time
— using ear plugs
— learning relaxation methods
— having a relaxing bath
— talking to friends
— playing a sport or exercising
— reading or watching television.

◆ Working with a trusted person to explore levels of control over voices.

◆ Working with a trusted person to test out beliefs about events or voices.

References

Beck A T, Rush J A, Brian F, Emery G 1979 Cognitive therapy of depression. Guilford Press, New York

Chadwick P, Birchwood M 1994 The Cognitive Assessment of Voices Schedule. In: Chadwick P, Birchwood M, Trower P (eds) 1996 Cognitive therapy for hallucinations, delusions and paranoia. Wiley, Chichester, pp 195–200

Chadwick P, Birchwood M 1995 The Beliefs about Voices Questionnaire. In: Chadwick P, Birchwood M, Trower P (eds) 1996 Cognitive therapy for hallucinations, delusions and paranoia. Wiley, Chichester, pp 201–202

Chadwick P, Birchwood M, Trower P (eds) 1996 Cognitive therapy for hallucinations, delusions and paranoia. Wiley, Chichester

Curson D, Patel M, Liddle P, Barnes T 1988 Psychiatric morbidity of a long stay hospital population with chronic schizophrenia and implications for future community care. British Medical Journal 297: 819–822

Garety P, Hemsley D 1994 Delusions: investigations into the psychology of delusional reasoning. Psychology Press, Hove

Hustig H, Hafner R 1990 Persistent auditory hallucinations and their relationship to delusions of mood. Journal of Nervous and Mental Diseases 178:264–267 (cited in) Chadwick P, Birchwood M, Trower P, (eds) 1996 Cognitive therapy for hallucinations, delusions and paranoia. Wiley, Chichester, p 203

Kingdon D, Turkington D 1994 Cognitive behavioural therapy of schizophrenia. Lawrence Erlbaum Associates, Hove

References (cont'd)

Kuipers E, Garety P, Fowler D, Freeman D, Dunn G, Bebbington P et al 1997 The London–East Anglia trial of cognitive behaviour therapy for psychosis 1: effects of the treatment phase. British Journal of Psychiatry 171:319–327

Zubin J, Spring B 1977 Vulnerability: a new view of schizophrenia. Journal of Abnormal Psychology 86:260–266

Annotated further reading

Bentall R (ed) 1989 Reconstructing schizophrenia. Routledge, London

This text examines the historical development and debate over the current relevance of the disease concept of schizophrenia. It provides part of the theoretical backdrop to the approaches described in this chapter.

Birchwood M, Tarrier N (eds) 1992 Innovations in the psychological management of schizophrenia: assessment, treatment and services. Wiley, Chichester

A thorough review of research that underpins psychological approaches to serious mental health problems. This review includes evidence relating to family work, early intervention and social skills. A whole section is given over to considering the development of services within which these approaches can be utilised.

Chadwick P, Birchwood M, Trower P 1996 Cognitive therapy for hallucinations, delusions and paranoia. Wiley, Chichester

Fowler P, Garety P, Kuipers L 1995 Cognitive behaviour therapy for psychosis, a clinical handbook. Wiley, Chichester

These two books are essentially treatment manuals. Either will be of use to the professional with training in CBT seeking to cross over to working with people experiencing psychosis. Alongside good supervision, either will provide a valuable guide to this process. The Fowler, Garety & Kuipers (1995) text is unique in that the approach described has been evaluated by randomised controlled trial.

Haddock G, Slade P (eds) 1996 Cognitive behavioural interventions with psychotic disorders. Routledge, London

A broad range of approaches under the umbrella of CBT is introduced in this book. It will be of use to the person seeking an introduction to the field.

Annotated further reading (cont'd)

Bentall R (ed) 1989 Reconstructing schizophrenia. Routledge, London

Hawton K, Salkovskis P, Kirk J, Clark D M (eds) 1989 Cognitive behaviour therapy for psychiatric problems: a practical guide. Oxford Medical Publications, Oxford

This is essential reading for the student of CBT. There is little on the approach described in this chapter. However, many aspects of CBT for psychosis were developed from the techniques that are described in this text. Of particular use is Kirk's chapter on assessment.

Kingdon D, Turkington D 1994 Cognitive behavioural therapy of schizophrenia. Lawrence Erlbaum Associates, Hove

Another treatment manual. One of the strengths of this book is the clear and practical description of the normalising approach. The whole text is clearly presented, providing an ideal first stop to the person developing a practical interest in this type of work.

Nelson H 1997 Cognitive behavioural therapy with schizophrenia: a practice manual. Stanley Thornes Publishers, Cheltenham

This very practical manual covers a wide range of strategies used within CBT. Again useful for a person with some experience or at least good CBT supervision. The text covers strategies for overcoming a range of common obstacles.

Wykes T (ed) 1998 Outcome and innovation in psychological treatment of schizophrenia. Wiley, Chichester

A more recent review of the state of the art in psychological approaches to serious mental health problems. The text describes emerging applications of CBT including problems arising from cognitive deficits and dissatisfaction with medication. The book will be of use to those interested in recent developments in the field as well as people involved in the development of services or training programmes.

10

Lack of motivation, confidence and volition

Geoff Brennan   Sue Kerr   Sally Goldspink

I developed a feeling of blankness and deadness which has stayed with me. To this day I have felt I have died inside and have lost all my inner energy. Because of this I thought I was going to die, which is very frightening

(Ch. 1)

Imagine the worst moment of your life. Extend it to an hour, a day, a year, years on end, moments stacked up and lost forever. This is the stultifying process of madness. This is why mental patients look, act and feel numb. To be in perpetual, suspended animation is better than never ending pain

(Unzicker 1989)

KEY ISSUES

◆ Theoretical understanding of negative symptoms.

◆ Assessment of symptoms and related problems.

◆ Acknowledgement of the impact of negative symptoms.

◆ Two case studies that highlight interventions used.

◆ Overview of therapeutic approach.

INTRODUCTION

The above quotes highlight an area that is often ignored or undervalued in conceptualising serious mental illness. To be 'mad' is to be 'raving', 'crazed', a 'lunatic' – all of which conjure images of dynamic movement, erratic, inexplicable and often violent behaviour, as if the person is removed from humanity through the grip of some terrifying alien force. These are the stereotypical images which first come to lay people's minds when they hear the words 'mental illness'. They do not include people who 'look, act and feel numb', or people who have 'lost all their inner energy'. They do not include the person sitting on a sofa smoking endless cigarettes and getting up only to make a cup of tea (and leaving milk, sugar and the used teabag in a mess afterwards). Neither does it include the individual who spends 2 hours getting out of bed, puts on the same clothes as worn for the last week and then falls asleep in the chair half an hour after getting up. Nor does it explain people whose families think they no longer have any feelings for them because they hardly talk and only reply 'yeah, I'm OK' in a flat and disinterested voice when asked how they are.

Bleuler (1983) eloquently describes these 'hidden' symptoms as 'The loss of feeling felt, the numbness perceived, the lifelessness experienced'. These hidden symptoms are the concern of this discussion. They are the so-called 'negative symptoms.'

Although mostly associated with a diagnosis of schizophrenia, negative symptoms cover a range of health and social factors. They are thought to apply to individuals with other mental health diagnoses and even some forms of physical ill health. For ease of description and discussion, however, this analysis will focus on the manifestation of negative symptoms within schizophrenia as most work has been carried out in this area.

WHAT ARE THE NEGATIVE SYMPTOMS?

Everybody has, and will, experience a lack of motivation, loss of interest and concentration, fatigue and a general sense of life being a grind. When discussing negative symptoms we are talking about more than a transient sense of apathy or fatigue. The severity and content of negative symptoms and difficulty in overcoming them fall into the same category as so-called positive symptoms (hallucinations and delusions), in that they grossly affect the individual's ability to function.

In Table 10.1 are a list of the five main negative symptom groups. As professionals usually suspect the presence of negative symptoms through observing changes in functioning and behaviour, these are included as a guideline.

THE DISTINCTION BETWEEN POSITIVE AND NEGATIVE

A diagnosis of schizophrenia is generally made when individuals experience

Table 10.1 Main negative symptom groups

Negative symptom	Observed behaviour/consequence
Blunted affect: 'Decreased range and intensity of emotional responsiveness'	◆ Diminished or absent facial expressiveness during interactions with others ◆ Unchanging, monotonous or inexpressive voice tone when conversing ◆ Lack of gestures when conversing
Alogia: 'Poverty of thought'	◆ Little or no spontaneous speech ◆ Little said during interactions ◆ Speech conveys little actual information ◆ Stopping in the middle of a conversation and forgetting what was said
Avolition: 'Loss of motivation or drive'	◆ Difficulty in following through on activities ◆ Lack of interest in doing things ◆ Sitting around doing little or engaged in activities requiring little effort (such as watching TV)
Anhendonia: 'Diminished capacity to experience pleasure'	◆ Lack of enjoyment from recreational activities ◆ Inability to feel close to others, such as friends and relatives ◆ Difficulty in experiencing pleasure from anything
Inattention:	◆ Becoming easily distracted during conversations ◆ Difficulty in focusing attention on a task, such as reading a magazine article or getting dressed ◆ Stopping midway through something, such as a task or conversation

Source: Adapted from Watkins (1996)

positive symptoms (hallucinations and/or delusions) at the onset and during the acute phase of their illness. Often these persist as residual symptoms. However, the severe positive symptoms are often transient, although a percentage remain despite treatment with neuroleptic medication. The positive symptoms are so called because they are 'outside the normal range of experience', although more recent debate on the symptoms of mental illness has quite rightly pointed out that some positive symptoms are experienced by a wider population than those diagnosed as mentally ill (see Chs 3, 9). Even so, hallucinations and delusion still remain a foreign experience to most people.

Negative symptoms, conversely, are defined as a 'failure' of everyday functions. They have the capacity to affect all aspects of functioning. Speech, behaviour, level of enjoyment, motivation and concentration can all be adversely affected. Unfortunately, as the features of negative symptoms are essentially an absence rather than an addition, they are harder to recognise as abnormal and can be misidentified as an aspect of sufferers' personalities or as wilful behaviour on their part. It follows that they could therefore be seen to be within an individual's control. It is this mistaken view of control that can lead to judgemental attitudes that adversely affect treatment philosophies and outcome. An example of this is someone who finds it difficult to get up in the morning being thought or described to be 'lazy', as the observer believes the person is wilfully staying in bed, rather than battling with symptoms. This mistaken view, that the sufferers are more in control and just need to 'pull themselves together', has been exhibited both by professional carers as well as by family and other informal carers (Oliver & Kuipers 1996).

In thinking about positive and negative symptoms in this way, we should be aware that the two can and do coexist within the individual's experience of illness. The manner in which they are related and coexist has been the subject of debate for some time. Although positive and negative symptoms are distinguishable in a number of ways (including possible biological processes and response to medication), our understanding of the interrelations between the two is mediocre (Smith, Mar & Turoff 1998). Indeed, present analysis of schizophrenia challenges the traditional breakdown of the syndrome into just the two symptom groups. As more is known about schizophrenia it would seem possible that there are different conjunctions of symptom types that can affect outcomes. Therefore, the area in need of greater exploration and expansion is not the positive but the negative symptom continuum (Liddle 1987, Smith, Mar & Turoff 1998). As mentioned earlier, serious mental illness is often associated with the presence of the positive symptoms and yet for some the first evidence of onset comprises behavioural changes, such as withdrawal, or a decrease in interest or hygiene. We therefore need to be careful that we do not give primacy to the positive symptoms in our treatment strategies. Negative symptoms have the capacity to cause long term distress to clients, professionals, family members or lay carers.

CAUTION AND CONFUSION

It would be wrong to proceed in our discussion of negative symptoms without considering the possibility of other factors explaining failures in functioning. We should be especially cautious as symptoms are often deduced through perceived deficits in behaviour and not, initially, through client report.

1. Link with positive symptoms

As discussed above, it is common for a person to have both positive and negative symptoms. What is also possible is that people's behaviour is defined by their natural reaction to positive symptoms rather than negative, although these behaviours correspond to those in Table 10.1. An example of this was when a young man was referred to one of the authors with suspected first onset psychosis. He was described as lacking in motivation and social skills as he 'hardly ever left his home'. Everyday tasks such as shopping and collecting allowances were carried out by other family members. On assessment the cause of this behaviour was that the young man experienced voices that told him that he would be killed and his family home burnt if he left the house. Within the home he was motivated, alert and sociable. His reaction to these voices was, understandably, to obey them.

This example further highlights the need for a sound assessment, which must explore the individual's reasoning for the observed behaviour. In this young man's situation the indicated treatment methods were medication to combat the auditory hallucinations in combination with cognitive–behavioural strategies to help him manage the voices.

2. Link with depression

There is a high prevalence between depression and schizophrenia, with as many as 25% of persons diagnosed with the latter thought also to exhibit clinical depression. While it is not the purpose of this discussion to hypothesise as to this high figure, it would require us to proceed carefully if we suspect the presence of negative symptoms as described above. The obvious presence of affective disturbance within bipolar disorders would indicate the same level of caution. This is because some of the symptoms in Table 10.1, such as lack of interest and pleasure, could be caused by a disturbance in affect, which may require special exploration and different treatment, either pharmacological or psychosocial. It is advocated that special attention be made to mood, anxiety and suicidality in any assessment strategy. The KGV described later (see also Ch. 5) includes these items and can be used to identify depression, or a specific tool such as Beck Depression Inventory (BDI) could be utilised. Even with the presence of depression we still need to ask if this is a natural result of the debilitating effect of the symptoms.

3. Neuroleptic medication

Professionals cannot ignore the fact that some behaviours and experiences described by clients are the result of taking neuroleptics, either from side-effects or sedation. It would seem that the new atypical neuroleptics do not cause as many problems in this regard. However, it should be acknowledged that medication may cause behaviours that appear to be negative symptoms. In general this possibility can be explored by considering medication levels and the side-effects of drugs being taken. These can be identified with the use of side-effect inventories such as the Liverpool University Side-Effect Rating Scale (LUNSERS, see Ch. 5). If in doubt, pharmacy departments can provide advice and alternatives.

4. Institutionalisation

Whilst positive symptoms, depression and medication are all factors that can blur the assessment of negative symptoms, institutionalisation was also thought to be a possible cause of the behaviours identified in Table 10.1. The move to community care has provided the opportunity to reassess the prevalence of negative symptoms outside of institutionalised settings. Indeed, it has been discovered that institutionalisation alone cannot account for the level of negative symptoms exhibited within the mentally ill population. It is also recognised that many individuals may have been functioning at a poor level prior to the perceived onset of their illness and before their involvement with the mental health system (Wykes 1994).

This does not necessarily mean that 'institutionalisation' occurs in, or is confined to, large hospital settings. Indeed, it is quite possible that family homes, hostels or even own accommodation can become places where the individual does not have the encouragement to maintain social skills (Brown, Birley & Wing 1972). Before professionals judge carers or the individuals themselves in this situation, it is important to remind ourselves that over-stimulation or high expectation can lead to an exacerbation in the positive symptoms! What is clear is that closing large psychiatric hospitals has not eradicated the presence of negative symptoms.

5. Protective factor of negative symptoms

Professionals need to be cautious of the assumption that lack of motivation, confidence and volition are always part of a 'deteriorating course' of mental illness. A study by Harding, Zubin & Strauss (1987) has disputed this by identifying windows of good functioning even with negative symptoms. These often last for some years. Some commentators feel that low levels of functioning may be a deliberate strategy on the part of the individual to have the space to learn to live with the illness (Strauss et al 1989). Close reading of Unzicker's comments at the beginning of this chapter highlights this possible protective function for negative symptoms in that they are 'better than being in never ending pain'. Venables & Wing (1962) reinforced this idea following electrophysiological evidence that withdrawal is associated with decreased ability to cope with sensory input and is, therefore, a possible defensive strategy. The possibility that sufferers are in some way cocooning themselves for a period of recuperation highlights the need for caution in all aspects of interventions. The individual with negative symptoms can often seem to be passive and compliant, which may induce a practitioner to become prescriptive and authoritarian. ('All he needs is a good shove! If you go soft on him, he won't do anything, believe me!', as was once said to one of the authors.) It is of great importance when planning any treatment not to fall into this trap. The impact of negative symptoms is so great that overzealous plans can exacerbate positive symptoms, drive the individual further into withdrawal and/or cause the individual to resort to other protective strategies such as avoidance of therapy or, in extreme cases, even physical violence.

AVOIDING THE PITFALLS

Research indicates that the characteristics of therapists are indicative of positive outcomes in therapy and are as important if not more so than the model of therapy itself (Luborsky et al 1985). Since schizophrenia generally, and 'negative' symptoms in particular, are thought to be the accumulative effect of genetic, biological, social and psychological vulnerability towards prevailing life stresses, understanding must include a broad framework of models and interventions that encompass all the aforementioned deficits experienced in everyday life as well as in the context of illness. Increased motivation, improved confidence and ability to act on their own volition are goals *all* individuals share, whether they suffer from mental illness or not. Therefore the focus of work must be to 'normalise' individuals' experiences and build on their desire to change, no matter how small that change may be.

Often professionals view individuals with mental health problems as collections of symptoms to be cured or deficits to be rectified. With regard to negative symptoms, it is important to view people as strengths and interests to be discovered and their environment as a goldmine of resources to be moulded and used. It is interesting how often an individual with negative symptoms (or, for that matter, depression or any of the cautions mentioned above) will be described in terms of negatives. Consider the statements below:

Mr Jones suffers from negative symptoms. The only time he ever leaves his home is to collect his benefit as he say's he 'can't be bothered' with any other daytime activity arranged by his care worker.

This statement gives you important clues as to how you are to consider Mr Jones. The basic message is that he is a difficult case, has little if no motivation and has rejected all the efforts of his care worker (poor soul) to improve his lot. Suppose, however, that the statement is changed to:

Mr Jones has negative symptoms. Despite this he retains the skills necessary to collect his benefit from the post office on the correct day. At the present time Mr Jones and the care team have not been able to expand on this skill base.

From this perspective the future becomes one of possibilities rather than predicted and expected failures. 'The only time' previously mentioned becomes a valuable exception and indicator of health to be explored. From here it becomes possible to identify skills, strengths and motivators.

To address any beliefs or behaviours that compound the effects of symptoms and be able to work therapeutically with individuals who experience negative symptoms, we must first explore our own attitudes. To understand the pitfalls from an individual's point of view, consider the scenario in Box 10.1.

GETTING STARTED

The assessment process discussed earlier in Chapter 5 is imperative in ensuring a solicitous account of persons' experiences and the impact on their daily life is obtained. To implement this effectively a pragmatic and supportive style is required. Indeed, to avoid the cautions and pitfalls mentioned earlier, the assessment should be a synonymous process that incorporates standardised assessment tools (Box 10.2) and clients' subjective descriptions of their experiences and daily difficulties.

These assessments provide standardised information of:

◆ the signs and symptoms shown by individuals
◆ the impact that these have on their social functioning
◆ the impact of neuroleptic medication on their physical well-being and their concentration.

Specific information regarding what the client experiences, when, why, where and with whom is gained from the functional analysis (see Ch. 6). You will need to explore clients' daily activity schedule, highlighting the positive aspects of their achievements, and noting any practical coping strategies that could be enhanced. Throughout this process it is important to look for *any* positives, as demonstrated by the case of Mr Jones earlier.

Box 10.1 How would you feel?

You are in hospital recovering from an acute relapse. Your hallucinations were very vivid and disturbing, yet despite these symptoms you realistically assessed your needs and entered hospital voluntarily. You have accepted medication, even though you doubt its effectiveness. As you have got 'better' the voices have lessened in volume and abuse, but you are constantly tired. The simplest thing exhausts you. It feels as if you have some sort of virus. You have had these feelings before, during after your last admission. You don't want this illness to get the better of you – you have a lot to gain from being well. You are determined to fight it!

Every morning the ward staff run a group from 9 a.m. to 10 a.m. You have decided to attend this as it provides a focus for the start of the day and may help you recover quicker. The first morning after you have made this decision you wake at 8.30 a.m., but can't seem to get up. You are tired and yet you've only just woken up. Finally, you manage to get out of bed. It's now 9.05 a.m. You drag yourself to have a wash. This makes you feel a bit better. It's now 9.20 a.m.

You postpone having a cup of tea and go straight to the group. You sit down. The group goes quiet. Everyone is looking at you. The staff member who's running the group waits a minute before addressing you. 'Good morning X. While I would like to welcome you to this group can I remind you that it starts at 9 a.m. and not 9.20 a.m. I mention this as it's not fair on other members and disruptive to the group if people come and go whenever they feel like it'.

How would you feel?

Box 10.2 Assessment tools to be used

KGV
Social Functioning Scale
Side-effects of medication (LUNSERS)
Functional analysis
Activity schedule
Mastery and Pleasure Inventory
Motivational interview
Negative Symptom Checklist

The principles of cognitive–behavioural therapy lend themselves to improving motivation and confidence, in that it is a flexible approach that aims to work collaboratively and foster individuals' control over their illness and to lessen and manage social disabilities. Due to the emotional nature of the presenting problems and the varying formation of individuals' beliefs about themselves and the world, any devised intervention will need to be tailor made to suit the individual, as the following case example shows:

Case study – Mark

Mark is a 32-year-old man with 3 year history of paranoid schizophrenia. He came to the attention of the psychiatric services following an incident in which he is believed to have jumped from a bridge while actively psychotic. At the time of the incident Mark believed he was being hunted. Subsequently, Mark sustained a number of fractures.

The diagnosis of schizophrenia was made following the incident described above. At this time Mark disclosed a 10 year history of social withdrawal, and family history of schizophrenia (father, brother and sister).

Mark was prescribed 30 mg of haloperidol and continued to take that dose for the following 2 years. He was seen on a monthly basis by a social worker. The social worker reported that, other than a lack of any social interests, Mark appeared to have recovered. A subsequent restructuring of services meant that he was reallocated and consequently reassessed by the rehabilitation services.

Observed behaviour *Mark slept for 16 hours each day. His waking time was spent 'staring at a newspaper or the TV'. He ate or drank what was put in front of him. His domestic chores were done by his mother. He appeared unable to initiate any conversation and his responses were monosyllabic. Mark denied any positive symptomatology, though he rated high on the Negative Symptoms Checklist.*

One important exception to the observed behaviour was Mark's consistency and punctuality when asked to attend appointments with the psychiatric services. This may be partly explained by Hatfield & Lefley (1987) who suggest that routine and order can be of particular benefit to people living with schizophrenia. In other words, by knowing where they are going to and what to expect, people can prepare themselves and thus exert a degree of control over events. It was felt to be important that professionals mirrored Mark's behaviour and were also consistent and punctual – old-fashioned behaviours mean a lot to this client group.

It was recognised that Mark was at risk with regard to self-neglect, and potential self-harm. This was felt to be due to the decline in his interest, confidence and overwhelming sense of hopelessness, along with an inability to express his thoughts and feelings. The aim of engaging Mark and monitoring any changes should be the focus of interventions.

One caution in Mark's presentation was that his medication may have been contributing to the behaviours diagnosed as negative symptoms. A LUNSERS was

Case study – Mark (cont'd)

carried out and Mark did score highly. These results highlighted the need for a formal review of neuroleptic medication. A case was presented for changing to an atypical antipsychotic. The multidisciplinary team were understandably cautious owing to Mark's history of self-harm and his difficulty in expressing the content of his inner world.

Specific areas of difficulty identified through the ongoing process of assessment were:

◆ difficulty with concentration
◆ lethargy
◆ excessive sleeping.

At this point it was not possible to carry out a functional analysis as described in Chapter 6. This was because of the disabling nature of Mark's illness and his inability to verbalise his problems. To attempt to carry out such an assessment at this stage may well have resulted in alienating him. It was therefore decided to proceed with the engagement process and try to develop an observed problem statement, as detailed in Box 10.3.

To reinforce and expand upon the positive, consistent, punctual behaviour already noted, a plan was drawn up to provide daily contact with the rehabilitation services. The idea to maintain social contact was discussed with Mark. He consented to the intervention as he said he liked the notion of having 'something to get up in the morning for'. He also liked the idea of seeing the staff as they were his only contact with the world and thus helped him stay in touch with reality.

This acceptance was the first indication that Mark had some insight into his situation. He later confided that he was, in fact, terrified of his psychotic experiences and had found that they had previously become worse when he attempted any social contact. As a consequence he had lost the ability to communicate even on the most basic of levels. Mark also believed that his slowness and difficulty in making decisions irritated people.

Mark's difficulties were discussed with him in the context of his illness. Within this his social isolation was reframed as coping strategies he had developed in order to maintain a safe and manageable environment. To improve the quality of his daily life he was encouraged to utilise and reframe other strategies.

As an addition to the assessments discussed earlier, the Allen Cognitive Disability Assessment (Velligan et al 1995) was carried out by an OT. This assessment identified the difficulties Mark was experiencing in planning activities and problem solving, along with a severe lack of social skills. Mark's care package was deemed to require input from a number of professionals. This was not only to ensure Mark had the benefit of a pool of skills, but also to expand his number of contacts. By providing a consistent approach they were able to address a number of problems and defined goals listed in Table 10.2.

One year on from the start of this process, Mark trusted the staff enough to tell his side of the story.

Case study – Mark (cont'd)

Mark's story *My life changed completely when I was 11 years old and my family moved into the town. My dad left us because he was ill. We had to be quiet when he was around. Then my brother became ill and he was just the same, then my sister became ill and I was just waiting for my turn. I was terrified all the time; everything was weird I couldn't understand what was happening and everyone seemed to be out to get me. I felt like a time bomb, I don't remember jumping off the bridge, but I remember waking up in hospital feeling like a 'numbskull'. My mind was empty. I thought that this was what the illness was all about. I didn't think of questioning anything, in fact I just didn't seem to think, because I wasn't as scared of feeling numb.*

Mark identified this time of feeling numb as a healing process, which resonates with the observation that some negative symptoms are protective and defensive. Mark is now engaged in an active rehabilitation programme and has set himself a number of short term and long term goals.

The clinicians involved with Mark have learnt a great deal from him. They summarise the salient points they have learnt to be:

◆ to avoid making assumptions
◆ to be pragmatic

Box 10.3 Interventions

Observed problem statement:
Mark exhibits low levels of motivation and social withdrawal leading to a lack of purpose or enjoyment in all activities.

Long term goal:
To engage Mark. Increase motivation, interest, enjoyment and improve social networks.

Action:
1. To offer a consistent, supportive, non-threatening environment for Mark.
2. To formulate a shared understanding of Mark's internal world and the threats proposed by the external world.

Table 10.2 Problems and goals – Mark	
Problems	**Goals**
◆ I have minimal conversation with people	◆ To have conversation with support worker for 15 minutes every day
◆ I am socially isolated	◆ To attend day centre communication classes for 1 hour a week ◆ To visit my mother for 2 hours each week
◆ I have minimal knowledge of what 'normal' behaviour is	◆ To attend mental health awareness sessions on Wednesday for 1 hour
◆ I find it difficult to plan things to do during the day	◆ To make an activity schedule on daily basis with occupational therapist

◆ to minimise expectations
◆ to accept the person as a person, not an illness
◆ to remember that we are novices with every client
◆ the client knows more about their illness than we will ever understand.

CONCLUSIONS

Individuals with serious mental illness often tread a fine line between overstimulation, which is likely to precipitate positive symptoms, and under-stimulation, which precipitates negative symptoms. Unfortunately, individuals with negative symptoms cause little fuss and are often suffering in undramatic ways; therefore they are easy to forget. This is wrong.

The sufferers of these symptoms are often criticised as being lazy, selfish and generally beyond help because they seem to have no inclination to help themselves. It is fundamental to the therapeutic relationship that clinicians explore their own beliefs and assumptions before attempting to work with clients; only then can the focus of the relationship be based on the expectations, beliefs and experiences of the individual sufferer.

A client-centred interpersonal relationship, which focuses on the conditions of accurate empathy, non-possessive warmth and genuineness, is a prerequisite to working collaboratively with individuals to enable them to identify personal strategies for improving their motivation and confidence and providing an informed vantage point to manage and live according to their own volition.

A truly longitudinal and flexible approach to the concept of lack of motivation, confidence and volition is needed if clinicians are to collaborate with individuals and their carers in managing the impact their illness has on their daily life.

Summary of practical strategies identified

◆ It is essential to take a longitudinal approach.

◆ Goals must be achievable and realistic for the client.

◆ Activity scheduling is an important method of instilling structure.

◆ Client and professional must focus on the future, not the past.

◆ We must negotiate together *how* change can be brought about, not just make assumptions about what the change should be.

◆ It is essential to work at the client's pace.

◆ Education about illness and normalising behaviour aids clients to gain insight and feel less 'abnormal'.

References

Bleuler M 1983 Schizophrenia determination. British Journal of Psychiatry 143(July):78–79

Brown G W, Birley J L T, Wing J K 1972 Influence of family life on the course of schizophrenic disorders: a replication. British Journal of Psychiatry 121:241–263

Harding C M, Zubin J, Strauss J S 1987 Chronicity in schizophrenia: fact, partial fact or artifact? Hospital Community Psychiatry 38(5):477–486

Hatfield A B, Lefley H 1987 Families of the mentally ill: coping and adaptation. Cassell, London

Liddle P F 1987 The symptoms of chronic schizophrenia: a re-examination of the positive negative dichotomy. British Journal of Psychiatry 151:145–151

Luborsky L, McLellan A T, Woody G E, O'Brien C P, Auerbach A 1985 Therapist success and its determinants. Archives of General Psychiatry 42(6):602–611

Oliver N, Kuipers E 1996 Stress and its relationship to expressed emotion in community mental health workers. International Journal of Social Psychiatry 42(2):150–159

Smith D A, Mar C M, Turoff B K 1998 The structure of schizophrenic symptoms: a meta-analytic confirmatory factor analysis. Schizophrenia Research 31:57–70

Strauss J S, Rakfeldt T J, Harding C M, Lieberman D 1989 Mediating processes in schizophrenia: towards a new dynamic psychiatry. British Journal of Psychiatry 155(suppl 5):24

Unzicker R 1989 On my own: a personal journey through madness and re-emergence. Psychosocial Rehabilitation Journal 13(1):16

References (*cont'd*)

Velligan D I, True J E, Lefton R S, Moore T C, Flores C V 1995 Validity of the Allen Cognitive Levels Assessment: a tri-ethnic comparison. Psychiatric Research 56(2):101–109

Venables P H, Wing J K 1962 Level of arousal and the subclassification of schizophrenia. Archives of General Psychiatry 7:114–119

Wing J 1989 The concept of negative symptoms. British Journal of Psychiatry 155(suppl 7):10–14

Watkins J 1996 Living with schizophrenia: an holistic approach to understanding, preventing and recovering from negative symptoms. Hill of Content, Melbourne

Wykes T 1994 Predicting symptomatic and behavioural outcomes of community care. British Journal of Psychiatry 165(4):486–492

Annotated further reading

Bellack A, Mueser K, Gingerich S, Agresta J 1997 Social skills training for schizophrenia: a step by step guide. Guilford, New York

This book provides a comprehensive guide on how to incorporate social skills training into everyday clinical practice.

Watkins J 1996 Living with schizophrenia: an holistic approach to understanding, preventing and recovering from negative symptoms. Hill of Content, Melbourne

This small, easy to read, thought provoking book provides the reader with an insight into the problems caused by negative symptoms. The author has wide experience in dealing with the subject matter. There are many logical and practical strategies given to aid any practitioner who wishes to work in collaboration with clients who experience negative symptoms.

Working with families and informal carers

Catherine Gamble   Geoff Brennan

For too long, mental illness has been kept in the shadows. Instead of rejection, we need acceptance. Instead of shame, we need love. Instead of despair, we need solid and unwavering support. It's time to come out of the shadows and into the light.

(Ann Deveson 1992)

Carers of people with mental health problems in particular were critical of how Social Services Departments and other agencies did not take their views and needs into account so that they would be left to manage very difficult situations on their own.

(Favin 1998)

KEY ISSUES

◆ Exploration of evidence-based family interventions.

◆ Reducing stress and burden in family environment.

◆ Identifying who to work with and why.

◆ Relating how to use family intervention in clinical practice.

INTRODUCTION

Historically, families have been as much burdened by the mental health system as by the illness. This may seem like a contentious statement but, as Ann Deveson (1992) illustrates, all too often they are and have been perceived as part of the problem, if not the cause, of serious mental illness. The reality is that the treatment of serious mental illness would not be tenable without them. Community care would be exclusive, expensive and unfeasible (Noland 1996). In the main, it is dependent on the participation of families and informal carers as they represent the major resource and support network.

This role has often been forced upon them with very little or no preparation. Unlike professional carers, they do not make an active choice to be involved with serious mental illness. In our experience, families when offered intervention immediately question why 'they were never given this at the start?' It is part of the professional's role to support and help the public, so what better place to start than within households where serious mental illness is an everyday reality? Practitioners of the future have a moral responsibility to alter the historical exclusion of this important caring role.

This chapter aims to outline the practical implementation of evidence-based family work interventions, which are outlined in Chapter 2. It also seeks to provide an insight into the skills and knowledge necessary to work effectively with informal carers.

WHAT CONSTITUTES A FAMILY?

This question is often raised when practitioners begin to explore the structures and systems within which their clients live. It is no longer applicable to see the 'family' as the traditional nuclear, two up two down, 2.2 children, mum and dad. Yet some practitioners continue to see this as the only system possible – hence the routine response 'there are no families where I work, all my clients live alone'. The authors of this chapter have used the interventions with gay couples of both sexes, step families, single lone carers, flatmates and significant others. We also believe that hostel workers who have long term relationships with clients could and should be constituted as 'family'. In addition we have noticed that 'family' is sometimes used as shorthand for mother. Mothers are often left with the emotional and practical responsibilities of care. However, if we unquestioningly accept this assumption, we are ignoring the influence and needs of siblings, fathers, grandparents and other extended family members. Serious mental illness reaches out into these people's lives and this should never be trivialised. As a general rule, if the question 'who should I work with?' is raised, the simple answer should be: 'whoever the client wants you to'.

So what about the case where a client says 'I don't want my family to know anything!' In this situation we need to ascertain whether the family will be taking an active caring role after our involvement. If so, how should we prepare and support them? Indeed, consider whether, if the above statement were reframed to: 'I don't want my GP to know anything', would this be accepted, if the client is to return to primary care and the community? If we are honest, this request would probably be questioned and even ignored. We would rationalise our actions by reinforcing the importance of a GP's role in aftercare – so they must have the information they need. Yet, clients never spend as much time with their GP as they do with their informal carers. In our experience as someone becomes more in control they often re-evaluate this position. If the family is involved in aftercare, professionals must assist and respond to this re-evaluation. Even in the event of the person maintaining their position the carer could access agencies external to the mental health system who would be in a position to assist them. Examples of such agencies are: the National Schizophrenia Fellowship, the Manic Depressive Fellowship, Saneline and numerous local carer organisations.

ENGAGEMENT ISSUES

After being confronted by the array of negative assumptions and historical beliefs that some professionals and systems hold, it is not surprising that many families are initially suspicious when family work is suggested. Indeed, contrary to popular myths, this work does not involve interpreting family dynamics or parent–child relationships. As mentioned, providing families with support is essential if community care is to be effective. It is therefore imperative that professionals introduce the idea of family work when practical help and information is asked for – that is, at a time of crisis. If the offer is taken up when it has been previously rejected this is not the time to think or say 'we told you so'. Instead, it is a time to listen and reflect on the families' experiences of service provision and ascertain what can be learnt and subsequently offered to address actual or perceived shortfalls. At this stage, some families may continue to refuse; however, this should not be perceived as rejection. The invitation must be left open, a lifeline given and contact maintained. In other words, families should be tentatively followed up. One advocated method is to write letters that seek to ascertain how the family is since you last met. Its content should contain a summary of what their situation was at the time of appraisal and an enquiry if they need anything more. For example:

> *We are currently in the process of reviewing the families on our books. We were therefore writing to ascertain how you are getting on and things are progressing. When we last met you described to your situation to be … if you no longer feel able to cope with these circumstances or if any additional issues have arisen we would be happy to meet up at the earliest possible convenience.*

To enhance the engagement process it is essential that the following guidelines are adhered to and provided:

◆ be flexible as to the time and venue – always be punctual and keep appointment
◆ give a clear and non-judgemental rationale for family intervention.

ASSESSMENT AND RATIONALE FOR IT

Considering that 'assessment' usually connotes a problem to be found or defined, we need to clarify what the process of assessment for family intervention means. To identify which family systems to work with, it could be argued that all you need to do is to use the rule of thumb shown in Box 11.1.

However, although this is a useful indicator of stress within the family system, it does not tell us much more about what practitioners may face after initial contact. In order to gain the fullest picture of the system and roots of stress, we should employ a more rigorous process. This does not mean to say that we are advocating for a long, drawn-out interrogation and questioning. Families are searching for recognition, support and help and we need to provide this at the earliest opportunity. It is important, however, that we have an identified framework within which to operate. There is nothing more insulting for families than to be given information they have found for themselves. In order to know how to link our knowledge with their experience and expertise, we need to assess what their experience and expertise is. Otherwise some of the areas identified in Table 11.1 will be missed.

From this exercise it is possible to deduce that we are not looking for 'problems to solve' but 'strengths to build on'. Formalised assessment strategies to help with this process are as follows.

Box 11.1 A 'rule of thumb'

◆ Carers living with clients who relapse more than twice a year despite taking regular medication
◆ Those who frequently contact staff for reassurance or help
◆ Home environments where there are repeated arguments, violence and/or the police are called
◆ Any carer who is looking after a client unaided

Source: Kuipers, Leff & Lam (1992)

Table 11.1 Family areas of expertise	
Participant	**Expertise in**
Client	◆ Symptoms ◆ Treatment effects from service and individual level ◆ Strengths in functioning ◆ Knowledge and understanding of own family, culture, values and philosophy ◆ History of illness
Informal carer	◆ History of prodrome and illness ◆ Early warning signs ◆ Assessment of stress ◆ Knowledge and understanding of own family, culture, values and philosophy ◆ Resource for client in family and wider systems
Professional	◆ Knowledge of illness and treatment strategies ◆ Advocating within professional systems ◆ Illness effects on wider population ◆ Interventions to reduce stress and burden

Relative assessment interview

The Relative Assessment Interview (RAI) aims to obtain information about the relatives' behaviours, beliefs and subjective feelings towards the client, their illness and its consequences. It helps to elicit clients' and carers' positive and successful coping strategies and resources as well as their difficulties. The RAI covers seven main areas (Barrowclough & Tarrier 1995):

◆ background to the patient and his/her family
◆ background information and contact time
◆ chronological history of the illness
◆ current problems/symptoms
◆ irritability or quarrels in the household
◆ relatives' relationship with patient
◆ effect of the illness on relatives.

Schizophrenia Nursing Assessment Protocol

The Schizophrenia Nursing Assessment Protocol (SNAP) adopts a holistic view of families. The devised, simplest formula covers four main assessment areas: personal history and significant life events, relationships within the household, psychiatric history, and understanding and knowledge of schizophrenia and medication (Brooker & Baguley 1990).

Whilst the above assessments have been targeted for use with schizophrenia, they need little adaptation for use with other diagnoses.

Assessment procedure

In clinical practice, an issue that often prevails is how, when and where to conduct the above interviews. This is a difficult question to be definitive about, as it always relies on the time, place and person. Ideally they should be conducted on a one to one basis in a quiet informal setting. It is also useful to gain consent to tape the interviews as it can be off-putting for the recipient if notes are constantly being made. An additional advantage of audio taping is that it is sometimes hard to remember everything that is said. Interviews can be time consuming and it is not always possible to interview all family members. However, in our experience and others, when attempts have been made to incorporate more than one family member at a time, the sessions become confusing and the ability to take notes is reduced. Some family members may also not feel able to disclose or discuss some of the points raised in Table 11.1. Ultimately, the whole process is a negotiated engagement trade-off between what ensures comfort and safety for the individual and professionals' need for information. When it comes to assessing client need, the same principles apply as those described in other chapters of this book.

GETTING STARTED

1. Dealing with the family as a group

When thinking about working with family groups, professionals often fear that they will be confronted with situations that they cannot manage (Leavey, Healy & Brennan 1998) They may feel overwhelmed or fear that they are going to be expected to sort everything out. This can be daunting and may be one of the reasons that families do not get seen regularly. Nevertheless, there are strategies to overcome some of these anxieties. First, no issue or problem can be formally addressed if everyone expects an overnight miracle, talks over each other and/or argues. Therefore, practitioners should not worry about lowering expectations and taking control. Many families express relief when they meet confident, knowledgeable, realistic practitioners who kindly but assertively deal with the prevailing issues. To achieve this, it is important to set simple, mutually negotiated ground rules within which all sessions can be conducted. These, as suggested by Kuipers, Leff & Lam (1992) could follow the guidelines outlined below, but you may wish to make them more idiosyncratic:

- Talk *to* people, not *about* them, and encourage the use of names, rather then using he/she.
- Speaking time should be shared out equally, so that each person's view can be heard, listened to and respected.
- Only one person may speak at a time, avoid interrupting each other and no one's – including the family worker's – opinion is any more important then the next person's.

2. Single practitioner or co-working pair?

One of the identifiable differences in models of family intervention is whether families are seen by single or co-working practitioners. Whilst there are obvious resource benefits for single practitioners to see families, it should not be underestimated how stressful this can be on a long term basis. The advantages of co-working tend to outweigh the disadvantages (see summary in Table 11.2). Furthermore, Leff & Gamble (1995) advocate that co-working should be considered for the following reasons:

Balancing alliances It is important for each family member to feel supported. This is difficult for a single person to achieve, especially if there are numerous family members present. A pair of family workers provide greater opportunity to form alliances with different members of the family. These alliances are not fixed but can shift between sessions or even within a session, according to the need.

Rescue operations Families are often in a state of emotional turmoil. It is easy for one family worker to get stuck in a maelstrom of emotions, or to be sidetracked and to lose the focus of the session. A second worker can help to maintain objectivity, rescue and intervene as necessary to bring the discussion back to the agreed topic.

Table 11.2 Advantages and disadvantages of co-working

Advantages of co-working	Disadvantages of co-working
Share the work and burden	Complicated to organise meeting times
Help when stuck	Rely on each other
Two views on the family	Too powerful for the family
Offer alliances to the family	
Advocate for the client	
Less overwhelming in pairs	
Role models	
Immediate evaluation of session possible	

Modelling the negotiation of differences Families in which conflict erupts find it difficult to resolve their differences thorough calm discussion. Family work pairs can openly discuss differences between themselves, thus modelling a rational approach to disagreements. (This strategy is recognised to be only successful if the family workers have developed a trusting, open working relationship with each other.)

Sharing the emotional burden Work with families should not be taken lightly, as it involves a considerable emotional burden. Raw emotions are close to the surface and are readily communicated to the family worker. It is a relief to be able to share these feelings with a co-worker.

Two heads are better then one Some of the problems generated are difficult to solve. Two workers increase the chances of finding solutions to the large array of problems experienced by families.

3. Providing education

All the practical handbooks in family work advocate that education should be provided first and foremost. This is because providing information about serious mental illness helps to defuse some of the myths and misunderstandings that may be around for carers and clients (Fadden 1998). This is important as practical advice and information sharing is something that carers have repeatedly asked for (Leavey, Healy & Brennan 1998). In addition, it is recognised to be a positive way of improving optimism and may help the carer appreciate clients' viewpoints and increase their insight into why some respond as they do (Kuipers, Leff & Lam 1992).

As mentioned previously it is often insulting for families to be told something they already know. Indeed, this is particularly the case for clients themselves – they rarely get the opportunity or permission to talk about what it's like to experience psychosis and yet, as we have seen, they are the experts. It is therefore strongly advised that a through assessment of knowledge is undertaken before embarking on an education session. The Knowledge about Schizophrenia Interview (KASI, see Box 11.2) was designed to be conducted informally (see Barrowclough & Tarrier 1995). It assesses knowledge, beliefs and attitudes about six areas of schizophrenia. Nevertheless, it is possible to adapt as necessary. Pre- and post-measures give an indication about how effective the sessions have been in achieving change to the areas in Box 11.2. Additional common problems when providing information can be summarised as in Table 11.3.

4. Problem solving

The core principle of family intervention is the ability to implement effective

Box 11.2 The knowledge about schizophrenia interview

- ◆ Diagnosis
- ◆ Symptomatology
- ◆ Aetiology
- ◆ Medication
- ◆ Prognosis
- ◆ Management

problem-solving strategies. Whilst all families have individualised coping strategies and must always be assumed to have strengths in this area, there are an array of challenges thrown up by the illness for which they may need assistance. Some families are stronger in this area than others. The majority really appreciate being given the opportunity to examine their current coping strategies and refine them to meet present and/or future situations. Indeed some families wish to revise some aspects of their management styles completely because they have found them to be ineffective and counter-productive. For example, a parent who constantly shouted at their relative to get out of bed ended up becoming so exasperated they pulled the person down the stairs on the mattress.

Problem solving is an art. It is inherent for some – but not for others. Before starting to think about helping families with their problems, it is worth considering our own attitudes to problems and the skills we have to deal with them (Mills, unpublished data, 1995). Some times we can sort problems out reasonably quickly. On other occasions we put decision making off. This usually occurs when we: (1) have already tried and the plan backfired horribly, (2) perceive the problem to be too large or (3) think it will upset others. Thus, it would appear that the ability to solve problems depends on: motivation, personal disposition, culture, past experiences, emotional involvement, and overcoming the fear of confronting difficult issues, others' expectations, losing control and change. Families' experiences are no different and it is important to realise that problems occur as a normal part of life and that finding ways to solve them is a skill that can be learnt and practised like any other. Indeed, learning to solve problems is a collaborative constructive process that involves having a clear idea of how to negotiate, set an agenda, priorities, agree on goals and practise tasks (Kuipers, Leff and Lam 1992).

The format given in Box 11.3 provides a useful structure to guide families through a six step problem-solving strategy.

Table 11.3 Problems and strategies in information provision

Common problems	Suggested strategies
1. Client is perceived as the poor sufferer – rather than the potential expert	Model a positive attitude to client's knowledge. If necessary make space and time for clients to describe their experience and interpretation of symptoms. Treat this input with respect – encourage other members to listen and ask direct but non-confrontational questions
2. Professionals expect those present to assimilate knowledge and literature as they do and therefore avoid a formal session	Plan to go through the literature in a formalised structured manner. But do not overload; break frequently for questions to clarify what has been covered
3. Carers and clients assimilate knowledge differently	Base the sessions upon their own experiences and subjective reasons for the occurrence of the illness. Provide information on an ongoing basis. Use clear non-jargonistic literature. Talk in lay rather than professional language
4. KASI reveals high level of knowledge in one member	Use this knowledge by directly referring to this expertise in session
5. Client does not agree with diagnosis	Use information on psychosis, relate to general experience and externalise rather than personalise on while asking client and carers to draw comparisons on the impact their experiences have on their lives. Avoid confrontation – and agree to disagree
6. Family produce practical issues that take priority over the session	Assess this need – is it likely that it will impede further progress if not immediately addressed? Act upon the practicalities if they are achievable and realistic in this time frame. Avoid brushing these issues aside – but reiterate that you will and can address them further on in the process
7. Not all members present	Continue with session. Leave leaflets for absent members. Ask who can relay the information from within the family. Check in subsequent sessions that this has been achieved
8. Carers and client feel awkward about saying things in front of each other	Conduct the sessions separately if necessary. Procure the consent of all to participate. Bring everyone together at a later date

---

Box 11.3 A six step problem-solving strategy

Step one: what exactly is the problem or the goal?
Talk about the problem until you can write down exactly what it is. Ask questions to clarify the issue. Break down into smaller parts.

Step two: list all possible solutions .
List all ideas, even silly ones. Try to get everyone to suggest something. Do not discuss merits of ideas at this stage.

Step three: highlight the main advantages and disadvantages
Briefly highlight the main advantages and disadvantages of each suggestion.

Step four: choose the 'best' solution
Choose a realistic, achievable one that can be most readily carried out with the resources available (time, money, skills).

Step five: plan exactly how to carry out the solution
Consider resources needed. Plan each step. Try to consider hitches and pre-empt them. Reduce expectations if necessary.

Date and time of review: _____

Step six: review progress in carrying out homework
Praise effort, not achievement. Review progress on each step. Revise the plan as necessary. Continue to solve problems until stress resolved or goal achieved.

Source: Falloon & Graham-Hole (1994)

WORKING WITH A FAMILY: EVALUATING THE PROCESS

The following case study encapsulates what can be achieved and learnt from family intervention work.

What was known about the family

The genogram in Figure 11.1 identifies the constitution of this family and who was living in the household at the time. Mum and dad were born in Africa, but all the children were born in England. The genogram indicates that mum and dad are divorced and have been amicably so for 7 years. They have two sons and two daughters. Steve, the eldest, lives independently. Although interested in his family's welfare, he had work commitments so he envisaged being unable to attend meetings. David, the second son, has learning

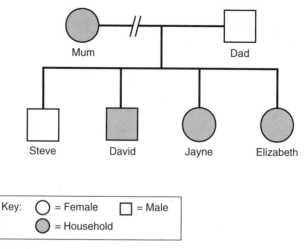

Figure 11.1 Genogram – case study of family intervention work.

difficulties. Jayne, the elder sister, also worked but was keen to attend meetings if they were held in the evenings. Elizabeth, the youngest, was the index client.

Family history of illness

- ◆ Elizabeth first described hearing voices shortly after her 18th birthday.
- ◆ Her first admission was at age 19 following the loss of job and partner.
- ◆ Her mother visited the ward for several hours every day to bring food and assist Elizabeth to wash; Elizabeth hit her mother during this admission and ward staff asked her not to visit as often.
- ◆ Elizabeth was discharged on depot medication; her mother was very concerned, and took over the caring role, accompanied her everywhere and began to assist her in all aspects of daily living.
- ◆ Elizabeth became psychotic again and hit her mother on numerous occasions. Consequently was readmitted to hospital 2 weeks later.

Getting started

On this second admission, the family were recognised to need more support than originally envisaged. Their needs fitted with a number of areas identified in the 'rule of thumb' (see Box 11.1) – that is, mum was a lone carer, whose responsibilities also included looking after someone with learning disabilities, and there had been violent episodes. The family accepted the offer of family work as part of the discharge plan. This work was advocated for by all members of the multidisciplinary team. This team ownership proved to be particularly important, especially in the light of the fact that the work would be conducted in the family home and that both family workers were full time members of the acute ward team.

The following outline is intended to explain the sequence of events and acquisition of skills.

Providing education

Formal interactive education sessions were carried out in the home with all members of the household. Education leaflets, such as the ones issued by the National Schizophrenia Fellowship, were provided. Everyone was encouraged to read them and discuss the salient issues. During these sessions it was noticeable that no one felt awkward about interrupting each other. At this stage, ground rules were negotiated, which took some time for everyone to own and respect. In particular, everyone had a tendency to talk over others, or for Elizabeth. In this instance the suggested strategy (no. 1) outlined in Table 11.3 was utilised. Furthermore, the family had a reasonable level of knowledge. This had been gained from a visit to the local library. Interestingly, they felt this was generally negative with regard to prognosis.

Additional specific issues unearthed during the education session

◆ **Grandmother had been mentally ill**: this information had not been elicited during admissions. It was highlighted that the mother was concerned that Elizabeth's life would follow the same path. However, the disclosure provided an opportunity to discuss the genetic and hereditary aspects of schizophrenia.

◆ **Mother thought that the illness had been caused by divorce**: this belief was probed and challenged, by asking questions such as: 'Why had only one sibling become ill as a consequence?' and 'Why did it take 7 years to manifest itself?' After this style of questioning it was clear that other family members did not share their mum's belief. However, mum continued to feel guilty.

◆ **Family unaware of negative symptoms**: the issues that caused the family most concern were caused by the negative symptoms Elizabeth experienced. It was therefore clarified that an inability to be bothered about things, lack of motivation, and loss of interest, enjoyment and concentration were all recognised symptoms of the illness. As with other families, this aspect of the illness proved to be the hardest thing for them to comprehend. Therefore, it was deemed important to revisit this part of the education process when issues such as 'laziness' and 'can't be bothered' were raised in subsequent sessions.

◆ **Family viewed schizophrenia outcome as the same as learning difficulties**: due to the information they had gathered, the family believed that Elizabeth was facing a process of deterioration that would require her to have similar treatment to her brother David. This had a major impact on their caring strategies and was directly related to mum's beliefs and behaviours.

◆ **Workers were aware and curious about the culture of the family as neither was from a similar background**: during these early engagement sessions, it was realised that there was a need to learn from the family about this important issue. Strategies used to aid this process were as follows:

— outside agencies and colleagues from the same culture were contacted for advice

— family workers reiterated how important it was for them to learn from the family about this issue; everyone was encouraged to share and inform them when any cultural issues came up. Interestingly, all the children described themselves as English and saw England as their home. One of the family workers, although white, was not born in England and felt an alliance with mother as a consequence. One area that the family did believe was culturally significant was the perceived power of the older sister who, in the absence of the parents, was often seen as the adult in charge. This did have an impact on how the family dealt with issues as Elizabeth, being the youngest daughter, was expected to respect her sister as she would her mother.

Enhancing communication

Specific issues

◆ **Using Elizabeth's 'expertise' and giving her room to speak**: as mentioned earlier, during education sessions it was apparent that Elizabeth found it hard to communicate how her symptoms made her feel. Room was made for Elizabeth to relate her experiences and how she perceived them. This proved to be very cathartic for the family; they began to shift from the perception of 'Elizabeth's problem' to 'the problems caused by schizophrenia'. One particular comment made highlighted this:

It was a good idea, us all meeting in the comfort of our own home to discuss my sister's illness. We were all able to say how it felt and for the first time I realised that I knew very little about what she was suffering from or how much – the word schizophrenia meant nothing to me before but it's much clearer now. I used to think she was just being lazy until she told me in the meeting what it was really like.

◆ **Reframing of mother's involvement**: as sessions progressed the family reassessed the mother's involvement. In one session the comment was made that she 'interfered too much', which seemed to be reinforced by the family's experience when mum was asked not to visit the ward. Family workers focused on this statement and reframed it to the mother 'working very hard and needing a break'. This was felt to be important as family members often criticise their previous care strategies without acknowledging their commitment to the individual. In this case, mum had indeed been working very hard and this was due to her obvious concern for her children.

◆ **Keeping dad and Steve informed of the sessions as they were not able to attend**: as dad and Steve were integral members of the informal care team, it was established that family members who could attend would take it in turns to relay what happened in the meetings to their brother and father.

Problem solving

Dealing with specific issues and problems generated by the illness is at the core of family work. As mentioned, one of the main areas of concern was the effects of negative symptoms on Elizabeth's functioning. Elizabeth's ultimate goal was to achieve some meaningful daily activity – that is, she wanted a positive social identity and a job. However, she was having difficulty in socialising and getting out of bed. Nevertheless, this ultimate goal proved to be an important key to gaining Elizabeth's and her family's cooperation. Family workers reiterated that in the long term this overall aim may be achievable. However, in these initial stages it was important to focus down on to a specific issue, identify objectives and plan small achievable tasks that could be practised by the family. The six step problem-solving framework was used to help frame their ideas. These are summarised in Box 11.4.

Subsequent problem-solving areas identified

Appropriate socialisation Elizabeth asked for this to be considered and the problem was subsequently solved. The family openly discussed mum's anxiety when Elizabeth was alone or outside of the family home. Eventually a solution was generated that involved Elizabeth going out with her sister and some friends. On these occasions they would take it in turns to ring home to say they were OK.

Combined with this solution was mum's awareness that Elizabeth was becoming less dependent on her. Such insights can exacerbate the feeling of losing control of the caring role; it is therefore important to generate ideas as to what this role could be replaced with. In this instance, however, mum was excited about returning to interests she had abandoned when Elizabeth had became ill. Had this not occurred spontaneously, the family workers had

Box 11.4 Application of the six step problem-solving strategy

Step one: what exactly is the problem or the goal?
Problem: 'Elizabeth is unable to get out of bed until after noon on most days.'
Goal: 'For Elizabeth to get up every morning from Monday to Friday by 10 a.m.'

Step two: list all possible solutions
The family were encouraged to generate solutions. An exploration of each solution was not formally listed, as the family wished to discuss them and solve problems informally.
At this point it became obvious that mum was volunteering to do everything. The family workers challenged this and, subsequently, the family began exploring supportive roles that other members could undertake.

Step three: highlight the main advantages and disadvantages
As these were discussed, the family began to incorporate different aspects of different solutions. This often happens in problem solving and workers need to be flexible enough to allow the ultimate solution to evolve. In this case, for example, it was clear that Elizabeth did not have an alarm clock. It was decided that she should have one, but that this should not be perceived as the ultimate solution.

Step four: choose the 'best' solution
Through the above process the family identified the following as a solution they were willing to implement.

◆ Jayne to wake Elizabeth at 9 a.m. when she gets up for her shower
◆ Family to leave Elizabeth and not scold her if she did not get up
◆ Mum to praise Elizabeth if she does get up.

Step five: plan exactly how to carry out the solution
It is clear from the above that the solution clearly outlines the role each person has to play in the solution. The solution also indicates what the family should do if Elizabeth was not able to get up.

Date and time of review
The solution, which was termed 'an experiment', was left with the family to practise for the next 2 weeks between sessions.

Step six: review progress in carrying out homework
Elizabeth did get up at 10 a.m. twice in the 10 days.
Whilst initially the family felt that the experiment had been of limited success, on examination it was felt by all that valuable lessons had been learnt. It became clear that Jayne had found consistency difficult, and that the solution had asked for too much from her as well as Elizabeth.

Box 11.4 (cont'd)

What was also clear, however, was the family's satisfaction with the two successes. Mum in particular described a feeling of joy on these two occasions and related this feeling to an increased sense of hope and relief.

Interestingly, when evaluating the session in which the solution had been formulated, the workers felt that they had contributed to the target being too high (i.e. for Elizabeth and family to be expected to achieve the goal on all ten occasions). This was fed back to the family and the workers focused more on the successful outcomes as valuable insights into effective problem solving.

From this it was identified that on the days the solution had been unsuccessful Elizabeth did not have anything meaningful to get up for. Therefore it should be focused on those days when she needed to be up to attend work training.

The family agreed to the change in goal to:

Goal: 'For Elizabeth to get up on Tuesday and Thursday by 10 a.m. in order to attend work training.'

planned to discuss mum finding replacement activities, such as visiting friends and relatives.

Elizabeth becoming independent As the family work sessions progressed this issue became increasingly important to Elizabeth. She wanted an antidote to the 'patient role' and a more positive social identity within the household. It was important at this stage to focus on helping Elizabeth with social-functioning deficits. A programme was devised for her to do her own laundry and cooking. Interestingly, mum, who had previously carried out these tasks for the entire household, now asked if Jayne could also be included!

Coming off medication As the family became more confident and Elizabeth regained control of her health, the issue of stopping medication arose. The workers discussed the need for maintenance medication and discussed the issue with the multidisciplinary team. Medication was eventually reduced to a small dose of oral medication.

Disengaging from family As Elizabeth and her family progressed the time between sessions was gradually extended. After 18 months the sessions were being held two monthly. It became clear that Elizabeth, who was now actively looking for a realistic work placement with her day service, viewed the family work as unnecessary as it reminded her of the period of illness. On one occasion the family workers went to the family home to find everyone out apart from mum. This was seen as a major change to initial visits where

---

Box 11.5 Early warning signs

Name: _____
I have a risk of developing episodes of schizophrenia.
My early warning signs are:
1 _____
2 _____
3 _____

If I experience *any* of these signs I/we will respond by:
a) _____
b) _____
c) _____

My doctor is _____ Phone: _____
My relative/carer is: _____ Phone: _____
If I/we have any concerns about my disorder I will contact _____
immediately.

Source: Adapted from Falloon & Graham-Hole (1994)

---

she talked of her anxiety of letting Elizabeth go out alone. One more session
was held to discuss family management in the case of relapse. To provide
them with a clear framework within which to voice any future concerns, an
early warning signs record was completed (see Box 11.5). Prior to formally
discontinuing, the family were given a lifeline and informed that they could
contact the team at any time in the future if they needed to.

Summary of practical strategies identified

◆ Education should be an ongoing, empowering process and
should encompass the following topics: aetiology, symptomatology,
diagnosis, medication course, prognosis and management
(Lam 1991).

◆ Cultural awareness and understanding must be acknowledged and
incorporated.

◆ The intervention should be offered over a substantial period and tasks
should be achievable, realistic and meaningful to clients' and families'
long term goals.

Summary of practical strategies identified (cont'd)

◆ Family workers should be flexible, knowledgeable and reliable and be able to access services and provide a range of options and opportunities.

◆ The philosophy of family work should be embraced and owned by the whole multidisciplinary team and be integrated into every treatment package (Smith & Birchwood 1990).

◆ Family work should be offered as and when it is required. Families who refuse should not be discriminated against (Budd & Hughes 1997).

References

Barrowclough C, Tarrier N 1995 Families of schizophrenic patients: cognitive behaviour intervention, 2nd edn. Chapman & Hall, London

Brooker C, Baguley I 1990 SNAP decisions. Nursing Times 86(41):56–58

Budd R J, Hughes I C T 1997 What do carers of people with schizophrenia find helpful and unhelpful about psychoeducation? Schizophrenia Bulletin 23:341–347

Deveson A 1992 Tell me I'm here. Penguin, London

Fadden G 1998 Family intervention. In: Brooker C, Repper J (eds) Serious mental health problems in the community: policy, practice and research. Baillière Tindall, London, pp 159–183

Falloon I R H, Graham-Hole V 1994 Comprehensive management of mental disorders. Buckingham Mental Health Service, Buckingham

Favin D 1998 A matter of chance for carers? Inspection of local authority support for carers. Social Care Group, Social Services Inspectorate. Department of Health, London

Kuipers L, Leff J, Lam D 1992 Family work for schizophrenia: a practical guide. Gaskell/Royal College of Psychiatrists, London

Lam D 1991 Psychosocial family intervention in schizophrenia: a review of empirical studies. Psychological Medicine 21:423–441

Leavey G, Healy H, Brennan G 1998 Providing information to carers of people admitted to psychiatric hospital. Mental Health Care 1(3):260–262

Leff J, Gamble C 1995 Training of community psychiatric nurses in family work for schizophrenia. International Journal of Mental Health 24(3):76–88

Nolan M 1996 Supporting family carers – the key to successful long term care? British Journal of Nursing 5(14):836

Smith J V, Birchwood M J 1990 Relatives and patients as partners in the management of schizophrenia: the development of a service model. British Journal of Psychiatry 156:645–660

Annotated further reading

Atkinson J M, Coia D A 1995 Families coping with schizophrenia: a practitioner's guide to family groups. Wiley, London

Outlines the importance of providing adequate services and resources to families. The appendices provide an excellent comprehensive guide to setting up relatives' education groups.

Barrowclough C, Tarrier N 1995 Families of schizophrenic patients: cognitive behaviour intervention, 2nd edn. Chapman & Hall, London

Describes the history of EE and family intervention research. Its most relevant chapters include those that describe how to work proactively with families. The assessments that are referred to in this chapter, such as the RAI and the KASI, are included in the appendices.

Fadden G 1998 Family intervention. In: Brooker C, Repper J (eds) Serious mental health problems in the community: policy, practice and research. Baillière Tindall, London, pp 159–163

This chapter provides a concise overview of the effectiveness of family intervention and discusses the current issues surrounding its effective implementation into routine clinical practice.

12

Coexistent substance use and psychiatric disorders

Iain Ryrie

KEY ISSUES

- Prevalence of comorbidity.
- Rationale for comorbidity.
- Patterns of drug use among individuals with mental illness.
- Clinical implications of comorbidity.
- Assessment procedures.
- Staged treatment approaches.

INTRODUCTION

The coexistence of severe mental illness and substance use disorder is an important clinical challenge for psychiatry. Although the UK has only recently begun to address this phenomenon, the USA has devoted well over a decade to studying its prevalence, clinical manifestations and treatment response. An evidence base has been established that is utilised throughout this chapter, whilst acknowledging any transcultural variations likely to affect its applicability.

The chapter is divided into three sections. The first provides a background to the condition and offers an overview of the nature and extent of substance use among individuals with severe mental illness. The heterogeneity of the client group, patterns of substance use and clinical sequelae are described to facilitate clinicians in their recognition of individuals with these dual conditions. The second section deals with assessment, which is presented as both an ongoing process and a therapeutic intervention, the focus of which will depend on a client's level of engagement with services. The final section deals with matters of treatment and describes a staged approach that incorporates different therapeutic interventions for each stage.

A case study is introduced at the end of Section 2, which is then elaborated further at the end of Section 3. It has been written to demonstrate the application of knowledge within these sections but also reflects the realities of current treatment provision and thereby highlights certain pitfalls that clinicians will face.

BACKGROUND

This section provides an overview of the prevalence, rationale, patterns and clinical implications of substance use among individuals with serious mental illness.

Prevalence

The true prevalence of comorbid psychiatric and substance use disorder is not yet known in the UK, although important epidemiological work has been conducted in the USA. The Epidemiological Catchment Area (ECA) study (Regier et al 1990) surveyed over 20 000 people living in both community and psychiatric settings. Substance use disorders were found to be more prevalent among individuals with mental illness than among the general population (Table 12.1). On average, mental illness doubled the chance of a comorbid substance use problem.

Table 12.1 Lifetime prevalence of substance use among a US sample

	Alcohol abuse disorder (%)	Drug abuse disorder (%)
General population	13.5	6.1
Individuals with psychiatric diagnosis	22.3	14.7

Source: Regier et al (1990)

Individuals with these coexistent disorders represent a heterogeneous group comprising people who have different types of mental disorder with differing degrees of severity (Franey 1996). The ECA study enabled differentiation within this group through analysis of substance use by psychiatric diagnosis (Table 12.2). Some commentators argue that, on this basis, clinicians who treat people with severe mental illness should expect

Table 12.2 Lifetime prevalence of substance use by psychiatric diagnosis among a US sample

Diagnosis	Substance abuse or dependence (%)
Schizophrenia	47.0
Any affective disorder	32.0
Any bipolar disorder	56.1
Any anxiety disorder	23.7
Antisocial personality disorder	83.6

Source: Regier et al (1990)

approximately 50% of their clients to have a positive history of substance use (Mueser, Bennett & Kushner 1995).

Although no equivalent epidemiological survey has been conducted in the UK, smaller scale studies have been undertaken. Menezes et al (1996) surveyed substance use among 171 individuals with psychosis who were attending a South London mental health service. Their results are presented in Table 12.3.

Table 12.3 Annual prevalence of substance problems among a UK sample of individuals with psychosis

Substance	Percentage
Alcohol	31.6
Other drugs	15.8
Any substance	36.3

Source: Menezes et al (1996)

Comparisons of Tables 12.1, 12.2 and 12.3 are difficult to make owing to their widely differing methodologies. The ECA study surveyed individuals in both rural and urban settings and assessed lifetime substance use. Menezes et al (1996) researched an inner city sample and examined annual substance use. A further problem is the variable thresholds selected by these teams to determine substance-related problems, abuse and/or dependence. It is clear that further work, using more representative samples, is required in the UK to determine prevalence accurately. However, on the evidence to date, Mueser, Bennett & Kushner's (1995) prediction that about half of those with severe mental illness will have a positive history of substance use may well hold in the UK, particularly in inner city areas. We should certainly expect substance use to be usual rather than exceptional among those with severe mental illness (Smith & Hucker 1993).

Rationale for comorbidity

A number of models exist to explain the increased rate of comorbidity. Although this remains a predominantly theoretical exercise, the models do provide an explanatory template that is of clinical utility. Optimal treatment will depend on a clinician's understanding of the most likely rationale for an individual's experience of comorbid substance use and psychiatric disorder. Such considerations should therefore form an integral part of the assessment process for this client group. Lehman, Myers & Corty (1989) have summarised the following four models.

Primary mental illness with substance use sequelae

Mental illness may increase an individual's vulnerability to substance use. This can arise from a desire to self-medicate negative affective states and/or positive symptomatology. Experiences of social marginalisation can also increase vulnerability owing to the perceived benefits of drugs as social facilitators. Their use may enable integration with a subculture whose identity is more acceptable than that attributed to mental patients (Lamb 1982). These rationale emphasise the value individuals can place on their substance use activities. In turn, clinical staff must take account of such positive expectancies, which may persist in spite of other deleterious consequences.

Primary substance use with psychiatric sequelae

This model posits that substance use has a role to play in the aetiology of mental illness. Whether it is a causative factor remains unclear since substance use may only precipitate a pre-existing vulnerability to mental illness. However, research has found drug and alcohol use to be predictive of subsequent psychotic disorders (Tien & Anthony 1990). What is more certain is the potential for substance use to cause transient symptoms of mental illness during either intoxication or withdrawal (Schuckit 1983).

Dual primary diagnosis

This model proposes that the disorders are initially unrelated and may develop independently of one another. It therefore recognises the multiple pathways by which comorbidity can occur, although, once established, the disorders are believed to be interactive and mutually sustaining.

Common aetiology

This model attributes coexistent substance use and mental illness to a common third variable. Genetic vulnerability is the most extensively studied factor although research findings remain equivocal. Socioenvironmental stress and poor social competence are also possible candidates, but each requires further research to determine its role (Mueser, Bennett & Kushner 1995).

Despite a lack of empirical data to support these models, Mueser, Bennett & Kushner (1995) suggest that their clinical utility may lie in a synthesis of different elements contained within them. More specifically, they believe that models that view substance use as secondary to mental illness, but acknowledge that the two can be mutually maintaining, hold the most promise for understanding the relationship between substance use and mental illness.

Patterns of use

Equivocal findings are evident in the literature regarding drug use patterns among individuals with mental illness. Schneier & Siris (1987), in their review of drug use in schizophrenia, identified a tendency toward the use of stimulants as a means of compensating for negative symptoms. Conversely, analysis of the ECA study data found alcohol and cannabis to be the predominant drugs of use in schizophrenia (Cuffel, Heithoff & Lawson 1993). These differences reflect the heterogeneity of the client group and may be related to demographic variables such as youth, which is a strong predictor of stimulant use (Mueser, Bennett & Kushner 1995).

It would seem unwise therefore to assume that individuals are prone to use one drug or another simply because of their psychiatric diagnosis. Multiple determinants are likely to be influential including the ready availability of substances in the local community. For this reason, in the majority of studies, alcohol is the substance most commonly used, followed by whichever illicit drug is most popular at the time (Mueser, Bennett & Kushner 1995). In the UK, the next most frequently cited drug of use has been cannabis (McKeown & Liebling 1995, Menezes et al 1996, Ryrie & McGowan 1998). However, empirical work has recently identified a resurgence in the use and availability of heroin within the UK (Eddington, Bury & Parker 1998). As this drug regains popularity and becomes ever more widely available we should expect its use to permeate many existing drug cultures including those with which psychiatric clients have contact.

It is also important to note that the American literature has found multiple drug use to be typical in urban samples of psychiatric clients (Chen et al 1992). This phenomenon has been found among inner city samples of British drug users (Hunter & Judd 1998, Ryrie et al 1997) but has not yet been assessed among those with a coexistent psychiatric disorder.

Clinical implications

Substance use among individuals with psychiatric disorders has been associated with significantly poorer clinical outcomes. Researchers in the USA have devoted considerable attention to monitoring these outcomes, which are summarised below in Box 12.1.

Box 12.1 Clinical implications of substance use among individuals with severe mental illness

◆ Poor medication adherence
◆ Increased rates of suicidal behaviour
◆ Increased rates of violence
◆ Homelessness
◆ Worsening of psychiatric symptoms
◆ Increased risk of HIV infection
◆ Increased use of institutional services

Sources: Carey, Carey & Meisler (1991), Drake & Wallach (1989), Kelly et al (1995)

Equivalent work has yet to be conducted in the UK although increased rates of violence (Smith, Frazer & Boer 1994) and an increased use of institutional resources (Menezes et al 1996) have both been found among UK samples. Additionally, clinical staff have consistently reported the full range of implications identified by US researchers (McKeown & Liebling 1995, Ryrie & McGowan 1998). Therefore, to overlook or neglect substance use in the course of psychiatric treatment will, at best, result in poor treatment outcome and, at worst, reflect the inappropriate use of scarce resources.

ASSESSMENT

Whenever possible, assessment should foster an educative process conducted in collaboration with clients and their significant others. Specific attributes of substance use, such as its often covert nature and its impact upon cognitive functioning, present challenges to this process. Clinicians must tailor their assessments according to clients' psychiatric stability and their level of engagement with services. Different approaches will be necessary during two stages of assessment (Drake & Mercer-McFadden 1995):

◆ detection
◆ specialised assessment.

Detection

A prima facie case exists for the routine screening of substance use among psychiatric clients. Failure to do so can result in misdiagnosis, overtreatment with psychiatric medications and the neglect of appropriate interventions such as drug education, treatment and relapse prevention (Drake, Alterman & Rosenberg 1993). In short, we will fail in our duty to care. It is also recognised that screening may be worthwhile only if clinicians feel they have the necessary skills and resources to respond appropriately. However, the opportunity to explore the experience of substance use and mental illness, in a sensitive and non-judgemental climate, can itself be therapeutic. More sophisticated interventions may require recourse or referral to specialist support, but at least these needs will now have been identified. Procedures that can aid detection include self-report methods, laboratory tests and collateral data.

Self-report

Eliciting a history of substance use can be undertaken in one of two ways: through completion of structured questionnaires or by offering simple exploratory questions. With the former, there is a lack of instrumentation that has been designed and validated for use with this client group. Those that have been validated among samples of drug users are plentiful and may have some clinical utility. The following are examples.

◆ **Michigan Alcoholism Screening Test (MAST) Selzer (1971)**: designed to detect problematic alcohol use by rating its effect on an individual's physical and social circumstances.
◆ **Leeds Dependence Questionnaire (LDQ) Raistrick et al (1994)**: designed to detect and rate the severity of illicit substance use; contains ten items which are rated on a four point scale.

Two problems arise when using such instruments. First, they require the client to acknowledge any substance use in order to complete them. Secondly, they are often designed to detect operationally defined levels of use such as 'problematic' or 'dependent'. However, it is known that individuals with psychiatric conditions can experience illness decompensation from infrequent substance use, which would not necessarily meet an instrument's threshold for 'problematic' or 'dependent' use (Drake et al 1990). Simple exploratory questioning may be a more suitable method for detection although the validity of the information will depend on the client's mental state and the interview style, which should be sensitive, non-judgemental and confidential (Drake and Mercer-McFadden 1995).

Laboratory tests

These will typically include blood and breathalyser assessments for alcohol, although the speed with which alcohol is metabolised in the body will limit their utility. Breathalysers, for example, are sensitive for only a few hours (Drake and Mercer-McFadden 1995). Urinalysis for other substances is more useful and, where resources allow, can be conducted on the spot without recourse to a laboratory. (Readers are advised to liaise with specialist drug services for the manufacturers of such products.) Box 12.2 presents approximate drug detection times in urine.

Box 12.2 Approximate drug detection times in urine	
Heroin	1–3 days
Methadone	1–2 days
Amphetamines	1–2 days
Cocaine	12 hours–3 days
Benzodiazepines	1 day (3 weeks if daily use)
Cannabis	2–7 days (up to 1 month if heavy use)
Ecstasy	2–4 days
Alcohol	12–24 hours

Collateral data

Collateral data are available from a number of sources including health records, 'significant others' and a range of professionals and agencies involved in a client's care. This information may lead to the detection of substance use but can also serve to validate any self-reports from the client.

Specialised assessment

Specialised assessment involves the detailed examination of substance use patterns, and forms the basis upon which subsequent treatment is planned. The success of treatment will therefore depend, in part, on the degree of collaboration between clinician and client during this assessment stage. The client should be involved in the review of clinical data, the formulation of hypotheses concerning the relationship between substance use and clinical symptoms, and the identification of appropriate interventions. The following areas reflect the scope of specialised assessments:

◆ severity of substance use behaviour
◆ problem analysis
◆ treatment planning.

Severity

This requires a method for detailing the duration, frequency and quantity of use, and its route of administration. Figure 12.1 presents a drug count chart for that purpose. It may be used in several ways. Typically clients would be encouraged to consider their drug use over the past 4 weeks. They would then be asked: which was the most frequent drug used during this time, whether it was prescribed or not, how often it was used during this time period, the amounts consumed per typical day/session, its route of administration, duration of this episode of use, and age when they first used this drug. They

	Drug name	Prescribed or not	How often	How much	Route	Duration	Age of first use
Main drug							
Drug 2							
Drug 3							
Drug 4							
Drug 5 /alcohol							

Figure 12.1 A drug count chart.

would then be asked for the next most frequently used drug, and so on. It is not unusual for clients to omit their alcohol consumption since they may feel the inquiry is directed toward illicit substances only. It is therefore important to prompt for this drug.

For clients who experience difficulty with memory recall the chart can be used prospectively to document drug use over an agreed time period. In many circumstances this is advisable, even when retrospective data are available, since it actively engages clients in the assessment process and will generally produce more reliable results.

Specialised assessments also explore the personal and environmental factors associated with use. The intention is to gain a more comprehensive account of individuals' drug use as it exists in a biopsychosocial context. Box 12.3 presents a schema that outlines specific areas of enquiry for this purpose.

Box 12.3 Schema for assessing context of use

Biological	◆ Evidence of tolerance to substances
	◆ Evidence of physical dependence and associated withdrawal risks
	◆ Physical problems and/or benefits arising from use
Psychological	◆ Positive and negative expectations of use
	◆ Evidence of psychological dependence
	◆ Psychological problems and/or benefits arising from use
Sociological	◆ Social context of use
	◆ Evidence of peer group attachments
	◆ Financial circumstances
	◆ Criminal activities
	◆ Perceived social problems and/or benefits arising from use

---

Collectively, these assessment data provide an indication of the severity of individuals' substance use. Drug count data might suggest experimental, recreational or dependent use, whereas associated contextual variables can indicate the degree of attachment to the behaviour. The severity of the condition can also be gauged against diagnostic criteria for substance abuse and substance dependence disorders. The Case Managers Rating Scale (Drake et al 1990) was specifically designed for this purpose. It contains a five point scale with each point operationally defined in terms of levels of substance use and their biopsychosocial consequences. The rating attributed to a client should reflect the evidence available from self-reports, interviews, behavioural observations and collateral reports. A score of three meets the Diagnostic Statistical Manual (DSM) III-R criteria for substance abuse and scores of four and five meet the criteria for dependence.

Problem analysis

At this stage the assessment data are summarised and reviewed with the client. This should be undertaken in a non-judgemental and matter of fact way. The intention is to present the facts and elicit interpretations from the client. This is a complex task requiring active listening skills and the suspension of a common desire among clinicians to offer their own interpretations. Often these are predicated on a fixed perception of substance use as a damaging activity that must be curtailed. Although abstinence may be an ideal outcome, it is unlikely to be realistic unless a desire for its attainment is shared by the client.

Staff should therefore acknowledge any positive associations that appear to exist between substance use and the client's circumstances, as well as highlight the negative associations. In turn, the client is encouraged to clarify and prioritise specific problem areas. A functional analysis can then be undertaken to explore the antecedents and consequences of the behaviours involved.

Treatment planning

Functional analyses provide the basis for treatment planning and the specification of target statements. Fundamentally, however, this process depends on a client's readiness and commitment to change. At times, for example, staff may feel unsure about pursuing certain goals that engender resistance in the client. A framework for understanding this process has been devised by Prochaska & DiClemente (1986). They have found that individuals who change substance use behaviours do so in a predictable pattern. Five key stages of change are identified:

- **precontemplation**: see no reason to change
- **contemplation**: aware of problem(s) and begin to consider change
- **determination**: decide to change and plan how
- **active change**: engage in change and implement plans
- **maintenance**: prevent relapse and consolidate change.

These stages are presented in the form of a cycle with a further stage of 'relapse' linking 'maintenance' to 'precontemplation'. Individuals who achieve and maintain change will exit from the cycle, whilst those who experience a relapse during treatment, or after achieving change, will return to a precontemplative or contemplative stage. Client resistance can therefore be understood as arising from an assessment or treatment intervention that is not congruent with the client's stage of change – for example, assuming a particular client is committed to tackling a problem area (determination) when in fact there is uncertainty as to its importance (contemplation).

Treatment planning therefore involves an assessment of the client's stage of change. Self-motivational statements are useful indicators for this purpose (Miller & Rollnick 1991). Problem recognition and expressions of concern suggest 'contemplation', whereas intentions to change and optimism about change suggest 'determination'. The absence of any self-motivational statement may be indicative of 'precontemplation'.

The specification of target statements and intervention selection can appropriately be undertaken with an individual in the 'determination' stage of change. For those in the 'precontemplation' or 'contemplation' stage, interventions should aim to build a foundation for treatment by strengthening the client's motivation. Motivational interviewing (MI) has been developed specifically for this purpose by Miller & Rollnick (1991). It is discussed in the final section of this chapter and matches the client's stage of change with different stages of treatment.

TREATMENT

Different models of treatment exist for the management of coexistent psychiatric and substance use disorders. Ries (1993) has identified three such models: serial, parallel and integrated treatment. In the former, treatment for one condition is given before progressing to treatment for the other condition. This approach is problematic in the case of severe mental illness and concurrent substance use since the two are mutually interactive. It would, for example, be difficult to stabilise an individual's psychiatric state if they continued to use substances. Equally, stabilising or ceasing substance use may be difficult if psychiatric symptoms are exacerbated during the process. The parallel model implies the concurrent but separate treatment of both conditions. This model is also problematic since the client is required to attend different services and is exposed to, and expected to engage with, different therapeutic structures and approaches. The integrated model implies the concurrent application of both psychiatric and substance use treatments by one service. Drake & Noordsy (1994) describe the development of hybrid case managers who possess this repertoire of skills. These authors have evaluated their work and conclude that integrated treatment is more effective than parallel or serial treatment for this client group.

Case study – Michael

Michael is a 37-year-old Caucasian man who lives alone in the inner city. His first contact with psychiatric services was in his early twenties when he was diagnosed as having paranoid schizophrenia. For the past 5 years his mental health has been stable. He is monitored every other month as an outpatient by his consultant psychiatrist and receives a monthly depot injection from a practice nurse in his GP surgery.

The practice nurse noted recent non-attendance for medication and reported this to his psychiatrist. At his next outpatient appointment a deterioration in his condition was apparent and, following lengthy discussion, Michael acknowledged his recent use of illicit drugs, which he believed were better for him than the psychiatric medication. Additionally, their use acquainted him with new friends whose company he enjoyed. The psychiatrist referred Michael to the local specialist drug service.

On referral the nurse undertook a retrospective drug count, which revealed Michael was using oral methadone and occasionally smoking heroin. The amounts taken depended on the drug's availability from friends and his ability to raise cash or 'do chores' for these friends. He tried to use the drug on a daily basis although over the last 4 weeks he had only been able to use it four or five times a week. This pattern of use has been ongoing for over 6 months and Michael experiences withdrawal symptoms on the days he doesn't use it, including lethargy, muscle aches, sweating and stomach cramps. At such times he drinks strong lager to try and ease the discomfort although he is not a regular alcohol drinker. Michael currently views his drug use as a solution to his mental problems and social isolation although he is anxious about difficulties in procuring the drug owing to finances and the unpredictable supply. This is the only problem he currently perceives himself to have.

The multidisciplinary team discuss Michael's case and conclude that he is vulnerable and in need of immediate treatment. They agree to titrate him on to a suitable dose of methadone (50 mg), which he collects daily from his local chemist. He attends the drug service for weekly monitoring.

Since substance use is a chronic relapsing condition it is important for clinicians to hold a longitudinal view of treatment, which contains different phases that correspond to the stages of client change. Osher and Kofoed (1989) have developed a four stage treatment model, which can be used for this purpose (Table 12.4). Each stage in the model implies the use of different therapeutic interventions.

Engagement

Engagement is concerned with the development of a therapeutic alliance between staff and client. This is an essential prerequisite for treatment among this client group, who demonstrate a tendency to drop out and disengage

Table 12.4 Stages of treatment and client change	
Treatment stage **(Osher & Kofoed 1989)**	**Client's stage of change** **(Prochaska & DiClemente 1986)**
Engagement	Precontemplation
Persuasion	Contemplation – determination
Active treatment	Active change
Relapse prevention	Maintenance

from services (Carey 1995). The strength of the alliance will depend, in part, on the value a client attributes to the service. This can be enhanced by the style of staff–client interactions and by endeavouring to meet the client's initial needs.

Style of interaction

A confrontative approach that requires the client to acknowledge the damaging consequences of substance use as a condition of treatment is likely to be met with resistance. At this early stage it is more important to employ a non-confrontative and empathic approach that acknowledges the validity of the client's perspective. Staff should also demonstrate commitment to working with clients to improve their lot. This will include assertive outreach for those who are isolated or disinclined to attend treatment centres.

Meeting need

The process of eliciting the client's perspective will provide staff with an idea of what clients need and value. The therapeutic alliance can then be strengthened by endeavouring to meet any initial need. These may include basic living requirements such as food, housing and clothing, or assistance with an application for benefit entitlements. It is not unusual for this client group to encounter legal difficulties associated with their substance use. Under such circumstances liaison with a solicitor to confirm an individual's involvement with treatment services can be a welcome intervention.

Clients may also complain of family overinvolvement. This is not unusual since substance use, if known to the family, can engender considerable anxiety. Paradoxically, this anxiety can also contribute to the substance use behaviours. Once again, liaison with 'significant others' to reassure them of your willingness to work with their loved one can allay much anxiety and enhance the foundations for treatment.

Persuasion

When first in contact with services, many clients are not ready to engage with treatment interventions. The persuasion stage endeavours to prepare clients by strengthening their motivation and commitment to change. The main counselling approach employed for this purpose is MI. This is described by its authors as 'a directive, client centred counselling style for eliciting behaviour change by helping clients to explore and resolve ambivalence' (Miller & Rollnick 1991).

Traditional treatment approaches in the substance use field have tended toward confrontation as a means of breaking down the user's denial. MI posits that client denial is actually a misinterpretation of client resistance, which arises when a provider offers an intervention that is not congruent with the client's stage of change. It also draws on the concept of ambivalence to understand the dilemma substance users face between indulgence and restraint. The expression, clarification and resolution of that ambivalence is necessary to create readiness for change.

It is beyond the scope of this chapter to provide a detailed account of MI. However, central to its purpose is the intention to develop discrepancy in clients between their current behaviour and any goals or hopes they have for the future. This represents the 'directive' element of MI contained within the definition above. A variety of simple techniques can be used for this purpose, including:

- education about drugs and the problems that may be associated with use
- presentation of objective assessment data (e.g. liver function tests, urinalysis results)
- balance sheets on which the client lists the pros and cons of continued use/abstinence
- exploration of barriers to the attainment of future goals
- reframe problems or past events emphasising the influence of substance use.

In each of these examples it is important to remember that the approach is non-confrontational and empathic. Information is not shared with the intention of frightening or coercing clients into recognising the need for change. They are invited to consider it and then offer their own interpretation. The therapist's task involves active listening and reflecting back to the client those aspects of use which appear problematic, thereby nudging the decisional balance in favour of change.

MI is particularly useful for clients who are in a precontemplation, contemplation or determination stage of change. Table 12.5 presents a number of MI tasks for these stages. This stage of treatment can be conducted in a

Table 12.5 MI tasks according to stage of change	
Stage of change	**MI task**
Precontemplation	◆ Provide education about substance use and mental illness to increase client's perception of risk ◆ Reframe problems or past events ◆ Present any objective assessment data
Contemplation	◆ Explore ambivalence ◆ Elicit reasons to change, costs of not changing ◆ Use reflecting listening to emphasise discrepancy ◆ Tip the decisional balance in favour of change
Determination	◆ Offer a range of treatment options for client to select from ◆ Promote clients' belief in their ability to achieve goals (self-efficacy)

group setting. Noordsy & Fox (1991) describe a persuasion group that was established to help clients perceive how substance use complicated their lives. Each week clients would meet with two facilitators, describe their substance use over the past 7 days and be encouraged to reflect on the antecedents and consequences of that behaviour. The group also had a psychoeducational function through the delivery of information by staff and the sharing of knowledge and experience among clients.

Active treatment

It may take several months of work with clients in the engagement and persuasion stages before they are ready to accept active treatment interventions for their substance use. Ideally these should aim toward abstinence although this can be difficult to achieve and may require several attempts. It is therefore important for clinicians to recognise the achievement of any intermediate goals and to maintain an optimistic outlook.

The selection of treatment interventions is informed by the process of assessment, during which specific problem areas and their target statements will have been identified. These might be associated with the self-medication of symptoms, affiliating with groups of drug users, managing psychosocial stressors or simply seeking pleasure. Alternative strategies for tackling these problem areas can be negotiated with the client and implemented as empirical trials or experiments. They should be regularly reviewed and modified according to their outcome. It is important throughout this process that any failures are used to reconsider the problem and selected intervention rather than to blame the client (Drake & Noordsy 1994).

Specific treatment interventions will vary for individual clients. However, two broad target areas are recommended in the literature: coping skills training and lifestyle modification (Carey 1995).

Coping skills training

Many clients will use substances as a way of coping with personal and environmental stressors. It therefore follows that the attainment of abstinence will require the learning of new skills. Carey (1995) emphasises the role of substances as social facilitators for individuals with mental illness. Social skills enhancement is therefore considered a necessary focus for training if individuals are to derive sufficient social support without resorting to the use of substances. Conversational and assertiveness skills are specifically recommended in this respect. Carey (1995) describes the following stages of a skills training model that is designed to enable individuals with mental illness to translate knowledge into behaviour change:

◆ definition of skills to be learned
◆ modelling of skills
◆ rehearsal of skills in vitro and in vivo
◆ corrective feedback on implementation of skills.

Another important area for coping skills training is medication management. Many clients will report the use of alcohol and illicit drugs as a method for combating uncomfortable symptoms. A thorough review of current medication, combined with educational interventions, is therefore necessary to reduce the likelihood of a reliance on substances.

Lifestyle modification

The cessation of substance use will necessarily involve a significant change in lifestyle. This can be difficult for clients to negotiate, particularly when substance use is central to their daily activities and social identity. Equally, it is unlikely to be achieved overnight and will require both clinician and client to hold a longitudinal perspective of treatment.

If we need, as Carey (1995) states, to encourage clients to avoid the people and places associated with substance use then we must also be able to offer them help in structuring time and engaging in drug-free leisure activities. This can be difficult to achieve with limited resources although successful strategies have been reported in the literature. Drake & Noordsy (1994) draw attention to the use of transitional or supported employment projects. Although these are only in their infancy in this country they do provide an invaluable structure that confers satisfaction and pride to the individual.

They also provide a context in which to establish non-substance-using friends.

Individuals' housing situation may also contribute to their substance use. Where this is indicated, and the client is in agreement, staff should be prepared to liaise with housing organisations and authorities to initiate the rehousing or transfer process. Typically this will involve the completion of relevant documentation, which should be augmented with a clinical report from the client's consultant stating the individual's condition, the motivation to change and the association between the medical condition and current housing circumstances. Since such interventions rarely result in immediate action, staff should be aware of the need to maintain their client's motivation and optimism.

Pharmacological considerations

A further treatment consideration is that of prescribed medications. Concerns often focus on the safety of prescribed neuroleptic and other drugs if a client is known to be using alcohol or illicit substances. More specifically, these concerns are associated with potentially harmful drug interactions and problems in achieving a therapeutic dose of prescribed medication. Generally, unless clients are known to be using a substance that has a negative interaction with their neuroleptic medication, the benefits of controlling psychiatric symptomatology would suggest that the prescribed regimen ought to be adhered to (Carey 1995). An excellent overview of these considerations is presented by Siris (1990).

Certain central nervous system depressants, including alcohol, barbiturates, benzodiazepines and opiates, can also lead to physical dependence syndromes if taken frequently over extended periods. Consequently, withdrawal can be a complicated process that carries certain risks. For example, abrupt cessation of alcohol, barbiturate and benzodiazepine use can result in seizures. Withdrawal therefore involves the substitution of these drugs with prescribed alternatives that are gradually reduced over a short time scale. A period of inpatient care for this type of treatment is advisable, particularly since the cessation of substance use may reveal or initiate the re-emergence of psychiatric symptoms.

Relapse prevention

Both substance use and severe mental illness are conditions for which relapse is to be anticipated (Carey 1995). Therefore, once a client has attained abstinence, or reduced substance use, therapeutic interventions should turn to the prevention and management of possible future relapses. The principles and strategies of relapse prevention have been documented by Marlatt & Gordon (1985). It aims to identify possible high risk situations and to develop and rehearse coping strategies proactively. Attention is also given to the development of action plans should the client return to substance use.

The experience of relapse can undermine individuals' motivation and their belief in their ability to succeed. Given the likelihood of its occurrence it is important for clinicians to utilise the event in a constructive way. Relapse prevention therefore views any relapse as a slip from which important insights can be gained and vulnerabilities identified, rather than as a failure. Carey (1995) also advises that progress and success should be gauged against reductions in the frequency of relapses or in their duration rather than simply in their complete cessation.

Case study – Michael (*cont'd*)

Michael's drug treatment had been ongoing for 3 months, during which time his attendance had become erratic and his mental state appeared to destabilise. He complained that the pharmacist diluted his methadone and 'had it in for him'. Consequently, Michael had been using street opiates to supplement his prescribed dose because of continued withdrawals.

During treatment Michael was arrested for shoplifting and his mental state deteriorated further. Following attendance at an appointment with his psychiatrist, in which he demanded a further prescription of methadone, an interagency meeting was convened involving psychiatric and substance use services to determine the most appropriate course of action. Michael did not attend although he had been invited.

It was agreed that Michael's current treatment was inadequate and that a more suitable approach would be to withdraw the methadone and re-establish him on neuroleptic medication. Ideally it was hoped this would be conducted as an inpatient and the consultant psychiatrist was happy to arrange a bed on an acute admission ward where staff had experience of working with these conditions. However, specialist drug staff reported his current disengagement with services and the likelihood of him refusing such interventions.

It was therefore decided that his methadone would be dispensed daily from the drug unit where he would meet with a specialist nurse who would work toward meeting any immediate needs that Michael identified whilst endeavouring to enhance his motivation for change. The nurse was able to compile a letter for the solicitor who was handling Michael's shoplifting charge and employed MI techniques to explore the dilemmas Michael faced. Gradually he reinterpreted past events that he believed were beneficial for him but, in fact, had generated additional problems. In particular, he acknowledged that his friends were not real friends but acquaintances who used him to their own ends and who contributed to his arrest for shoplifting. Together with his nurse, Michael listed the pros and cons of continued drug use and gradually began to express a desire to change his circumstances.

Case study – Michael (cont'd)

Several treatment options were offered including outpatient and inpatient withdrawal. Michael was anxious about inpatient care and chose to pursue a reduction programme as an outpatient. However, he found it difficult to distance himself from his drug-using associates and this method of treatment was curtailed. Michael asked if the inpatient option was still available and what it might entail. His nurse arranged a joint meeting with one of the inpatient staff, who reassured Michael and informed him of the aftercare service that was available. This involved twice weekly meetings at the hospital with other clients who had experienced problems with substance use but who were currently abstinent or working toward abstinence.

Six months after initiating drug treatment Michael was admitted into psychiatric care and over a 2 week period withdrew from his methadone. He has been re-established on neuroleptic medication and is a regular attender of the twice weekly group. He has had two brief lapses of drug use since being discharged 4 weeks ago but has found the group supportive and is currently working with other clients and staff to identify and implement alternative coping strategies when faced with risk situations.

Summary of practical strategies identified

◆ Substance use among individuals with severe mental illness is usual rather than exceptional.

◆ Clinical outcomes for this client group are poor, when compared with non-substance-using psychiatric clients.

◆ All clinicians have a duty to screen for substance use and initiate (or refer on for) a specialised assessment.

◆ Self-report procedures, laboratory tests and collateral data sources are methods for initial screening and detection.

◆ Specialised assessments generate data on substance use patterns and severity, and the personal and environmental factors associated with use.

◆ Assessment data are summarised and reviewed with the client, who is encouraged to clarify and prioritise problem areas.

◆ Effective treatment requires the integrated delivery of concurrent substance use and psychiatric interventions by one service or case manager.

Summary of practical strategies identified (*cont'd*)

◆ Treatment planning is based on an assessment of clients' readiness to change and the use of MI to enhance their commitment to change.

◆ The process of treatment moves through four stages of engagement, persuasion, active treatment and relapse prevention with each stage requiring different interventions.

◆ Clinicians should foster a longitudinal view of treatment with their clients, which is congruent with the chronicity of the condition and within which optimism about the possibility of change is maintained.

References

Carey K 1995 Treatment of substance use disorders and schizophrenia. In: Lehman A, Dixon L (eds) Double jeopardy: chronic mental illness and substance use disorders. Harwood Academic, Chur, Switzerland, pp 85–105

Carey M, Carey K, Meisler A 1991 Psychiatric symptoms in mentally ill chemical abusers. Journal of Nervous and Mental Disease 179:136–138

Chen C, Balogh R, Bathija J, Howanitz E, Plutchik R, Conye H 1992 Substance abuse among psychiatric inpatients. Comprehensive Psychiatry 33:60–64

Cuffel B, Heithoff K, Lawson W 1993 Correlates of patterns of substance use among patients with schizophrenia. Hospital and Community Psychiatry 44:247–251

Drake R, Mercer-McFadden C 1995 Assessment of substance use among persons with chronic mental illnesses. In: Lehman A, Dixon L (eds) Double jeopardy: chronic mental illness and substance use disorders. Harwood Academic, Chur, Switzerland, pp 47–62

Drake R, Noordsy F 1994 Case management for people with coexisting severe mental disorder and substance use disorder. Psychiatric Annals 24:427–431

Drake R, Wallach M 1989 Substance abuse among the chronic mentally ill. Hospital and Community Psychiatry 40:1041–1046

Drake R, Osher F, Noordsy D, Hurlbut S, Teague G, Beaudett M 1990 Diagnosis of alcohol use disorders in schizophrenia. Schizophrenia Bulletin 16:57–67

Drake R, Alterman A, Rosenberg S 1993 Detection of substance abuse in persons with severe mental disorders. Community Mental Health Journal 29:175–192

Eddington R, Bury C, Parker H 1998 Heroin still screws you up: responding to new heroin outbreaks. Druglink 13(5):17–20

Franey C 1996 Managing patients with dual diagnosis in Ealing, Hammersmith and Hounslow. Centre for Research on Drugs and Health Behaviour, London

References (cont'd)

Hunter G, Judd A 1998 Women injecting drug users in London: use and views of health services. Executive Summary no. 60. Centre for Research on Drugs and Health Behaviour, London

Kelly J, Heckman T, Helfrich S, Mence R, Adair V, Broyles L 1995 HIV risk factors and behaviours among men in a Milwaukee homeless shelter. American Journal of Public Health 85:1585

Lamb H 1982 Young adult chronic patients: the new drifters. Hospital and Community Psychiatry 33:465–468

Lehman A, Myers C, Corty E 1989 Assessment and classification of patients with psychiatric and substance abuse syndromes. Hospital and Community Psychiatry 40:1019–1024

McKeown M, Liebling H 1995 Staff perceptions of illicit drug use within a special hospital. Journal of Psychiatric and Mental Health Nursing 2:343–350

Marlatt G, Gordon J 1985 Relapse prevention: maintenance strategies in the treatment of addictive behaviors. Guilford, New York

Menezes P, Johnson S, Thornicroft G et al 1996 Drug and alcohol problems among individuals with severe mental illnesses in South London. British Journal of Psychiatry 168:612–619

Miller W, Rollnick S 1991 Motivational interviewing: preparing people to change addictive behaviour. Guilford Press, New York

Mueser K, Bennett M, Kushner M 1995 In: Lehman A, Dixon L (eds) Double jeopardy: chronic mental illness and substance use disorders. Harwood Academic, Chur, Switzerland, pp 9–25

Noordsy D, Fox L 1991 Group intervention techniques for people with dual disorders. Psychosocial Rehabilitation Journal 15:67–78

Osher F, Kofoed L 1989 Treatment of patients with psychiatric and psychoactive substance abuse disorders. Hospital and Community Psychiatry 40:1025–1030

Prochaska J, DiClemente C 1986 Toward a comprehensive model of change. In: Miller W, Heather N (eds) Treating addictive behaviours: processes of change. Plenum, New York, pp 3–27

Raistrick D, Bradshaw J, Tober G, Weiner J, Allison J, Healey C 1994 Development of the Leeds dependence questionnaire (LDQ): a questionnaire to measure alcohol and opiate dependence in the context of a treatment evaluation package. Addiction 89:563–572

Regier D, Farmer M, Rae D et al 1990 Comorbidity of mental disorders with alcohol and other drug abuse. Journal of the American Medical Association 264:2511–2518

Ries R 1993 Clinical treatment matching models for dually diagnosed patients. Psychiatric Clinics of North America 16:167–175

Ryrie I, McGowan J 1998 Staff perceptions of substance use among acute psychiatric inpatients. Journal of Psychiatric and Mental Health Nursing 5:137–142

Ryrie I, Dickson J, Robbins C, MacLean K, Climpson C 1997 Evaluation of a low-threshold clinic for opiate dependent drug users. Journal of Psychiatric and Mental Health Nursing 4:105–110

Schneier F, Siris S 1987 A review of psychoactive substance use and abuse in schizophrenia: patterns of drug choice. Journal of Nervous and Mental Disease 175:641–652

Schuckit M 1983 Alcoholic patients with secondary depression. American Journal of Psychiatry 140:711–714

Selzer M 1971 The Michigan Alcoholism Screening Test: the quest for a new diagnostic instrument. American Journal of Psychiatry 127:1653–1658

References (cont'd)

Siris S 1990 Pharmacological treatment of substance-abusing schizophrenic patients. Schizophrenia Bulletin 16:111–122

Smith J, Hucker S 1993 Dual diagnosis patients: substance abuse by the severely mentally ill. British Journal of Hospital Medicine 50:650–654

Smith J, Frazer S, Boer H 1994 Dangerous dual diagnosis patients. Hospital and Community Psychiatry 45:280–281

Tien A, Anthony J 1990 Epidemiological analysis of alcohol and drug use as risk factors for psychotic experiences. Journal of Nervous and Mental Disease 178:473–480

Annotated further reading

Lehman A, Dixon L 1995 Double jeopardy: chronic mental illness and substance use disorders. Harwood Academic, Chur, Switzerland

This book provides a comprehensive account of the epidemiology, assessment, diagnosis and treatment of substance use among persons with chronic mental illness. It is written by US contributors who have extensive experience of working with this client group. The book is practice orientated and provides a sound basis upon which to initiate interventions.

Jarvis T, Tebbutt J, Mattick R 1995 Treatment approaches for alcohol and drug dependence: an introductory guide. John Wiley, Chichester

This is an Australian text that arose from a series of meta-analytical reviews, supplemented with the views of experienced clinicians, to provide an evidence base for drug and alcohol treatment. It logically progresses through assessment, goal setting, specific interventions and maintenance of change. Each chapter offers descriptions of the interventions, their key concepts and applications, as well as practice exercises and client handouts.

Department of Health 1999 Drug misuse and dependence – guidelines on clinical management. The Stationery Office, London

Intended primarily for medical practitioners, these guidelines provide a valuable resource to all clinicians working in the drugs field. They represent a consensus view of good clinical practice, which is presented across seven chapters that loosely follow the process of treatment. The guidelines are annexed with 19 appendices that cover additional issues including drug use and comorbid mental illness.

13

Working with people with serious mental illness who are angry

Paul Rogers   Andrew Vidgen

KEY ISSUES

◆ Working with people who have a serious mental illness and who become angry.

◆ A brief review of anger research and conceptualisation.

◆ A discussion of the relationship between anger and aggression.

◆ A discussion of the relationship between anger and serious mental illness.

◆ The principles of working with such clients.

◆ A pragmatic approach to the assessment and intervention of clients with anger and serious mental illness.

◆ Strategies that will assist in the formulation of such clients' problems.

◆ Intervention strategies for such clients.

This chapter focuses on working with people who have SMI and become angry. It aims to challenge professional rhetoric, and some traditional practices, and provide a pragmatic evidence-based approach to working *with* as opposed to working *against* people who are angry.

INTRODUCTION

Anger is a common emotion, which is frequently experienced several times a week (Averill 1983). Ekman's (1972) anger study found that it is one of the six emotions with identifiable facial expressions across cultures. Historically, the power of anger is well documented and recognised: 'The lord is full of compassion and mercy: long-suffering, and of great goodness. He will not always be chiding: neither keep his anger for ever' (Psalm 103: 8). Yet, despite early recognition of the power of anger and its long textual history (Kemp & Strongman 1995), it remains one the most understudied of emotions (DiGiuseppe, Tafrate & Eckhardt 1994). Furthermore, Deffenbacher (1996) notes that diagnostically 'even though there are well defined groups of anxiety and depressive disorders there is no group of disorders for which anger is the primary defining characteristic (i.e. necessary for a diagnosis)'. A number of researchers have repeatedly called for a new 'anger disorder' to be included in the Diagnostic and statistical manual (Deffenbacher 1996, DiGiuseppe, Tafrate & Eckhardt 1994, Novaco 1985); however, to date this has not happened.

The problem of definition compounds this problem further. Finding an ultimate definition is fraught with difficulties and to date no consensus of agreement exists (see Russel & Fehr 1994). So, what does 'anger' actually mean? We can all gauge what anger means for us personally and how it makes us feel, but can we lay claim to knowing what it means for others, and how this emotion effects them?

Undoubtedly, we have all at one time or another observed, or been on the 'receiving end' of, another person's anger that we have felt was unjust or unwarranted. We may have concluded that the angry person must be ill informed, jumping to conclusions or being unreasonable. Alternatively, we may have found ourselves agreeing with people for being angry and their perceptions of injustice. Whichever of the above conclusions are drawn, we are making judgements as to the validity of another person's 'right' to experience anger. As mental health professionals we are often told (through implication or training) to be non-judgemental, because making judgements about clients is inherently wrong. However, 'being judgemental' is a common experience. The most important issue about judgements is how they are interpreted. If a judgement about anger is not drawn, how are we to respond?

For example, consider the common professional response clichés, which we have probably all used at some time or another: 'You're obviously quite outraged at what's happened to you' or 'I can see that you're feeling very angry right now'.

If you have been angry and these above two responses were used, you would probably be even more annoyed as a result, because these statements reduce the likelihood of the emotion being resolved. Indeed, they could be perceived as putting the ball back into the angry person's court and being interpreted as 'So what?' Let's imagine, for example, that someone at work tells you that a trusted colleague and friend is breaking a close confidence – one that you did not want others to know, no matter what the circumstances. You immediately feel angry and confront your friend with: 'How could you?', 'I thought we were friends?' or 'I trusted you with that information and you've gone and told everyone!!!' You're feeling outraged, and expect an apology, a commitment to stop disclosing, an explanation as to why this has been done, even a means as to how this wrong is going to be undone. You eventually stop and wait for the reply, only to be faced with: 'I recognise that your feeling angry right now...'.

As mentioned earlier, being judgemental, or making judgements, is not in itself inappropriate. It is alright to believe that *actions* are wrong (e.g. stealing or punching someone). But you should resist making generalisations about *people* (e.g. they are a thief, they are assaultative) as these are not helpful. Asking questions about behaviours is more useful: 'What function does stealing and punching serve?', 'What were the circumstances?' or 'What was the person thinking at the time?'

ANGER, AN EMOTIONAL RESPONSE: A BRIEF OVERVIEW

The main themes underlying most diagnoses of anger is that it is an emotional state, which consists of cognitions, behaviours and physiological arousal. A number of descriptive models of anger exist. The work of Navaco (1985) is probably the most well known. Novaco proposes that anger is a dyscontrol phenomena made up of three loosely related components activated by an aversive event or environmental stressor. Novaco's model has three main components (Box 13.1).

Box 13.1 Components of Novaco's Model

◆ **Physiological arousal:** activation in the cardiovascular and endocrine systems causing somatic tension and irritability
◆ **Cognitive structures and processes:** antagonistic thought patterns such as attention focus, suspicious ruminations and hostile attitude
◆ **Behaviour reactions:** such as impulsive reactions, verbal aggression, physical confrontation and indirect expression

---

Therefore, the model suggests that anger is associated with thoughts that are related to behaviour and faulty appraisal. When a person is exposed to continual demands of a stressor or environment they experience physiological arousal; they consequently become tense and irritable. As exposure continues, antagonistic thought patterns induce faulty appraisals of the situation or behaviour. If the person has inappropriate coping strategies they react impulsively, becoming either verbally or physically aggressive. On evaluation, if this action produces relief or respite from the stress or aversive event, the response is more likely to be used again. The aim of anger management is to break this cycle, and methods to achieve this will be described in the latter part of this chapter.

Differentiating between anger and aggression

As mentioned, definitions of anger are fraught with difficulties. The same problem is evident for aggression. It is important, however, to consider the differences between them. Friedman & Booth-Kewley (1987) provide some clarification: anger is an immediate emotional arousal; whereas hostility is a more enduring negative attitude and aggression is the actual act of or intention of harming another. We can be angry without becoming aggressive and we can also be aggressive without being angry (e.g. during war). Averill (1983) reported on the responses of 160 subjects when angry, with direct physical aggression or punishment occurring in only 10% of the subjects as a result of anger. Furthermore, DiGiuseppe, Tafrate & Eckhardt (1994), when reporting on their clinical experience of aggressive and angry clients, noted that only '2%–5% of client's angry episodes co-occur with aggressive behaviour'. Thus, it could be concluded that most people maintain some coping strategies in relation to anger and behavioural control.

Thus, anger and aggression are not the same, but a relationship between anger and aggression does exist. This inferred relationship has consequences. Novaco (1979) notes that 'the association between anger and aggression engenders the belief that anger is negative or harmful because it is expected to result in "harmdoing"'.

The problems of violence and aggression are all too real for health care practitioners in today's services, and the importance of having meaningful policies, training and support cannot be understated. However, all too often there is a preoccupation with prevention, physical control and management of the aggressive incidents and the violent client (Bjorn 1991, Cahill et al 1991, Carton & Larkin 1991, Visalli et al 1997). Little if no attention is paid to helping clients to develop new methods of managing their anger, especially those who also have a serious mental illness. Although we are do not mean to criticise individual practitioners who are involved in the day to day management of some very assaultative clients, there is insufficient education, training and research into the problems faced by the violent client. In essence, we suggest that mental health generally pays little or no attention to clients' secondary problems, with time, resources and research being instead targeted towards clients' main, primary diagnosis, regardless of co-occurring difficulties (see Rogers & Vidgen 1997).

Anger and SMI

Whilst it is recognised that anger problems can co-occur with other mental health disorders, for example Post Traumatic Stress Disorder (Chemtob et al 1997a,b, Garlic 1994, Really et al 1994). The relationship between anger and SMI has been largely ignored, and there are only a few case studies and discussions of anger and SMI available (Rogers & Gronow 1997, Rogers & Darnley, in press). However, despite this lack of evidence, it is important to consider the impact that SMI can have on lifestyle, as there are numerous potential triggers for anger. Let's first briefly consider the symptoms some clients experience.

Symptoms

Hearing voices that are unpredictable in nature (i.e. in their content, meaning, frequency, volume and duration) can be extremely distressing. Even the most patient of us can become highly irritable if we are constantly interrupted, fearful that someone is making us look a fool or deliberately trying to annoy us. Also, clients' delusional symptoms, although often fantastical, are sometimes held with the same conviction, validity and meaningfulness as devout religious beliefs. Our beliefs are personal areas, whether it be religion, politics, morals, etc. that we hold dear. Ridiculing these beliefs can trigger a range of emotions, not least anger.

The impact of symptoms on lifestyle

The impact of symptoms on a client's lifestyle has been well documented (see Ch. 3). However, the emotional impact has been less recognised. Clients are generally expected to face and cope with unemployment, limited social lives and/or intimate relationships and intrusion from mental health services. Therefore, there are undoubtedly going to be times when they feel frustrated, victimised through prejudice, irritated by slow progress and aggrieved by the loss of autonomy and freedom of choice.

Being a patient and 'the psychiatric system'

The effects of being a 'patient' in the psychiatric system have been long recognised, with issues such as disempowerment, lack of autonomy and loss of control all regular features. Furthermore, the control strategies used (e.g. seclusion, restraint, sections, enforced medication and aftercare) can have a significant impact on whether someone becomes angry,

PRINCIPLES OF WORKING WITH CLIENTS WHO HAVE A SMI AND ARE ANGRY

Before any attempt is made to work with a client's anger, a number of guiding principles must be considered. Failure to incorporate the following recommendations and others identified throughout this book will undoubtedly reduce the chances of a positive outcome being achieved.

◆ **Engagement**: the need for collaboration and negotiation throughout cannot be overemphasised. All work is based upon partnership and exploration of difficulties and potential solutions.

◆ **Flexibility**: you must remain flexible. The assessment may throw up something important that has not been identified before, or the client's goal may change from week to week. Flexibility will assist in fully meeting the needs of the client.

◆ **Problem identification**: all work must be based on an accurate problem identification. The success of any intervention relies on the appropriateness of the problem identified. Your intervention idea may be perfect but, unless you choose the 'right' problem in the first place, you probably won't change a thing.

◆ **Goal focused**: all work must be directed towards predetermined and agreed goals. These goals must be the client's and not ours. Goal focusing involves a long term goal so that the client get a clear picture of how the work has been completed. Furthermore, weekly goals will be agreed as homework.

◆ **Pragmatism**: the focus of this work is based on pragmatism as opposed to the application of learning theories. What matters is what works for the individual client.

◆ **Homework**: all work will inevitably involve homework tasks. Session focuses on looking at ways at solving the agreed problem and then deciding on what is the best way to practise these in real life situations.

◆ **Regular evaluation**: Two principles underlie any successful therapy: (1) the problem assessment is accurate; (2) the interventions used are appropriate to the identified problem. However, even the most experienced therapists will sometimes get these wrong. Regular evaluation (e.g. every 4 weeks) will ensure that if the problem is not changing then it can be picked up early and reassessed. Everyone makes mistakes in the above two areas and regular evaluation guards against continuing with something that is not relevant or achievable.

◆ **Case management**: when involved with clients who have anger problems, effective communication and multidisciplinary working are essential. To aid accurate risk assessment and management, enlist the support of other key professionals.

◆ **Short term**: aim for a maximum of 20 sessions. By this time you will know whether therapy is making a difference. Therapy does not necessarily aim to treat clients from start to finish; it should provide them with new skills or approaches to situations that they can practise and incorporate into their daily lives.

Specific engagement issues

The issue of engaging clients is the crux of all successful interventions. Clients who are angry and have a SMI are no exception. Unless you can develop a collaborative relationship you will have little or no success. It may be possible to work with clients without their cooperation but this will be imposed *upon* them as opposed to *with* them. Working on clients' anger usually involves behavioural management, which will not generalise, as well as treatment aimed at reducing the underlying problem. The main obstacle is that clients may not feel that their anger is a problem, unlike other clinical disorders (e.g. phobias, depression, obsessive–compulsive disorder and post-traumatic stress disorder). Principles include the following:

◆ Develop a collaborative relationship – be aware that, unlike other clinical disorders, most clients do not feel that anger is their main problem.
◆ Agree that a problem exists – try to identify and agree the correct one.
◆ Agree the goals of the treatment.

All too often clients will not engage owing to one of the above three areas. In addition to those characteristics previously described (see Ch. 8) to aid the engagement process, a number of positive attitudes/beliefs are required (Box 13.2).

An example of how problems can occur in the engagement process is presented in the case study of Mike.

After obtaining clinical supervision and with the benefit of hindsight, it is clear that the therapist's insistence to examine both areas was a major barrier to engagement. It was the therapist's goals for treatment, not the client's. The insistence that the second problem was worked on rather than the first led to the client refusing treatment. It is therefore likely that the client's behaviour would continue. If the therapist had worked on the main problem as the client saw it, he may have been more willing to work on the second some time in the future. Also, the skills that the client would have learned by working on the first may have generalised across both situations.

Box 13.2 Positive attitudes/beliefs required in engagement

◆ **Normalisation:** anger is a common emotion; it affects us all. Internal and external triggers cannot be assumed for any one person and its effects can be both positive and negative.

◆ **Coping:** anger is powerful – it controls, frightens and intimidates. Giving this up can be threatening especially if it is the person's main coping strategy.

◆ **Ability to change:** motivation to work on problems fluctuates within all of us. People with anger problems are no different. Just because they may not want to change this week does not mean that they won't be interested next week.

◆ **Self-management:** recognise that working with such clients can cause us a number of emotions including anger, frustration, exasperation and annoyance. Clinical supervision specifically negotiated to discuss, manage and utilise these emotions positively is invaluable (see following case study).

◆ **Expectations:** you both may have a number of expectations about your relationship, the work you hope to do, when benefits will occur and so on. These expectations may interfere with engagement and it is useful to discuss these at the beginning of any interventions and at regular intervals.

 Case study – Mike

When one of the authors (PR) was training as a nurse behaviour psychotherapist, the first client assessed with an anger problem was a 32-year-old male taxi driver. Mike's anger affected him in two areas: (1) at work he had arguments with work colleagues, and (2) at home he committed a number of assaults on his wife. Mike was motivated to work on one area of his anger, but not the other. When discussing the goals of treatment, Mike was very clear – he wanted help to deal with his anger at work and refused to consider the other issue. The therapist could not understand Mike's reluctance to work on his problems at home and after 30 minutes of both parties disputing and disagreeing about what the focus of the work should be, Mike stopped the interview, stating 'it's my problem not yours', and left.

Whilst these latter points are hypothetical, they highlight some of the issues involved during the engagement process. The case study of John illustrates some of these.

Case study – John

John was a 24-year-old man who was detained in a medium secure unit. John's diagnosis was paranoid psychosis. He had intermittent bouts of anger, which on 50% of occasions resulted in physical aggression. John was referred by his clinical team for anger management. He felt his actions were justified and denied that he had problems. He was asked if he would be happy to discuss the referral as there was disagreement between his and his clinical team's views of the problems. He agreed. On assessment, John explained that he became angry and violent owing to being medicated against his will. He did not believe that he was mentally ill. To him the voices he heard were from a benevolent spirit who informed him of whom he could and could not trust.

It appeared that John's violence was linked to issues of detention and being involuntarily medicated. To offer him anger management would therefore have been inappropriate. Targeting the problem causing his anger became the focus for future work. This was that he and the clinical team had not agreed his difficulties, treatment and management. John was not in agreement; however, he was ready to accept that this lack of collaboration was a trigger for his anger and violence.

Initially, John said his goals were: (1) to be let out; (2) not to have to take medication. This was obviously important but unfeasible, as this decision was beyond the control of both parties. After negotiation his goal was restated as 'To live in the community, and fully engage with my aftercare arrangements, which both the clinical team and I will have negotiated, recorded and agreed prior to my discharge'.

Assessment

The process of assessment of anger in people with SMI is of paramount importance as any intervention will only be as good as the data it is based upon. The assessment process has five key structures: preparation, anger assessment, SMI assessment, personal history and current circumstances.

1. Preparation

Prior to beginning any assessment, you will need to prepare fully. The aim of preparation is to identify the areas where you may need to focus on particularly and to plan the goals of the assessment (Richards & McDonald 1990). Preparation includes:

◆ a full review of the information already available
◆ discussion with 'significant others' (i.e. care workers and, where possible, family)

◆ identifying any issues that may effect engagement prior to the interview and planning strategies of how you can overcome these.

2. Anger assessment

The assessment process will usually take three to four sessions, but can take more depending on the client. The focus of assessment is to identify those domains of anger that are current. For the purposes of treatment the anger must be both current and predictable. 'Current' means that the problem is currently affecting the client's lifestyle. 'Predictable' means that triggers for anger can be identified across aspects of time, situations and social interactions. The principles of problem assessment identified in 'Chapter 6 are the same (beginning with open questions then funnelling down to specifics).

Specific areas to focus on when assessing anger are:

Behavioural These include the following questions. What is the client's main problem? Where does the anger happen more or less? With whom does the anger occur or is lessened? What is the frequency of anger (hourly/daily/weekly), intensity on a 0–8 scale (0 = calm, 8 = rage), and duration of anger?

Behavioural excesses These can be identified through asking clients what things they do 'more of' when angry. These may include: verbal expressions of anger (shouting, screaming, or swearing), physical expressions (smashing things, hitting out, or throwing things), or cognitive events (plotting revenge, or planning a future interaction, which may involve violence).

Behavioural avoidances These can be identified by asking what things clients avoid doing. These may include prior avoidances (having arguments, certain people, or certain places) as they are likely to trigger anger. They may also include post avoidances (talking to the person who they are angry with, or being in the same place as the person), which occur after the angry event. By identifying behavioural excesses and deficits you will be able to identify how clients respond when angry and what strategies they use to cope.

Cognitive Once these behavioural triggers have been identified you can use them to detect the cognitions at play. Begin by asking clients to explain why their anger is triggered. Then explore their explanations – for example, 'the last time this happened to you, what were you thinking?' By raising this question it is possible to identify what cognitive triggers the client has. The case study of Joe is an example of cognitive assessment.

At this stage of the assessment process no attempt is made to challenge such cognitions as it could have resulted in alienation as opposed to collaboration.

Autonomic The physiology of anger affects people in different ways. Indeed, there are a number of commonly used sayings that we all use to describe the physiology of anger and its relationship with the cardiovascular

Case study – Joe

Joe's anger was behaviourally triggered more in hospital than when he was at home. This information provided an indication that Joe had angry thoughts about being in hospital. When asked 'why do you feel your anger is worse in hospital?' Joe responded with a number of reasons:

1. *'I hate injections.'*
2. *'There is nothing wrong with me.'*
3. *'I'm unable to do the things that I want to, when I want to.'*

These explanations provide an indication of what exacerbates Joe's anger. The first indicates that Joe does not like injections, but tells us nothing more, bearing in mind that some clients dislike needles, hate side-effects or the manner in which injections are given. It is useful to validate first and foremost which particular aspects of the injection process a client dislikes. When asked, Joe said that 'his rights were being violated', 'the chemicals were poisonous' and he 'no longer felt in control of his life'.

system – for example, 'it made my blood boil', 'I was fuming', 'he's a hot-head', 'he's hot under the collar' and 'he's letting off steam'. Other sayings such as 'I'm wound up' and 'he's ready to explode' are indications of somatic tension. Asking clients about the first physical signs they notice and what happens to their bodies when angry will give an indication of individuals' autonomic symptoms. Indeed such information can be used later to help them detect early signs of anger (early anger signs monitoring).

Functional analysis The ABC analysis (see p. 137) is of paramount importance when assessing anger. It allows you to conceptualise how the previously assessed areas interrelate and affect each other and provides you with an indication as to the person's patterns of anger. Furthermore, it should tell you whether your assessment to date has included all the relevant areas brought up in the functional analysis. It is important to conduct an ABC analysis on as many episodes as possible. This will ensure that you don't focus on just one area of a client's anger as there may be more than one trigger, behaviour and consequence.

3. SMI assessment

The assessment of SMI is described in Chapter 4. In relation to anger and SMI, however, a number of specific areas will require further assessment.

Clients' views of their problems Issues such as clients' agreement or disagreement about whether they have mental health problems and whether they need treatment are crucial. The authors have found that clients who feel that there is nothing wrong with them and who do not want treatment are much more likely to become angry and assaultative. Such clients will often view the actions of mental health professionals as unwarranted and as an intrusion into their lives.

Symptoms Do symptoms of SMI cause anger? In assessing any relationship between voices and anger, you will need to ascertain what the voices are saying, and who the client believes the voices belong to? the reason why the voices are talking to the client and the client's engagement with voices – for example, does the client resist them or want them? Do the voices talk about others, or their intentions? Do they annoy the client? Do they make the client irritable? do they distract the client?

In assessing beliefs, you will need to examine whether client's have delusional symptoms that may make them more prone to feeling angry. For example clients who are paranoid that others are out to hurt them may be more prone to feeling angry at their perceived tormentors. It is also useful to examine whether clients discuss their beliefs with others and the responses that they have had. Sometimes the belittling of a belief may exacerbate anger. If clients believe 100% that they are going to be murdered in their sleep they will obviously be frightened. Consequently, they may become angry when others dismiss their fears and either want to hit out or get out, even if this means escaping from a secure unit.

Once these areas have been assessed, it is useful to ascertain the relationship between clients' symptoms and their anger by conducting a further functional analysis (ABC). Collecting data from as many experiences as possible will aid you in understanding the relationship between stressors and anger. This will enable you to define any particular pattern that is unique to the individual.

4. Personal history

There are a number of personal history issues that are important to ascertain. These should include:

1. exposure to anger or violence throughout clients' lives (social learning)
2. the positive and negative impact of anger upon their lives
3. whether their anger has caused them major problems (police contact, court appearances, loss of freedom)?

5. Current circumstances

Obtaining the client's view about current circumstances helps to identify what life stressors may be contributing to the anger – for example, difficulties with finance, housing, neighbours, family members or employment. Stress has a significant relationship with anger (Novaco 1979). Indeed, in normal circumstances clients may be able to cope with their symptoms of SMI. However, if they are experiencing any one or more than one of the afore-mentioned, these extra stressors may be too much to cope with; consequently the probability of becoming angry increases.

Assessment measures

It is important to stress that the measures used should always be an aid to assessment and not the priority or a replacement. Discriminate use of measures without consideration of clients' abilities can sometimes adversely effect engagement. Therefore the measures should not be exhaustive or exhausting. Measures that are useful include:

◆ Problem and Target Ratings (Marks et al 1986)
◆ Work and Social Adjustment Ratings (Marks et al 1986)
◆ Reaction to Provocation (Novaco 1990)
◆ Beck Depression Inventory (Beck et al 1961)
◆ General Health Questionnaire – 28 (Goldberg 1972; Goldberg & Williams 1988)
◆ Cognitive Assessment of Voices: Interview Schedule (Chadwick & Birchwood 1994)
◆ Beliefs About Voices Questionnaire (Chadwick & Birchwood 1995).

Formulation

After completing the above assessments the next stage is to formulate the client's anger. The formulation exercise is usually best completed separately and it may sometimes take two sessions to complete fully. During the formulation, a number of possible variations of relationships may arise.

In assisting the formulation stage, a 'relationship chart' is a useful format to follow. Its purpose is to establish how the client's anger relates to the other variables assessed. By placing anger in the middle, you and the client can then decide which of the other variables are related to the client's anger and draw links between them as appropriate (see Fig. 13.1).

Once this has been completed you can then map out any anger patterns that have been identified (Box 13.3).

The more frequently this exercise is practised the easier it is to examine relationships and the more sophisticated it becomes. It is often helpful for clients if they are given a copy of the formulation exercise. They can then take it away to either look at or refine it if they wish. This process of collaboratively looking at potential links can be very engaging.

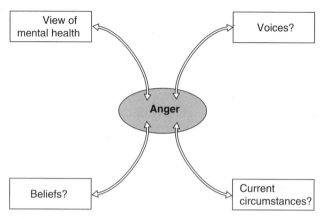

Figure 13.1 Example of a relationship chart.

Once the formulation exercise has been completed and agreed by both parties, the next step is to agree some problems and goals (see Ch. 6).

Interventions

So far we have engaged, assessed and formulated with our clients, the penultimate process following formulation is that of intervention. The

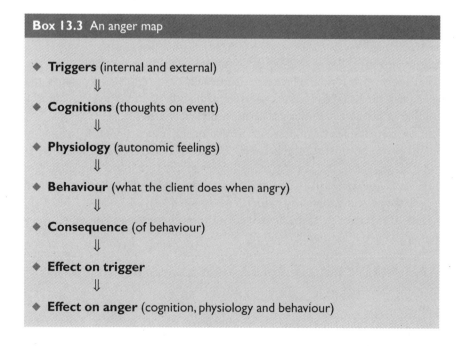

Box 13.3 An anger map

◆ **Triggers** (internal and external)
⇓
◆ **Cognitions** (thoughts on event)
⇓
◆ **Physiology** (autonomic feelings)
⇓
◆ **Behaviour** (what the client does when angry)
⇓
◆ **Consequence** (of behaviour)
⇓
◆ **Effect on trigger**
⇓
◆ **Effect on anger** (cognition, physiology and behaviour)

intervention(s) chosen will depend on the assessment and formulation. The application of the right intervention in the right place will greatly enhance the efficacy of the total treatment.

Self-monitoring

The first stage of most anger treatments involves varying degrees of self-monitoring. Self-monitoring aims to assist clients assimilate their actual anger experiences into the formulation framework. A number of strategies are available to aid self-monitoring, the most common being the anger diary (Fig. 13.2). However, we have sometimes had to alter the method of self-monitoring. For example, for those who have difficulties with reading or writing,

Week commencing............................ Name............................

Anger levels

```
0     1     2     3     4     5     6     7     8
├─────┼─────┼─────┼─────┼─────┼─────┼─────┼─────┤
None        Slight      Moderate        Marked        Rage
```

When		Trigger	Anger levels (0–8)			Thoughts	Behaviour	Outcomes
Date	Time and duration	What happened	Before	During	After	What were you thinking? Before? During? After?	What did you do? Before? During? After?	What were the positive benefits? What were the negatives?

Figure 13.2 An anger diary.

we have successfully employed a dictaphone and used it to record and elicit the details outlined in the homework diary.

When asking clients to record diaries, it is important to encourage them to fill the details out as soon as possible, so that they don't forget. Based on the themes that emerge, the information obtained can be used to refine the formulation process further and develop a collaborative treatment plan. As mentioned earlier, the aim of anger intervention is to break the cycle between behaviour, physiology and cognitions. Intervention can involve a number of different treatment strategies. However, the crux should be that they are solution focused, practical and encourage clients to take active responsibility for carrying out their own treatment, thus encouraging self-efficacy and minimising dependence on the therapist.

Physiological strategies

Relaxation strategies aim to reduce the physiological component of anger, as these learnt strategies can affect clients' cognitions and behavioural responses. Indeed, it is advocated that anxiety management training should be adopted in most cases of anger, and there are detailed procedure descriptions available (see Deffenbacher 1996 for review). The process of applied relaxation will not be described in this text as many descriptions are available (see Suinn 1990, Suinn & Deffenbacher 1988). However, we have found that relaxation can be an effective and powerful method of engaging clients prior to moving on to some of the more challenging work (i.e. cognitive interventions). If clients gain some success in this stage then their belief in the credibility of subsequent therapy can be enhanced.

Behavioural strategies

'Preanger' strategies Preanger strategies focus on identifying anger cues/triggers and then developing strategies with clients as to how these cues can be avoided or better managed. This can often be helpful for clients who feel 'out of control' or whose lack of control is potentially about to cause significant problems in terms of offending. In our clinical experience, we have found that the greater the range of avoidance strategies clients have to hand, the more they can choose methods to suit themselves. For example, one client had overwhelming anger towards his employer and was fearful that the latter would seek him out and assault him. He agreed that, if all other identified strategies proved ineffective or failed, he would attend his local police station as a last resort. This was never actually required, but it did give this client a sense of relief to know that he had this external option, and allowed him to avoid viewing his own self-control strategies as 'all or nothing'.

'Current' anger strategies These involve identifying behavioural methods that clients can use once their anger has been activated. These are more successful if the strategies are tailored to the individual and may include:

◆ immediately leaving the scene and retiring to a place where the client can calm down without interruption
◆ interrupting the anger response by identifying an alternative behaviour that 'competes' with the usual anger response.

Other more 'alternative' individualised strategies have included:

1. 'Getting naked': This was employed by one client – an inpatient in a medium secure unit suffering from post-traumatic stress disorder. Every time he had flashbacks he became immediately aroused and tended to smash up the ward, and once assaulted a member of staff who had attempted to intervene. After the event he felt very guilty and wanted an immediate strategy to stop him assaulting staff again. He identified that if he were naked he would not be able to come out of his room. So, as soon as he identified the first signs of anger, he would go to his room and strip off his clothes.

2. 'Headstands': one outpatient client who again wanted to control his explosive outburst towards staff agreed that if he were in the headstand position it would be difficult to continue with the assault.

Assertion training In some cases, clients' anger may be directly related to a lack of ability to assert themselves with other people who have transgressed them (Defenbacher et al 1987, Frederiksen et al 1976, Rogers & Darnley 2000, Rogers & Gronow 1997). Consequently, they find that their anger continues after the transgression and they ruminate for long periods thereafter. We have found that assertion or social skills training early on in therapy can have excellent results. Indeed, it appears to help improvements in behaviours, self-esteem and motivation to continue.

Cognitive strategies

Identifying cognitions Through the assessment process and the use of anger diaries, it is possible to identify which cognitions may be linked to anger. Also, this process of self-monitoring can assist the client in examining internal relationships to anger as opposed to purely external events. Novaco (1979) identifies two types of cognitive processes that are related to angry cognitions: appraisals and expectations.

Appraisals The way we appraise a situation greatly affects our responses and differs significantly from individual to individual. For example, suppose that a senior manager mentions to two staff that he likes their ties. One readily accepts the compliment, whereas the other becomes annoyed and irritated, believing it is a reference to the fact that he was not wearing a tie the day before. Thus, in this context, appraisals have a historical connection and are the meanings we attribute to previous events.

Expectations Personal expectations can often be a cause for anger. If we expect that something will happen or will be done in a certain manner and later find that it isn't, we can become angry. We blame someone else for something not happening, when in fact it was our original expectation that was the problem. For example, if two clients attend their GP's surgery without making a prior appointment, one may expect a delay whilst the other may expect to be seen immediately. The person expecting to be seen immediately is more likely to become more irate at having to wait.

Interventions – special issues

We urge caution against attempting to challenge a client's faulty appraisals or expectations immediately. As in all cognitive therapy, the process of examining thoughts is a collaborative process. Professionals should *always* avoid 'seeing' the problem cognition and 'going straight in' to help the client see their wisdom Box 13.4 contains some cautions.

Box 13.4 Challenging cognitions – some cautions

◆ 'Problem cognitions' – don't jump straight in with identifying and pointing out faulty cognitions. Examine the thoughts collaboratively.

◆ Don't challenge faulty assumptions immediately. Looking at the evidence for appraisals or reasonableness of expectations may be counterproductive at this early stage. Map out the relationships between thoughts, affect and behaviour.

◆ Don't expect clients to see relationships immediately. It is more beneficial to assist people to identify and examine their own cognitions.

The process of cognitive interventions for misappraisals and expectations requires:

◆ validating clients' experiences as upsetting and difficult
◆ treating anger experiences as events to be explored – in terms of what happened
◆ recording and/or drawing these experiences on paper can help clients to visualise what is happening so they are more able to draw their own conclusions
◆ avoiding questions like 'What's the evidence for and against?', and using

questions like 'Could we map out what happened and then look at all the events more closely?' instead; this 'mapping out' process helps clients think about and record the internal thoughts that they were having in relation to the external events

◆ not expecting a client to see the relationship immediately; after 'mapping out' exercises have been completed a few times in a variety of different settings, clients may be more able to identify that the factor which remains constant is their expectations or appraisals as opposed to the event, the other person, the time of day, and so on.

CONCLUSIONS

In this chapter, we have examined the assessment, engagement and treatment of clients with SMI and who are angry. These clients are difficult to engage, are frustrating to work with and are often perceived to have the most difficult and complex problems. Your colleagues may at times suggest that these experiences and multiple problems cannot be changed. Indeed, we have frequently come across such attitudes, but believe the way forward is to try and get colleagues 'on side' by helping them to understand the client better and by focusing on the potential benefits and the 'what if's?'

This chapter provides only a brief outline of the stages involved, but does offer a firm starting point. It can be highly rewarding to work *with* these clients as opposed to *against* them. Nevertheless, irrespective of whether 'novice' or 'expert' we *strongly* advocate that before embarking with any of the outline strategies you seek out a suitable clinical supervisor.

Summary of practical strategies identified

◆ Anger is an emotional state consisting of cognitions (thoughts), behaviours and physiological arousal.

◆ Interventions should focus on helping clients cope with anger – not stop them feeling anger.

◆ Engagement and assessment should be flexible and client centred.

◆ Intervention can focus on any of the constituents of anger to effect change.

◆ Anger mapping is a useful tool in the process.

◆ Clinical supervision from an experienced professional is strongly advised.

References

Averill J R 1983 Studies on anger and aggression: implications for theories of emotion. American Psychologist 38:1145–1160

Beck A T, Ward C M, Mendelson M, Moch J, Erbaugh J 1961 An inventory for measuring depression. Archives of General Psychiatry 4:561–571

Bjorn P R 1991 An approach to the potentially violent patient. Journal of Emergency Nursing 17(5):336–338

Cahill C D, Stuart G W, Laraia M T, Arana G W 1991 Inpatient management of violent behaviour: nursing prevention and intervention. Issues in Mental Health Nursing 12:239–252

Carton G, Larkin E 1991 Reducing violence in a special hospital. Nursing Standard 5(17):29–31

Chadwick P, Birchwood M 1994 Cognitive assessment of voices: interview schedule. In: Chadwick P, Birchwood M, Trower P (eds) Cognitive therapy for delusions, voices and paranoia. Wiley, Chichester, pp 195–200

Chadwick P, Birchwood M 1995 The omnipotence of voices II: the Beliefs About Voices Questionnaire (BAVQ). British Journal of Psychiatry 166:733–776

Chemtob C M, Novaco R W, Hamada R S, Gross D M 1997a Cognitive–behavioural treatment for severe anger in post-traumatic stress disorder. Journal of Consulting and Clinical Psychology 65(1):184–189

Chemtob C M, Novaco R W, Hamada R S, Gross D M, Smith G 1997b Anger regulation in combat related posttraumatc stress disorder. Journal of Traumatic Stress 10(1):17–36

Deffenbacher J 1996 Cognitive–behavioural approaches to anger reduction. In: Dobson K S, Craig K D (eds) Advances in cognitive–behavioural therapy. London, Sage, 31–62

Deffenbacher J, Story D A, Stark R S, Hogg J A, Brandon A D 1987 Cognitive–relaxation and social skills interventions in the treatment of general anger. Journal of Counselling Psychology 34:171–176

DiGiuseppe R, Tafrate R, Eckhardt C 1994 Critical issues in the treatment of anger. Cognitive and Behavioural Practice 1:111–132

Ekman P 1972 Darwin and facial expression: a century of research in review. Academic Press, New York

Frederiksen L W, Jenkins J O, Foy D W, Eisler R M 1976 Social skills training to modify abusive verbal outbursts in adults. Journal of Applied Behavioural Analysis 9(2):117–125

Friedman H S, Booth-Kewley S 1987 The 'disease-prone personality': a meta-analytical view of the construct. American Psychologist 42(6):539–555

Garlic 1994 Veterans' responses to anger management intervention. Issues in Mental Health Nursing 15:393–408

Goldberg D P 1972 The detection of psychiatric illness by questionnaire. Oxford University Press, London

Goldberg D, Williams P 1988 A user's guide to the General Health Questionnaire. NFER-Nelson, Windsor

Kemp S, Strongman K T 1995 Anger theory and management: a historical analysis. American Journal of Psychology 108(3):397–417

Marks I M, Bird J, Brown M, Ghosh A 1986 Behavioural psychotherapy: Maudsley pocket book of clinical management. Wright, Bristol

Novaco R W 1979 The cognitive regulation of anger and stress. In: Kendall P, Hollon S D (eds) Cognitive–behavioural interventions: theory, research and practice. Academic Press, New York, pp 241–285

References (*cont'd*)

Novaco R W 1985 Anger and its therapeutic regulation. In: Chesney M A, Rosenman R H (eds) Anger and hostility in cardiovascular and behavioural disorders. Hemisphere, Washington DC, pp 31–84

Novaco R W 1990 Reactions to provocation (NAS). Irvine, University of California

Reilly P M, Westley Clarke H, Shopshire M S, Lewis E W, Sorenson D J 1994 Anger management: critical components of post traumatic stress disorder and substance abuse treatment. Journal of Psychoactive Drugs 26(4):401–407

Richards D, McDonald B 1990 Behavioural psychotherapy: a pocket book for nurses. Heinemann, Oxford

Rogers P, Darnley S 2000 Behavioural psychotherapy in forensic mental health. In: Burnard P, Tarbuck P, Topping-Morris B (eds) Aspects of forensic mental health nursing: policy, strategy and implementation. Whurr, London, in press

Rogers P, Gronow T 1997 Turn down the heat. Nursing Times 93(43):26–29

Rogers P, Vidgen A 1997 Social phobia: the consequence of 15 years as an inpatient in forensic institutions – a case study. Psychiatric Care 4(6):250–252

Russel J, Fehr B 1994 Fuzzy concepts in a fuzzy hierarchy: varieties of anger. Journal of Personality and Social Psychology 67(2):186–205

Suinn R M 1990 Anxiety management training. Plenum, New York

Suinn R M, Deffenbacher J L 1988 Anxiety management training. Counselling Psychologist 16:31–49

Visalli H, McNasser G, Johnstone L, Lazzaro C A 1997 Reducing high risk interventions for managing aggression in psychiatric settings. Journal of Nursing Care Quality 11(3):54–61

Annotated further reading

Kassinove H, Sukhodolsky D G 1995 Anger disorders: basic science and practice issues. In: Kassinove H (ed) Anger disorders: definition, diagnosis and treatment. Taylor & Francis, Washington DC, pp 1–26

This book provides a very useful overview of the basic practice issues when working with clients who have anger disorders and the chapters are set out in such a manner which allow for useful reference. Unfortunately, this book is not specifically for those clients with serious mental illness and anger disorders and we would strongly recommend the following two books for further pragmatic cognitive–behavioural guidance when working with such clients:

Chadwick P, Birchwood M 1994 Cognitive therapy for delusions, voices and paranoia. Wiley, Chichester

Birchwood M, Tarrier N 1994 Psychological management of schizophrenia. Wiley, Chichester

14

Working with people with serious mental illness at risk of offending

Andrew Vidgen   Paul Rogers

KEY ISSUES

- ◆ Introduction to some of the legal and clinical issues arising out of working with this client group.
- ◆ Assessment issues relating to individuals who have committed offences using a broad cognitive behavioural and functional analysis approach.
- ◆ Intervention approaches covering a range of options aimed at reducing offending.

INTRODUCTION

This chapter provides an overview of the relationship between mental health and offending behaviour. It aims to focus on the more serious offences and the interface between symptoms, psychological functioning and criminal behaviour. In order that the relationship issues are better understood, part 1 examines conceptual and theoretical viewpoints, whereas part 2 examines engagement, assessment and treatment issues.

PART I – CONCEPTUAL AND THEORETICAL VIEWPOINTS: OFFENDING BEHAVIOUR AND SMI

The main problem for those who wish to unravel the available evidence on offending behaviour and diagnosis is that the literature is fraught with definitional problems. This hampers the study of the relationship between people with serious mental health problem and offending behaviour and often makes comparison across studies difficult. The points below highlight this anomaly:

❖ mental illness is not defined in the Mental Health Act (DOH 1983)
❖ no single definition of criminality exists (Feldman 1993).

In addition, offending by people with SMI often leads to them being involved with a number of formal systems, such as the criminal justice system and mental health services. This is important; to understand the relationship between SMI and criminality we must consider more than the causal relationship between them (Blackburn 1993). Their relationship is also influenced by social factors and the interfacing within and between the mental health and criminal justice systems. This confusion can extend from ideas of the relationship to actual provision and planning of services for both the population and the individual. Examples of this confusion can be shown in considering the following questions:

❖ are persons with SMI who offend 'criminals' or not?
❖ who makes this decision?
❖ if care is needed, who should provide it and where?
❖ if the SMI is in remission, should the person move from a care to a custodial setting or back to the community?

Historical, social and high media profile responses have also undoubtedly influenced the view of politicians and designers of mental health policy. In addition, these have helped frame the general public's stereotypical view of mentally ill people, which one could argue also has an influence on mental health policy decisions. The following are assumptions expressed with regard to people with SMI:

❖ they are dangerous and commit violent crimes (Richie 1994)
❖ they are unpredictable – at risk to themselves and others
❖ they are 'untreatable' – so why not just lock them up and throw away the key? (Hall et al 1993, Hiday 1995, Levey & Howells 1995)

Although these views would indicate that the stereotypical viewpoint has no difficulties in linking SMI and offending, the exact nature of the relationship between 'mental disorder' (including serious mental health problems) and 'crime', especially violence, remains controversial (Blackburn 1993, Monahan & Steadman 1983). Studies that have attempted to examine the relationship have been challenged as being methodologically flawed, as they have placed a heavy reliance on hospital and prison populations (therefore introducing bias) and have lacked suitable comparison and/or control groups (Hiday 1995, Shah 1993, Taylor & Hodgins 1994, Wessely & Taylor 1991).

Nevertheless it has been argued that people with diagnoses of mental illness are more likely to commit offences compared with the general population and that a significant proportion of these crimes involve offences against people (Côté & Hodgins 1992, Mulvey 1994). However, it is important to acknowledge that people with serious psychiatric disorders may be statistically overrepresented in committing more serious offences such as murder. For example, in the UK, psychiatric disorder has been implicated in approximately 30–40% of murders over the last century (Blackburn 1996). However, when examining the mental states of 600 English prisoners Gunn et al (1978) found that rates of depression and anxiety were higher than rates of schizophrenia. Spry (1984), when reviewing occurrence rates of schizophrenia in offender populations, found an incidence of only 1%, which is comparable to that found in the general population. Thus, it could be argued that the vast majority of this group are no more likely than members of the general public to commit serious offences. Thus, it remains difficult to draw any firm conclusions, especially if consideration is given to the following factors, which would produce an increase in the number of persons with SMI appearing in statistical analysis:

◆ **The Home Office (1990) circular 66/90**: Provisions for mentally disordered offenders – now advises that offenders with a recognisable mental disorder should be diverted away from the criminal justice system.

◆ **Police detection and arrest rates**: 'compared with "mentally stable" offenders this group may "choose more difficult targets, plan an offence less carefully or carry it out less skilfully – all failings increase the risk of detection, arrest and official statistics". The police may arrest or charge a disturbed person more readily than others' (Feldman 1993).

All these factors indicate that we should be very careful in our formulation of SMI and offending as there are many pitfalls.

Working with this client group

When working with people with SMI and offending behaviour it is all too easy to assume a direct causal relationship between the person's mental state/psychiatric diagnosis and the offending behaviour. In our experience, this is particularly so within specialised mental health secure facilities where some of the more extreme ends of the mental illness spectrum receive services (stereotypically this would include the paranoid schizophrenic who has committed a very serious offence against a member of their family or the general public).

However, we should concede that a large degree of variation exists between people's mental health and offending behaviour. When working with this client group a comprehensive and careful assessment has to be carried out to ascertain the nature of people's mental health in relation to their offending history (and risk of committing future offences). It is insufficient to treat someone's psychiatric problems solely (with medication) without directly addressing offending behaviour and psychological functioning. It is useful to bear in mind that people commit offences for a variety of reasons, including financial gain, when angry, influence of peer or group pressure or as a result of behavioural responses to hearing voices or beliefs regarding the victim (some of which may be delusional). Furthermore, attention must be paid to previous offending and age (McCord 1990). Obtaining a person's full criminal history is particularly useful when predicting future risk areas. Focusing on a person's range of criminal activities will add to the richness of the assessment as well as providing a number of pointers for intervention. For example, someone's criminal behaviour may be exacerbated by drug taking; by addressing specific offences such as violence there may be scope to intervene at the level of the substance misuse. A further point to bear in mind is that criminal behaviour is versatile. Indeed, 'those who steal and commit burglary are pretty much the same people who engage in violence, vandalism and drug abuse, who drink excessively, drive recklessly and commit sexual offences' (Stephenson 1992). Thus, as mental health workers we should not automatically assume that a causal relationship exists between clients' mental health problems and their offending behaviour, but look instead at the offending behaviour and its relationship with mental health functioning.

It is also important to recognise that people with psychotic disorders are not a comparable group. Diagnosis alone does not clarify why a particular individual has committed an offence. In addition, the variety of symptoms that people experience, namely hallucinations and idiosyncratic patterns of thought, have traditionally been seen as increasing the risk of offending when present. Indeed, over the past decade, there has been an increased interest in the phenomenology of symptoms and how these relate to people's experiences and offending behaviour (Chadwick, Birchwood & Trower 1996, Johnson et al 1997, Junginger 1995, Taylor & Hodgins 1994, Wessely et al 1993). For example, Wessely et al (1993) found that approximately 50% of their inpatient sample ($n = 88$) had acted on delusional beliefs on at least one occasion; however, violent behaviour was uncommon. To examine further the relationship between type of delusions and subsequent behaviour, a subsample of this group (approximately 10%) were studied. They found that delusions of catastrophe were significantly associated with aggression. Interestingly, no association was found in those people experiencing other types of delusions including those of reference, religion, jealousy, persecution, grandiosity, guilt or those with a sexual content. However, this suggests only that some delusions may facilitate certain behaviours, as opposed to certain delusions being more likely to be acted upon. Attention has also to be paid to the type of hallucination experienced. It is a common, but mainly unsubstantiated, belief that people experiencing command hallucinations are at risk of committing violent acts.

The need to pay attention to the content of hallucinations in order to formulate the relationship between them and behaviour (including offending) has recently been noted (e.g. Chadwick, Birchwood & Trower 1996). This can be done in two ways: firstly, by referring to the events preceding a person's offence(s) and, secondly, by gaining an understanding of the types of situations where people experience hallucinations (e.g. voices), as well as their beliefs about voices and their behavioural responses to them. In our opinion, too much attention is paid to voices as triggers for behaviour. The importance of environmental and/or psychological triggers has been neglected. The advantage of paying attention to such antecedents of voice hearing is that it provides another level for possible intervention. The following case study helps to illustrate this point:

Case study – Joan

Joan, a 19-year-old woman, had threatened staff with a knife in the local supermarket. She was admitted to hospital for assessment under the Mental Health Act. Joan was given a preliminary diagnosis of paranoid schizophrenia, her primary symptoms being auditory hallucinations (a male voice telling her to get a knife) and paranoid beliefs regarding members of her family (that they were trying to poison her). Joan's risk of violence increased when she heard the 'male voice' instructing her to obtain a knife. On the ward, Joan reported hearing this voice on a number of occasions. On further analysis, these symptoms increased either after her mother departed from visiting her or when she telephoned to say that she would be unable to visit. This left Joan feeling vulnerable and lonely. Thus, although Joan's risk of threatening others did increase when she was experiencing her voice, they were significantly related to her mother leaving or informing Joan that she could not visit.

Traditionally, mental health practitioners have been taught to distract clients when they experience voices or when they wish to discuss their beliefs. This approach was largely influenced by the Jasperian view that delusions cannot be altered by discussing them (Allen & Kingdon 1998). The framework of behaviourism lent support to this view, when it was demonstrated that, if nurses did not respond, clients were observed to state their delusional beliefs less frequently (Allyon & Haughton 1964). This view has been very difficult to shift and it is only recently that the validity of such an approach has been fully challenged. The disadvantages of taking such a dismissive approach undoubtedly affect the engagement process, especially when clients become aware that their most distressing experiences are being actively avoided (Allen & Kingdon 1998). Indeed, whilst such practice continues it will remain difficult to develop trust and demonstrate genuine concern for a person's distress, and in this context potential risk areas will go undetected (see Ch. 7).

PART 2 – ASSESSMENT, INTERVENTION AND RELATED ISSUES

Working with people in secure environments

When examining offending behaviours in people with SMI in a secure setting there are a number of points worth consideration. Below are some of the more regular issues faced.

Engagement issues

Disclosure can affect disposal

Close consideration must be paid to general and more specific factors that may influence engagement. Clients usually learn fairly soon how a system works and its pros and cons. One of the main problems facing them is that often disclosure of offence details can (and usually will) influence final disposal. This is particularly apparent in people who have been transferred from prisons to secure units. Disclosure of symptoms in a prison environment can often lead to transfer to secure health facilities. However, once this has occurred, 'not disclosing symptoms' can often lead to people moving through the system, especially if the index offence has been largely attributed to a person's mental health status.

Faking good and faking bad

As mentioned above, there may be global reasons why people would alter their presentation of symptoms within a secure environment. However, there may be blocks to therapeutic engagement on a more specific level. People may overaccentuate symptoms or psychological distress as a way of minimising their involvement and responsibility in their offending behaviour (faking bad), in the same way that some offenders attribute the responsibility of their actions to being intoxicated at the time of their offence. To present a more favourable picture of themselves, people can also underplay the role of psychological factors (faking good).

Confidentiality

This can be one of the major blocks to engagement. Whether working in a clinical team or with outpatients, it should be made *explicit* that the information discussed will be disclosed if it impacts on the safety of others, clients themselves, or has direct relevance to their clinical care. This does not mean that you have to disclose the exact details of your work; however, the main themes, issues and content of sessions may be available to a wider audience than can be normally agreed within a therapeutic relationship.

Labelling

Assessment has to take into consideration the role of the labelling process in relation to engagement. The negative stigma attached to people who offend and have a SMI may block therapeutic work. Indeed, this can also be affected if clients do not hold the same views of their current mental health status as their clinical team. Also, careful consideration has to be paid to the language used when addressing issues that the assessment process has raised. A brief case example serves to highlight this.

Case study – Robert

Robert (26) had a diagnosis of paranoid schizophrenia that had responded well to medication. However, on the ward, he was observed to be quiet in social situations and avoided approaching staff to meet day to day needs. The clinical team made a referral to one of the authors for an assessment of his social skills and 'weaknesses'. Following assessment it was suggested that Robert would benefit from social skills training. However, Robert did not consider himself to have any problems in this area despite the clinical team's opinion that he would benefit from this work. Robert did not engage with this intervention and now believes that others see him as having a major psychiatric condition and social skills deficits.

We have found that clients often have entirely different ideas about their problems and what needs to be done by their clinical teams. By helping them to work on their priorities, rather than the teams', clients are more willing to trust you, and subsequently some of the 'wider issues' can be dealt with. It is useful to remember that some clients will trust someone to help them with their more difficult problems only if they have helped them with some of their current needs first.

Mental illness = offending

As mentioned, it is often common to hold the belief that people's offending behaviour is a direct result of their mental illness. This has two implications for engagement. First, this position is often reinforced by health care professionals and by the criminal justice system, in that clients may receive a health service disposal owing to their mental state at the time of his/her offence. Consequently, clients may not wish to engage (even at assessment level) because they fear that, if they disclose symptoms, this will influence the clinical team and make them believe the presenting mental state will increase the risk of future offending. Secondly, future engagement may be hampered by those professionals who solely rely on psychotropic medication to settle a person's mental state and leave clients believing the major cause of their offending behaviour has been addressed – 'I'm not going to offend – I'm not ill'.

Professional overinvolvement early on

It is likely in a secure setting that, following a person's admission, there will be a flurry of activity from a number of professionals (nursing, psychiatry, psychology, social work, OT, probation, etc.) who are all attempting to gain their own perspective on the person's presenting problems, mental health, offending behaviour, risk areas and current functioning. It should therefore not come as a great surprise if this bombardment of questioning and scrutiny meets with some resistance from the person on the receiving end. Thus, we have to achieve a balance between fulfilling professional requirements with the need to be sensitive regarding time and the amount of information the person is required to provide at the time of admission.

Paranoia, voices and delusions

It can be very difficult to engage with clients when they are actively experiencing voices or hold beliefs that induce feelings of paranoia or vulnerability. Also, clients' beliefs about their voices (see Ch. 9) may hamper the assessment process – for example, if they believe the source of their voice to be extremely powerful or omniscient, or if they believe that disclosing information about the source of the voice will lead to harm coming to themselves or 'significant others'.

For additional material on engagement issues see the following.

1. Chadwick, Birchwood & Trower (1996) discuss some issues in engaging with people who are experiencing voices, delusions and paranoia as well as strategies to overcome these.

2. Gresswell & Kruppa (1994) provide a number of strategies to enhance engagement, communication and the assessment process in relation to working in secure environments.

3. Perkins (1991) looks at working specifically with sex offenders in secure environments.

Assessment

In essence, the underlying guiding principles that should enhance the engagement process are those where both client and practitioner collaborate, are flexible and where the practitioner communicates understanding. These are detailed in Box 14.1.

Box 14.1 Attitudes and skills ensuring engagement

◆ **Collaborative**: both parties agree the goals and processes involved.
◆ **Empathic**: including providing feedback when you do and do not understand.
◆ **Short frequent**: work in manageable chunks with the person. Do not attempt to cram a full assessment into two interviews.
◆ **Pragmatic**: be willing to adapt your work to suit the person's interpersonal style, cognitive ability and, most importantly, you do not have to follow intervention strategies by the book!

Before meeting the client you will always need to review all relevant materials and obtain background information. As mentioned in Chapter 13, the purpose of assessment is to identify those areas that need particular attention and to plan the focus and goals of the assessment (Richards & McDonald 1990). Preparation will include:

◆ review of previous case notes, including depositions of offences, where available
◆ review of relevant literature
◆ discussion with 'significant others' (e.g. family and previous professionals involved in care)
◆ as well as those engagement issues outlined above, preparation will allow the identification of specific issues as well as strategies of how to overcome these.

Agreeing the problems and the goals of assessment

Agreeing the problems to focus on is paramount to a good assessment and subsequent interventions. As previously discussed, if we attempt to push the person towards issues that we perceive to be central to their difficulties in the absence of them owning them or agreeing with this perception then we will run into problems. Work has to be collaborative. Interventions should be broken down into manageable steps and goals should be divided into short, medium and long term outcomes. Explicitly agreeing these and clarifying the expectations will partly overcome some of the engagement problems outlined.

Assessment will usually take approximately three to four sessions, but may take longer if there is a number or range of offences.

Functional analysis (FA)

There are a number of models of functional analyses, which largely have their underpinnings in behavioural theory (see Sturmey 1996). Largely, these involve some form of analysis of the consequences of the behaviour for the person in relation to reinforcements and punishments within a framework of antecedents, behaviours and consequences (or ABC – see Ch. 6) (Table 14.1).

Table 14.1 ABC analysis of offence

A = antecedents	**Distal:** ◆ Offence history ◆ Significant life events ◆ Previous behaviour patterns **Proximal just before offence(s): where? when?** ◆ Thoughts ◆ Feelings ◆ Arousal level ◆ Physical condition (drunk?)
B = behaviour	◆ Detailed description of offence ◆ Previous patterns of behaviour
C = consequences	**Positive/negative reinforcements:** ◆ Thoughts ◆ Feelings ◆ Material gains ◆ Avoidances **Positive/negative punishments:** ◆ Fine/sentenced ◆ Loss of family contact ◆ Decrease in positive affect ◆ Increase in negative affect

Although a considerable amount of controversy regarding functional analysis (FA) exists (McDonnell & Samson 1992, Owens & Jones 1992, Samson & McDonnell 1990), FA remains a useful tool. It helps us to understand and conceptualise patterns of behaviour and how each element of the person's difficulties fits together. When attempting to look for points to intervene with clients and/or you need an aid to formulate problems identified, FA can also help to:

♦ provide material to weigh up the pros and cons of their offending behaviour (in relation to consequences)
♦ provide clients with self-monitoring strategies in relation to their own offending behaviour.

In relation to offending the FA can be extended to include the following categories.

Behavioural These include the following questions:

♦ Which offence does the person see as most serious or more accessible to change?
♦ Did the person act alone or in a group?
♦ If there was a victim or victims, who were they?
♦ Was a weapon used?
♦ If a sexual offence? Which offence did professionals or 'significant others' make most fuss about?
♦ Why that particular victim?
♦ What were the chief motivations to offending?
♦ How do environmental events activate behaviour?

Rating scales can be developed in relation to how serious the person considers some offences over others and how many times approximately the client believes each offence was carried out.

Cognitive These include:

♦ attitudes towards the offence
♦ thoughts prior to, during and following offence
♦ justifications – including victim blaming or perceiving the crime as victimless (as in the case of armed robbery or burglary).

In relation to sexual offending, thoughts that minimise the seriousness of the offence or blame the victim are usually termed 'cognitive distortions'. These can include general attitudes towards the role of women in society, rape myths (Burt 1980) or beliefs about children and sexuality. More specific beliefs regarding clients' victims can be accessed by asking them to talk through their offence(s). Prior to this, a review of the depositions may also highlight potential distortions to be followed up during face to face assessment.

Attempts to challenge distortions at this point may lead to the person feeling alienated from the process and should be avoided.

At a more specific level, assessment can be made of thoughts prior to, during and following the offending behaviour. Benefits include:

♦ a thorough functional analysis provides rich information
♦ focusing on the antecedents – it can provide the person with preliminary indicators that certain thoughts are associated with offending behaviour
♦ it provides a good opportunity to discuss the role of thoughts and their influence on behaviour within a cognitive–behavioural framework.

Affective Gaining a clear idea of the mood of the person at each stage of the offence(s) will also enhance your assessment and provide information in relation to the function served by the offence. For example, did the person report getting a 'buzz' from the offence? Also, pay attention to the affect displayed by clients when recounting their offence. For example, do they appear: aroused, angry, upset or indifferent?

Determining the relationship between mental health functioning and offending

As mentioned, there are a variety of reasons why someone with a mental health problem may commit an offence. Knowing clients' diagnoses may contribute somewhat to understanding why their offending behaviour has occurred; however, it will offer little information in relation to the function it serves for them. Nevertheless, there will be symptoms and psychological consequences of mental health problems that will influence motivation, planning, commissioning and consequences of offending (including detection as mentioned above). For the purposes of assessment, we have divided these up into primary and secondary factors.

1. Primary factors Primary factors include symptoms directly associated with diagnosis (e.g. delusional beliefs and voices). Assessment should focus on symptoms as an influence to the offending behaviour. Again, working within a framework of functional analysis helps focus the person's experience of these symptoms at the antecedent, behavioural and consequence level. A person may hold specific beliefs about their victim that can be understood in terms of the diagnosis – for example, that the client's partner is having an affair, or the person is being poisoned by a 'significant other', or that a close family member has been replaced by aliens.

2. Secondary factors These include psychological and emotional problems that are not part of the primary diagnosis, but may contribute to the offending behaviour – for example, memory, attention and concentration problems, irritability and anger. Talking through the offence(s) with the person should 'tease out' these factors. Focusing on these factors during the assessment period also enables a broadening out of the factors that may contribute to offending apart from those directly associated with diagnosis.

Thus people's symptoms may influence their offending at the antecedent, behavioural and consequence level. Table 14.2 illustrates this.

Table 14.2 ABC analysis of mental health and offending

	Leading to
Antecedents (e.g. voices)	◆ Anger ◆ Beliefs about voices ◆ Anxiety/fear ◆ Isolation ◆ Difficulty gaining employment
Behaviour	◆ Psychological experiences during offence, e.g. beliefs about voices
Consequences	◆ Positive reinforcement – attention from services ◆ Decrease in feelings of isolation (negative reinforcement) ◆ Increase in medication (positive punishment) ◆ Loss of liberty (negative punishment)

Assessment measures

Questionnaires and measures should be used in conjunction with clinical interview to aid the assessment process and also to evaluate interventions. Apart from assessing mental health (see Ch. 4), some specific measures that are useful include:

◆ Sexual Fantasy Questionnaire (Wilson 1978)
◆ Reactions to Provocation Scale (Novaco 1990)
◆ Situations–Reactions Hostility Inventory (Blackburn & Lee-Evans 1985)
◆ Internal–External Scale (Rotter 1966).

Formulation

Formulation usually takes between two and three sessions to complete. The main purpose of formulation is to reach a shared understanding of people's difficulties and functions served by their offending. Collaboration in this process facilitates ownership and will aid engagement when there is more focus on intervening. More basically, clients will often have some idea

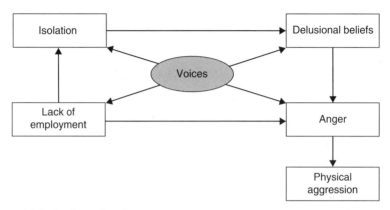

Figure 14.1 A relationship chart.

of how their difficulties relate to each other, and an understanding of the development of, and reasons for, their offending. As discussed earlier (see Ch. 13), a relationship diagram (Fig. 14.1) is a useful tool for exploring these relationships, using either clients' mental health problems or their offending as a starting point.

Once this has been agreed with clients you can begin to identify which issues they feel are central to their understanding of their difficulties. It may happen that you as a worker will not share the same view as clients regarding the main influences on their offending behaviour or future risk. However, this is not entirely necessary; what is more important is that you both agree which problems are practical and productive to work on. Also, with sensitivity, your differences and reasons for these different viewpoints can be discussed.

Providing clients with a copy of the formulation is good practice and they can take this away with them and think about these potential relationships in their own time between sessions.

Interventions

As with the assessment procedure, intervention strategies have to be developed collaboratively. There is little point in getting straight in with a punishment schedule if the person does not agree with or own this process.

General interventions regarding severe mental health problems are outlined throughout this book (e.g. Ch. 9). We will therefore outline only strategies pertaining to offending issues and relate these where applicable.

Offending behaviour does not occur in a vacuum and there are multiple influences on this behaviour and therefore there are a number of levels where interventions can take place, including arousal, cognitive, behavioural, interpersonal and social.

Cognitive–behavioural strategies

Cognitive–behavioural and behavioural strategies have been successfully applied to a variety of offences, including sexual offending (Daniel 1987, Laws & O'Neil 1981). There are a number of techniques available including:

1. **Stimulus control** The initial assessment should highlight some triggers to offending. Avoidance of these could be the first step to reduce the person's risk of committing future offences. Therefore, until a full assessment of the function of behaviours has been completed, it could be agreed that behaviours will be managed in this way in the interim.

2. **Problem-solving strategies** A person's offending behaviour may relate to a particular problem (e.g. financial or interpersonal). Hence a person's risk of offending may be reduced through coaching in the skills of problem solving, including:

◆ identifying when problems arise
◆ generating alternative behaviours/strategies
◆ identifying steps to reach an alternative goal (e.g. getting money legally).

You can work with clients on generated solutions to problems, pre-empting triggers, predicting what is likely to happen in a high risk situation and role playing with them until they feel more confident that they have gained some of these skills.

3. **Response cost strategies** This involves working with clients on identifying the consequences of their actions and has much in common with the problem-solving approach above. It is helpful to work from the standpoint of: the person not only has to reduce the risk of reoffending but must be seen to be doing this. For example, people with a history of sexually offending may be working extremely well identifying the triggers and consequences of their offending; however, they could live with a family that included children or close to a school.

4. **Offending behaviour chains** Any offence is a sequence of behaviours – for example, from the planning stage to making off after the event. Work can be done on identifying this sequence and developing ways of disrupting it. This can be completed for a single type of offence or a range of offences.

5. **Social skills and assertion training** Training should focus on verbal and non-verbal cues and behaviours. It should be comprehensive enough to include a variety of adaptive behaviours that a person can employ when circumstances and situations alter – for example, communication skills, anger management (see Ch. 13), problem-solving training and behavioural relaxation. A person may also benefit from more specific skills such as training in job interview skills.

6. **Working on identified cognitions** Those cognitions identified during

the assessment and formulation stages can be extended to using techniques such as diary keeping to enhance awareness of habitual or automatic thinking and its influence on behaviour. From this, patterns of high risk thinking and behaviours can be identified, for example:

◆ 'I feel lonely; I'll just go for a walk in the park' (sexual offending).
◆ 'This guy is taking me for granted; I'll sort him out' (violent offending).

There are a number of techniques available to alter cognitive distortions in sexual offenders. However, these are probably best addressed in a group setting where other difficulties can be explored – for example, victim empathy training and relationship problems (Epps 1996).

7. Taking responsibility for offending There are two main ways of working with clients' cognitions regarding their offending behaviour that may reduce the likelihood that they will continue offending:

◆ victim empathy awareness
◆ passive to active account of offending.

Victim empathy The literature on sexual offending has been instrumental in raising awareness of the role of victim blaming attitudes and cognitions and the part played by these in offending (Hildebran & Pithers 1989, Stermac & Segal 1990). Running through the offence(s) with clients and getting them to generate possible thoughts, feelings and experiences of their victim(s) is a way of raising awareness of the distress and damage caused by their actions. Even offences that are considered 'victimless', such as burglary or armed robbery, can be explored to highlight cognitions regarding the experiences of the victims and cognitions associated with offending – for example, 'no one gets hurt; it's the banks I'm taking from – they can afford it'.

Passive to active accounts Related to the above is the issue of passivity in clients' accounts of their offence. Moving the person from the notion of being a passive recipient to an active responsible participant is the goal of this intervention. Below are a few examples of passive and active accounts of sexual offending:

Passive: *'The kid sat on my lap. I tried to stop him.'*
Active: *'I asked him to sit on me. I was horny.'*
Passive: *'I started taking her blouse off and she never asked me to stop.'*
Active: *'She was so drunk I could do what I wanted.'*

In other words this is attempting to move from an external to an internal locus of control (Rotter 1966). This can be achieved by getting clients to talk through their offence(s) and recording those explanations and accounts that are passive.

8. Seemingly irrelevant (unimportant) decisions Offending involves a number of behaviours that result in the final act. The literature on sexual offending has been instrumental in highlighting those decisions in an offence chain that appear irrelevant to the offending behaviour. To understand this concept, consider the following:

Case example

A person who is attempting to abstain from alcohol is walking through the centre of town. He reaches in his pocket for his cigarettes and discovers that he has run out. He sees a pub in front of him and thinks 'I'll just nip in here and buy some cigarettes'. He goes in and discovers that he has no change for the machine. He buys a half pint of beer to get change. Once he finishes this half pint, he buys another pint, takes his newspaper and settles down to read it.

This person has made a number of decisions in order to get to the stage where he is drinking alcohol in the pub. Working from the standpoint that offending follows the same pattern of seemingly irreverent decisions/choices leading to the final act, targeting and changing these seems logical and essential to managing the risk of reoffending.

Challenging cognitions

On a one to one basis, direct challenging of cognitive distortions may be too confrontational if the timing is wrong. If this is the case (which is usually dependent upon experience and good supervision) getting clients to identify their own pro-offending attitudes and thoughts or working with the problems and contractions that people's own belief systems present them with may be a more productive strategy. Another strategy is following the chaining of how cognitions can lead to behaviours that have serious consequences for clients as they see it – for example, losing contact with family and friends.

CONCLUSIONS

This chapter has provided an outline to the issues faced when working with this client group. It is hoped that it has provided an introduction to stimulate further interest. The work is challenging; many clients have often committed very serious offences, which undoubtedly raises a number of professional as well as personal issues. We have stressed the importance of obtaining supervision, and working collaboratively with users, which includes not only agreeing problems and goals to focus on, but also working on the difficulties as the person sees them.

Summary of practical strategies identified

◆ Negative stigma may block therapeutic work, therefore always endeavour to work on the client's priorities rather than your own or the team's.

◆ Don't rush the assessment process; plan to take it over 3–4 sessions or longer if there is a range or number of offences.

◆ Work on the problems as the client sees them. Both parties should agree the goals and processes involved.

◆ Using a functional analysis helps to frame, understand and conceptualise patterns of offending behaviour.

◆ Utilise cognitive–behavioural interventions as these have been successfully applied within a variety of offences.

References

Allen J, Kingdon D 1998 Using cognitive behavioural interventions for people with acute psychosis. Mental Health Practice 1(9):14–21

Allyon T, Haughton S 1964 Modification of symptomatic verbal behaviour of mental patients. Behaviour Research and Therapy 2:305–312

Blackburn R 1993 The psychology of criminal conduct: theory, research and practice. Wiley, Chichester

Blackburn R 1996 Mentally disordered offenders. In: Hollin C R (ed) Working with offenders: psychological practice in offender rehabilitation. Wiley, Chichester, p 128

Blackburn R, Lee-Evans J M 1985 Reactions of primary and secondary psychopaths to anger-evoking situations. British Journal of Clinical Psychology 24:93–100

Burt M R 1980 Cultural myths and supports for rape. Journal of Personality and Social Psychology 38:217–230

Chadwick P, Birchwood M, Trower P (eds) 1996 Cognitive therapy for delusions, voices and paranoia. Wiley, Chichester

Côtè G, Hodgins S 1992 The prevalence of major mental disorders among homicide offenders. International Journal of Law and Psychiatry 15:89–99

Daniel C J 1987 Shame aversion therapy and social skills training in an indecent exposure. In: McGurk B J, Thornton D M, Williams M (eds) Applying psychology to imprisonment: theory and practice. HMSO, London, pp 245–254

Department of Health (1983) Mental Health Act. London, HMSO

Epps K 1996 Sex offenders. In: Hollin C R (ed) Working with offenders: psychological practice in offender rehabilitation. Wiley, Chichester, pp 150–187

Feldman P 1993 The psychology of crime. Cambridge University Press, Cambridge, p 172

References

Gresswell D M, Kruppa I 1994 Special demand of assessment in a secure setting: setting the scene. In: McMurran M, Hodge J (eds) The assessment of criminal behaviours of clients in secure settings. Jessica Kingsley, London, pp 35–52

Gunn J, Robertson G, Dell S, Way C 1978 Psychiatric aspects of imprisonment. Academic, London

Hall P, Brockington I F, Levings J, Murphy C 1993 A comparison of responses to the mentally ill in two communities. British Journal of Psychiatry 162:99–108

Hiday V A 1995 The social context of mental illness and violence. Journal of Health and Social Behaviour 36 (June):122–137

Hildebran D, Pithers W D 1989 Enhancing offender empathy for sexual abuse victims. In: Hildebran D, Laws R (eds) Relapse prevention with sex offenders. Guilford, New York, pp 236–243

Home Office 1990 Circular no. 66/90: provision for mentally disordered offenders. HMSO, London.

Johnson B, Martin M L, Guha M, Montgomery P 1997 The experience of thought-disordered individuals preceding an aggressive incident. Journal of Psychiatric and Mental Health Nursing 4:213–220

Junginger J 1995 Command hallucinations and the prediction of dangerousness. Psychiatric Services 46(9):911–914

Laws D R, O'Neil J A 1981 Variations on masturbatory conditioning. Behavioural Psychotherapy 9:111–136

Levey S, Howells K 1995 Dangerousness, unpredictability and the fear of people with schizophrenia. Journal of Forensic Psychiatry 6(1):19–39

McCord J 1990 Crime in moral and social contexts. The American Society of Criminology, 1989, presidential address. Criminology 28:1–26

McDonnell A A, Samsom D M 1992 Explanation and prediction in functional analysis: a reply to Jones and Owens. Behavioural Psychotherapy 20:41–43

Monahan J, Steadman H 1983 Crime and mental disorder: an epidemiological approach. In: Morris N, Tonrys M (eds) Crime and justice: an annual review of research. University of Chicago Press, Chicago, pp 1–19

Mulvey E P 1994 Assessing the link between mental illness and violence. Hospital and Community Psychiatry 45(7):663–668

Novaco R W 1990 Reactions to provocation. (NAS) Irvine, University of California

Owens R G, Jones R S P 1992 Extending the role of functional analysis in challenging behaviour. Behavioural Psychotherapy 20:45–46

Perkins D 1991 Clinical work with sex offenders in secure settings. In: Hollin C R, Howells K (eds) Clinical approaches to sex offenders and their victims. Wiley, Chichester, pp 151–179

Richards D, McDonald B 1990 Behavioural psychotherapy: a pocket book for nurses. Heinemann, Oxford

Ritchie J 1994 The report of the inquiry into the care and treatment of Christopher Clunis. HMSO, London

Rotter J B 1966 Generalised expectancies for internal versus external control of reinforcement. Psychological Monographs 80 (no. 609).

Samson D M, McDonnell A A 1990 Functional analysis and challenging behaviours. Behavioural Analysis 18:259–272

Shah A K 1993 An increase in violence among psychiatric inpatients: real or apparent? Medicine, Science and Law 33(3):227–230

References (cont'd)

Spry W B 1984 Schizophrenia and crime. In: Craft M, Craft A (eds) Mentally
abnormal offenders. Baillière Tindall, London
Stephenson G M 1992 The psychology of criminal justice. Blackwell,
Oxford, p 11
Stermac L E, Segal Z V 1989 Adult sexual contact with children: an
examination of cognitive factors. Behaviour Therapy 20:573–584
Sturmey P 1996 Functional analysis in clinical psychology. Wiley,
Chichester
Taylor P J, Hodgins S 1994 Violence and psychosis: critical timings. Criminal
Behaviour and Mental Health 4:267–289
Wessely S, Taylor P J 1991 Madness and crime: criminology versus
psychiatry. Criminal Behaviour and Mental Health 1:193–228
Wessely S, Buchanan A, Reed A, Cutting J, Everitt B, Garety P, Taylor P J
1993 Acting on delusions. I: prevalence. British Journal of Psychiatry
163:69–76
Wilson G 1978 The secrets of sexual fantasy. Dent, London

Annotated further reading

Blackburn R 1993 The psychology of criminal conduct theory, research and practice. Wiley, Chichester

Comprehensive coverage of mental health and psychological functioning in relation to offending.

McMurran M, Hodge J (eds) The assessment of criminal behaviours in secure settings. Jessica Kingsley, London

Provides an excellent coverage of assessment techniques and issues in relation to secure settings. Especially see Chapter 2: special demands of assessment in a secure setting.

Sturmey P 1996 Functional analysis in clinical psychology. Wiley, Chichester

Bolton D, Hill J 1996 Mind, meaning and mental disorder: the nature of causal explanations in psychology and psychiatry. Oxford University Press, Oxford

Excellent but extended philosophical discussion of causal explanations of behaviour including psychiatric diagnosis.

15

Chemical management of psychotic symptoms

*Geoff Brennan   Cliff Roberts   Catherine Gamble
TF Chan*

KEY ISSUES

- ◆ Neurochemistry and brain function.
- ◆ The role of neuropharmacology and antipsychotics in the treatment of schizophrenia.
- ◆ Typical and atypical antipsychotics.
- ◆ 'Real life' case study.

INTRODUCTION

Despite the fact that many innovative treatment strategies and interventions have been developed over the last few years, antipsychotic medication is still widely recognised to be the treatment of choice for persons with a psychotic illness (Lieberman 1993). User groups, however, have found that few clients receiving antipsychotics have been educated with regard to their medication (Rogers, Pilgrim & Lacey 1993). Practitioners (especially mental health nurses) are often placed in a difficult position as they are responsible for administration, monitoring, or prescribing medication without the confidence of a firm knowledge base (Jordan, Hardy & Coleman 1999). There is a need, then, for practitioners to be more aware of the effects, use and potential abuse of medication with regard to individual clients.

The aim of this chapter is not to produce experts in the complex subject of psychopharmacology, but it seeks to inform the reader about:

1. neurochemistry and brain function

2. the role of neuropharmacology and antipsychotics in the treatment of schizophrenia
3. areas such as the assessment of side-effects
4. eliciting clients' subjective experience of their medication via a worked example of a case study.

Although individuals with serious mental illness receive a wide range of medications to assist with additional issues such as depression, this chapter will predominantly explore medication used in the control of psychotic symptoms. The focus of discussion is, therefore, on the management of schizophrenia rather than any of the affective disorders.

UNDERSTANDING NEUROCHEMISTRY

To understand how antipsychotic medication works, we must first consider neurochemistry, the general workings of the brain and how chemicals affect it.

The brain functions owing to the specialised effects of *nerve cells* or *neurons*. The special nature of neurons means they are capable of interacting with each other. To signify this they are termed 'excitable cells'. Neurons normally have one *cell body*, from which an *axon* may give off many side branches or may terminate on a dendrite. This gives them the ability to communicate with thousands of other neurons. Consequently neurons tend to develop during embryological development into pathways or circuits. They conduct electrical impulses sometimes over long distances. Neurons 'communicate' by passing this electrical impulse from one cell to another. This is done by releasing *neurotransmitters* at their terminal. The gap between neurons, over which the neurotransmitter communicates its chemical message, is called the *synaptic cleft* or *synapse* (Fig. 15.1).

Neurotransmitters are selective in the message they transmit. Indeed, many different neurotransmitters carry out different functions. To imagine this, picture a household plug. It has one cable going in, but internally it is divided into three different but equally important sections: earth, neutral and live. Neurons are like this in that they rely on all the conditions being perfectly 'wired' before communication can take place. Therefore, in neurons, the impulse will be transmitted only through the 'right connection'. This means that a neurotransmitter needs to be released, move across the synapse and find an appropriate socket that is able to receive it. Neurotransmitters can only be received and interpreted by specific nerve circuits – that is, the nerve circuit must have a reciprocal receptor for the neurotransmitter.

Communication across the synaptic cleft results in information transfer. Information transfer in the brain is made up of two processes. First, as mentioned, the neurotransmitter is released into the synaptic cleft. (This is

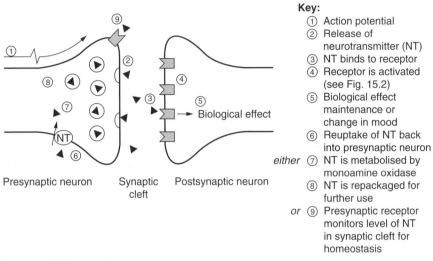

Key:
1. Action potential
2. Release of neurotransmitter (NT)
3. NT binds to receptor
4. Receptor is activated (see Fig. 15.2)
5. Biological effect maintenance or change in mood
6. Reuptake of NT back into presynaptic neuron

either 7. NT is metabolised by monoamine oxidase
8. NT is repackaged for further use

or 9. Presynaptic receptor monitors level of NT in synaptic cleft for homeostasis

Figure 15.1 Model of synaptic communication.

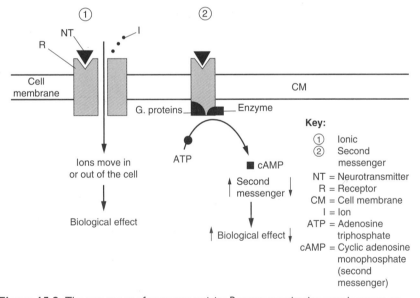

Key:
1. Ionic
2. Second messenger

NT = Neurotransmitter
R = Receptor
CM = Cell membrane
I = Ion
ATP = Adenosine triphosphate
cAMP = Cyclic adenosine monophosphate (second messenger)

Figure 15.2 The two types of receptor activity. Receptor activation may increase or decrease the turnover of cAMP, depending on the type of G-protein involved. This results in an increase or decrease of the biological effects respectively.

referred to as the *first messenger*.) Now this neurotransmitter binds with its specific receptor on the postsynaptic neuronal cell membrane. Intracellular processes or enzymes (referred to as the *second messenger*) are altered, which change the function of the postsynaptic neuron (Fig. 15.2). For the individual, this can result in a change in function such as a change of mood or alteration in level of alertness.

Another factor influencing communication across the synaptic cleft is what is happening in the cleft itself. We should not think of this gap as a vacuum, but as a constantly changing electrochemical environment. A neurotransmitter may enter the cleft but not connect to a receiver. This failure can be due to many of the receptors being occupied, or the environment destroying neurotransmitters before they reach their target. To complicate matters, the function of communication across the synaptic cleft can be to *inhibit* the receiving neuron. In other words, rather than excite the receiving neuron to pass on the message, synaptic communication can tell it to remain dormant.

So far, the brain is known to contain around 40 transmitters. There are probably more, but they have yet to be identified. The key neurotransmitters thought to influence mental health appear to be dopamine, serotonin and noradrenaline, as will be discussed below.

INFLUENCING NEUROTRANSMITTERS: THE PART HUMANS PLAY

So far the basic brain functions have been addressed. It has been possible to identify that the aforementioned transmitters can influence mood, mental health and emotions. Psychopharmacology is concerned with the controlled regulation of medication upon the chemical and electrical environment of an unpolluted brain. Yet, as highlighted in Chapter 12, practitioners work in an uncontrolled environment – that is the real world. Therefore, we also need to briefly consider the part humans play in influencing their own neurotransmitters and altering brain chemistry. Substances that are ingested and have a discernible effect on mood are termed *psychoactive*. For the majority of our clients, and indeed ourselves, licit psychoactive substances such as caffeine, nicotine and alcohol are used routinely and are an everyday fact of life.

Alcohol is probably the most recognisable; it induces well-being, promotes sleep and has *depressant* and *anxiolytic* properties. However, the effects of other chemicals on human behaviour have been known for thousands of years. Indeed, we need only to look at ancient civilisations to get an idea of how ingenious human beings are when it comes to finding mood-altering substances.

The Inca civilisation, for example, chewed leaves from the coca bush to improve performance and resilience. The use of the leaves, whose active substance is now taken as cocaine, spread through Europe via the Spaniards and Italians who returned from exploring South America. It became popular because of its ability to improve alertness, instil vigour, and reduce weakness and starvation. Its popularity increased when it was combined with alcohol and it became the panacea to relieve all aches and pains, often being added to medicinal liquids. In 1892 the Coca-Cola company was founded and the beverage for 'intellectuals' became widespread throughout Western society. Cocaine was eventually substituted by caffeine. Interestingly both cocaine and caffeine are stimulants; these substances are referred to as *psychostimulants* and their effect on mood can clearly be described by the user. Psychostimulants have a positive effect on mood because of their mechanism of action. They also affect the cardiovascular and autonomic nervous system, and chronic use is known to induce strokes or myocardial infarction in 20–30 year olds.

The peyote cactus *Lophophora williamsii* provides us with another interesting substance called mescaline. The Mexican Indians utilised extracts from this cactus in religious ceremonies. Mescaline belongs to a group of drugs known as *psychedelic*. These are 'mind-altering' substances, which are capable of inducing hallucinations, both auditory and visual. They include lysergic acid diethylamide, better known in this country as LSD. With this drug, experiences of being able to see sound are described and temporal changes are common, with seconds becoming minutes, hours or even months.

We can finish this examination of the diversity of substances and the ingenuity of the human mind to manipulate its environment by discussing the use of opiates. Writings dating back to 4000BC indicate the use of poppy extracts in areas of the Middle East. In the second century (and probably before that) Galen, a physician, utilised the pain-relieving properties of opium; in contrast to the psychostimulants it elicited a state of euphoria and calmness. In the early part of the nineteenth century morphine was extracted from opium. It wasn't until the mid nineteenth century that the syringe was invented, which in terms of the relief of pain was a godsend, but in terms of addiction was a demon. Heroin, a simple chemical manipulation of opium, was subsequently developed. It was able to pass into the brain more rapidly than morphine, thereby bringing faster pain relief. Heroin produces a 'rush', and this is probably why it has become a popular illicit drug.

The use of psychoactive chemicals in society, both licit and illicit, shows no sign of declining. Any substance that is psychoactive is liable to overuse or misuse and therefore very likely to be used as part of a coping strategy (Winger, Hofman & Woods 1992). It is perhaps, then, not surprising that many clients use psychoactive chemicals to deal with their experiences of life. Their use alters internal biochemical activity in the brain with the result that individuals' perception of their external environment changes. Problems do not go away but they do seem less significant, at least while the ingested chemical has its initial effect. Some users refer to their problems being smaller

Table 15.1 Groups of psychoactive substances

Drug	Effect on mood
Cocaine, caffeine	Psychostimulants: elevate mood, stimulate energy, improve alertness and instil vigour
Alcohol, opiates	Depressants: produce a state of euphoria and calmness
LSD, mescaline	Psychedelic (hallucinogens): 'mind-altering' substances that are capable of inducing hallucinations, both auditory and visual

or further away under the influence of drugs, like looking down a telescope the wrong way round.

There are many different groups of substances that are psychoactive. Before moving on it is helpful to reflect on the three groups discussed. These are listed in Table 15.1.

NEUROPHARMACOLOGY: ANTIPSYCHOTICS AND SCHIZOPHRENIA

The difference between inducing a change in mood and/or sensory experience by taking some of the psychoactive substance outlined above, and having it forced upon you through the presence of a mental illness, is immense. Most people consume chemicals for the short term feeling it gives. Individuals who have psychotic symptoms are in no way comparable as they are not in control of the experience and often suffer long term consequences. Most wish for the experiences and symptoms to stop.

Within pharmacology, the drugs that are designed to assist clients' psychotic symptoms are called *antipsychotics*. When neuropharmacists first began to examine how and why individuals suffered from psychotic symptoms, they thought that the neurotransmitter dopamine was responsible. Excessive dopamine transmission seemed to be a key to the individual experiencing symptoms. The researchers reasoned that controlling the dopamine levels should, therefore, alleviate these symptoms.

Antipsychotics act as an antagonist at dopamine receptors (see Fig. 15.3). This means that they significantly interfere with the binding of dopamine to dopamine receptors. This results in a reduction in postsynaptic activity. As the dopamine hypothesis indicates that dopamine transmission in schizophrenia is overactive, antagonists of dopamine transmission will reduce this hyperactivity, thereby reducing the florid symptoms of schizophrenia. There is a problem, however. We actually want to target specific areas of the brain with regard to reducing the levels of dopamine. This is not possible. Therefore, while we may

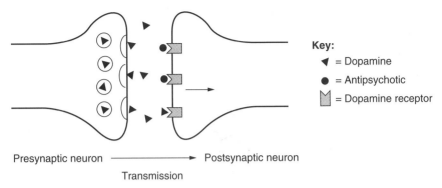

Key:
◀ = Dopamine
● = Antipsychotic
⬔ = Dopamine receptor

Presynaptic neuron ⟶ Postsynaptic neuron

Transmission

Figure 15.3 Antagonistic effects of antipsychotics at dopamine receptors. This is a simple diagram: antipsychotics produce their effects through interaction at dopamine and other receptors such as serotonin.

well get a positive result in one area of the brain, we may also induce a negative effect in another. It has been this non-specificity of antipsychotics that has led to the presence of side-effects. Also, dopamine transmission may increase or decrease transmission in other transmitter pathways.

Dopamine receptors are situated in central pathways of the brain containing high numbers of dopaminergic receptors (see Table 15.2). Antipsychotics have their effect on these pathways, and result in both *therapeutic effects* and *side-effects* (see Tables 15.2 and 15.3).

Table 15.2 Therapeutic effects and side-effects of antipsychotics

Tract	Pharmacological effects
Mesolimbic and mesocortical: which have fibres originating in the ventral tegmental area and spreading to the limbic system, frontal cortex and other regions	Therapeutic action of antipsychotics
Nigrostriatal tract: which has fibres projecting into the caudate nucleus, the putamen and the basal ganglia	Extrapyramidal side-effects such as: parkinsonism, acute dystonias, akathisia and tardive dyskinesia
Tuberoinfundibular tract: which has fibres originating in the arcuate nucleus of the hypothalamus and projecting to the median eminence (pituitary) (hypothalamic–pituitary axis, or HPA)	Endocrine side-effects such as: gynaecomastia (enlarged breasts), amenorrhoea (absence of menstruation), weight gain, lactorrhoea (milk production from breasts), impotence and false pregnancy tests

Table 15.3 Identifying side-effects and selecting an intervention

Side-effect	Description/definition	Action/intervention
Extrapyramidal symptoms Parkinsonism	Parkinsonian symptoms can be mimicked by antipsychotic antagonism of dopamine transmission. Akinesia (slowing of movement and expression), rigidity, tremor	Administration of anticholinergic drugs and close monitoring
Acute dystonias	Fixed upward or lateral gaze. Torsion dystonia and torticollis (muscle spasms, particularly neck) may occur	Systemic administration of anticholinergic drug will restore the balance between dopamine and acetylcholine
Acute dyskinesia	Involuntary movements of head and neck. These symptoms are possibly caused by an imbalance of dopamine and acetylcholine in favour of the latter	As for dystonias
Akathisia	Motor restlessness, agitation, dysphoria (bad feelings and thoughts), leg shifting and/or tapping of the feet	Propranolol
Tardive dyskinesia	Involuntary movements of orofacial and buccal–lingual muscles. Uncoordinated movements of upper and lower limbs. Tics, abnormal postures, grunting and vocalisations may occur	Conflicting management strategies. Discontinuation of antipsychotic by gradual withdrawal provides better prognosis than continuation. Introduce clozapine as antipsychotics are withdrawn
Antipsychotic malignant syndrome	Hyperpyrexia (increase in temperature), severe rigidity, tachycardia (rapid heart beat), fluctuating level of consciousness. Complications such as renal failure can develop	Discontinue all antipsychotics, administration of dantrolene, or dopamine agonists L-dopa, apomorphine or bromocriptine

Table 15.3 (cont'd)

Side-effect	Description/definition	Action/intervention
Anticholinergic effects	Delirium, dry mouth, blurred vision, tachycardia (rapid heart beat), paralytic ileus (paralysis of the small bowel), constipation, erectile dysfunction and urinary retention	Many patients will develop tolerance to some of these side-effects. If persistent and affecting quality of life, change to a more selective drug
α-adrenergic blockade	Orthostatic hypotension (positional fluctuations in blood pressure) and reflex tachycardia (rapid heart beat). Dizziness	During an acute episode lie the client down and elevate their legs. Advise to rise slowly; tolerance may develop to these side-effects
Antihistamine effect	Sedation	Can be beneficial, take medication at night if appropriate. Change to a more selective drug
Allergies	Jaundice, urticaria (rash), dermatitis, photosensitivity, optic neuritis, pigmentary retinopathy (visual changes in retina), agranulocytosis (lowering of white blood cells), aplastic anaemia (abnormally structured, non-functioning cells leading to blood disorder)	Careful monitoring of client for these symptoms is essential and discontinuation of the drug will be essential for a significant reaction

(**Note:** *In the following discussion there is reference to 'Parkinsonian symptoms'. While Parkinson's disease is caused by reduced levels of dopamine and the use of certain antipsychotics produces effects that mimic Parkinson's disease, they do not cause it. The side-effects are entirely drug induced and therefore reversible.*)

As more information began to emerge about the actions of neurotransmitters, the idea that dopamine alone could be responsible for psychotic symptoms became suspect. It was realised, for example, that more than one type of dopamine exists with, subsequently, different receptor subtypes. At the moment there are known to be at least five receptors, denoted by the letter 'D' followed by the subscript 1, 2, 3, 4 or 5 (i.e. D_1–D_5). Clinical potency of older antipsychotics such as chlorpromazine is due to their ability to antagonise the normal effects of dopamine at D_2 receptors. This action is supportive of the dopamine hypothesis of schizophrenia.

Newer antipsychotics have an antagonistic effect at both D_2 and receptors of the neurotransmitter serotonin (often represented by 5-HT). The inclusion of serotonin receptor antagonism achieves a therapeutic effect on negative symptoms in some individuals. Given the role of serotonin in psychotic experiences, we now consider that the dopamine hypothesis of schizophrenia is too simplistic. Discovery of the role of serotonin and the targeting of specific serotonin receptors, in addition to dopamine receptors, has enabled the development of drugs that give less side-effects as they are more specific in their actions. The 'older' drugs, which were developed to target dopamine alone, are called the 'typical antipsychotics'. The newer drugs, which are more specific in their targeting, are called the 'atypical antipsychotics'.

It is impossible at the present time to design an antipsychotic that will be therapeutic and have no side-effects. One of the major challenges for psychopharmacology remains the search for medications that give the maximum benefit, with regard to reducing symptom experience, with the minimum drawback, with regard to side-effects. It is obvious from the side-effects (Table 15.2) that many physical problems can be caused by medication. It is therefore essential that practitioners completely review clients' physical health. This is an area often neglected. Reviews should not be 'one-off' but a routine aspect of care.

Typical and atypical antipsychotics

As mentioned above, antipsychotic drugs can be subdivided into typical (older), and atypical (new). We should be careful not to think 'new' always means 'just developed' as some drugs have been around for some time now. Clozapine, for example, was first manufactured in 1962 (Healy 1997).

Typical antipsychotic drugs include:

◆ chlorpromazine
◆ trifluoperazine
◆ thioridazine
◆ haloperidol
◆ flupenthixol.

These drugs are sometimes also referred to by the name 'major tranquillisers'.

Typical antipsychotics are very good at treating the positive symptoms of schizophrenia but unfortunately induce side-effects in 75% of clients. This is due to the reasons cited above. Typical antipsychotic drugs are often prescribed on initial diagnosis of schizophrenia. If intolerable side-effects are experienced or there is no response to treatment an atypical antipsychotic drug may be the next choice.

Atypical antipsychotics include:

◆ amisulpride
◆ clozapine
◆ risperidone
◆ sertindole
◆ olanzapine
◆ quetiapine.

The atypical antipsychotics have less severe side-effects and are good at treating the positive and negative symptoms of schizophrenia. They are also of benefit in clients who do not respond to typical antipsychotics. Significantly, at low doses they produce a therapeutic effect without the suffering incurred by extrapyramidal symptoms (see Table 15.3). At higher doses extrapyramidal symptoms can be a problem. One serious drawback is that some atypicals (e.g. clozapine) can cause agranulocytosis; therefore careful haematological monitoring must be included in the care of these clients.

Atypical antipsychotics are much more expensive than typical anti-psychotics and this leads to a dilemma in terms of cost. Whilst the cost of antipsychotics is an important factor in the care of clients with schizophrenia, this has to be balanced against the savings made on the provision of inpatient and community care, not to mention the benefit to the client and carers of an improved quality of life.

The following case study has been devised to expand and explore further the issues raised. Issues such as compliance and polypharmacy are included within it.

 Case study – John

(This case study, unlike the others in this book, poses questions for the reader as well as providing information. This is meant to facilitate readers' thinking with regard to psychopharmacology. In order to explore as many areas as possible, 'John' is in fact an amalgamation of several real life histories rather than one specific client.)

Initial information *On coming into contact with services, John and his family relate the following history. John was born in Africa and emigrated to the UK at the age of 12 with his parents. He settled here well, attended school and went into full time employment following his A levels. Following his 20th birthday, however, John's family noticed subtle changes in his behaviour. The situation gradually deteriorated*

Case study – John (cont'd)

until the family could see that something was seriously wrong. John had begun to mix urine with cooking oil, and seemed to be deliberately incontinent and aggressive toward his mother. The family noted that John appeared to be 'having conversations with someone who is not there'. Occasionally John would also burst out laughing or shout obscenities for no apparent reason. His work performance deteriorated to the point where he lost his job.

Despite encouragement from his mother, John made no attempt to look for another job. At this time he began to lock himself in his room for long periods and could be heard to be talking, laughing and shouting when alone. The family also noticed John constantly wearing a baseball cap to 'keep people from reading my thoughts'. When family members attempted to talk to John about their concerns, he became verbally aggressive and smashed a window. At this point help was sought from his GP.

◆ What would be your initial thought if you were John's GP and asked to give an opinion on his case?

Whilst it is always difficult to be definitive about pinpointing diagnosis to specific illness, we can make an educated guess that John, as described, is suffering from some form of psychotic breakdown. With regard to symptoms, there is reported presence of thought interference and behaviour that is indicative of hallucinations.

The evidence would point to a tentative diagnosis of schizophrenia. The indicators here are not only the symptomatology, but also the fact that the family report the behaviours to have been apparent for some time now (see Ch. 4).

◆ What factors would you want to rule out as possible problems for John?

The main factor we should be aware of is the possible use of illicit drugs. As mentioned previously in this chapter, these can also cause an individual to present as John is described.

As the GP, you should also be concerned with regard to possible organic causes such as brain tumour, head injury, etc.

Case study

In this case, John was physically examined and a drug screen was carried out. All results were negative and both John and his family were clear that John had not used drugs and had not had any injuries or other signs of physical ill health.

◆ Do you think John's future prospects are good or poor? What factors contribute to possible outcomes?

It is difficult to predict how things will go for John as this is his first presentation. On the positive side, John's family appear to be supportive and caring. As discussed in Chapter 11, this is very significant. The fact that John has been able to work for several years prior to this breakdown is in his favour; it indicates a previous high level of functioning. The fact that John does not use drugs will also help him in his recovery.

Nevertheless, we should be concerned that John is a young man and that a prolonged bout of psychosis at this stage in his life could have a major impact. While there is no 'good time' to have a psychosis, John has not got a job or a stable relationship, both of which could help to maintain social functioning and self-esteem. The fact that there appear to be no precipitating factors would also cause us concern, as should the aggressive presentation of John's illness behaviour.

◆ Would you recommend a trial dose of antipsychotic medication?
◆ If John had been found to have had previous episodes of illness and been prescribed medication in the past, what aspects of this would you be interested in when considering the above?

The decision to administer antipsychotic medication should be made as a team. If we were in the GP's position, we should take advice from the local psychiatric services. If we were a practitioner in this service, the discussion should be taken at a multidisciplinary level.

It would seem, however, that antipsychotic medication is appropriate at this time as John has well-recognised psychotic symptoms. He appears to be a 'risk' in the sense that he has been aggressive towards members of his family. The choice of medication is determined by any previous response, tolerance to side-effects, compliance history, clinical presentation and sedation required. In this instance it would be justified to treat John with a low dose of an antipsychotic such as droperidol or haloperidol.

 Case study

John was eventually admitted into the hospital and was given an intramuscular injection of chlorpromazine. This caused him to become sedated and he slept. The next morning he could be aroused only with difficulty. When he attempted to stand up, he fell over. He looked pale, felt cold and, when checked, his blood pressure was very low.

◆ What may be causing John to present in this way and how would you help him?

Chlorpromazine is what is known as a 'dirty' drug. As well as affecting the receptors that may give some relief from psychotic symptoms, it also antagonises a wide range of other receptors. If we think of our previous analogy of the neurotransmitters being like electrical connections, it is as if we are turning off a light in a house by switching off the mains. This does indeed turn off the light, but it also affects many other connections. Blockage or closing down of the other receptors (α-adrenoceptors) causes side-effects such as hypothermia and hypotension.

To manage these adverse effects, John should be laid down with his feet raised and moved to a warm environment. His blood pressure should be closely monitored. His notes should *clearly* record his reaction to chlorpromazine.

◆ A locum psychiatrist reviews John's medication and feels he can receive regular chlorpromazine. Would you agree?

Absolutely not. It would be our duty to inform the psychiatrist of John's previous experience and draw his attention to the documented records. Even if the psychiatrist were to insist, it would also be our duty to advocate on John's behalf and facilitate a multidisciplinary discussion in an appropriate forum such as ward round or team meeting. In view of his previous response to chlorpromazine, a drug selected from a different chemical group is advisable.

 Case study

> *Haloperidol 5 mg was initiated and John's behaviour improved over the next few days. On day four of this medication regimen, John complained of a spasm sensation in his neck and his speech was slurred.*

◆ What might be the cause of this? How would you respond?

As mentioned earlier, most antipsychotics work by blocking the dopamine receptors (i.e. the neuron receptors sensitive to the neurotransmitter dopamine). We actually want to target this to areas of the brain known as the mesolimbic and mesocortical areas. Haloperidol is not this selective and also affects dopamine receptors in the nigrostriatal region. This gives rise to extrapyramidal side-effects (see Tables 15.2 and 15.3).

John is suffering what is known as an acute dystonic reaction, which is characterised by sustained muscle contractions, usually in the face, neck, mouth, tongue and occasionally the eyes. Dystonia is unpleasant, painful and extremely frightening.

This reaction can usually be resolved by the use of an anticholinergic drug such as procyclidine or orphenadrine. In an acute situation, parenteral anticholinergic may be required for rapid relief. Anticholinergics are not routinely prescribed these days as they too can have side-effects such as blurred vision, dry mouth, constipation and urinary infrequency. Another option is to change medication to the newer atypical antipsychotics in an attempt to reduce side-effects.

Case study

Eventually John is discharged home. His family continue to be supportive and John is allocated a skilled CPN. Despite this, his symptoms re-emerge after 2 months. His personal hygiene deteriorates and he again becomes incontinent. He now eats large amounts of food 'to feed the snake in my stomach'. His weight is now 20 stones. Eventually, despite the best efforts of his care team, he is readmitted. On readmission, it becomes apparent that he had discontinued with his medication shortly after discharge.

◆ What may have led to John's stopping his medication?

Non-compliance with medication is not isolated to the clients of mental health systems. In many areas of general health care, such as epilepsy and diabetes control, there are issues of people not being able or willing to comply with medication. Within mental health, it is thought that as much as 80% of clients become non-compliant (Corrigan, Liberman & Engel 1990).

There are many possible reasons for non-compliance. These include:

◆ lack of insight
◆ side-effects
◆ horrible taste of medication
◆ pain due to injection (if administered as a depot)
◆ cultural belief
◆ stigmatisation
◆ forgetfulness
◆ affordability.

◆ How could medication compliance be improved?

As you can see from the above, there can be a number of reasons for non-compliance. We would need to clarify with John which of the above, if any, are influencing his non-compliance.

Helping clients with their non-compliance has become a major focus of attention as it is a preventable cause of relapse. Accordingly, a regimen of therapy called compliance therapy has been devised (see Key principles of compliance therapy p. 284) (Kemp, Hayward & David 1997). Despite some criticisms (Perkins & Repper 1998) compliance therapy is broadening in appeal as it is being shown to have a positive effect on client outcomes and is based on cognitive psychoeducational principles. This is a broad subject, however, so it is not possible to do justice to it here. A summary of the key principles and phases of therapy with indications of input is shown at the end of this chapter.

Case study

John's symptoms settle down and now he is due to return home. He wants to avoid taking lots of medication but, after this second experience in hospital, both John and his family are keen to avoid another relapse.

◆ Concurrent use of medication is common. How would you respond if John was placed on more than one medication at a time?

Polypharmacy – that is, concurrent use of medication – is common, but *really* should be used only when necessary and with caution. The British National Formulary should always be consulted and the guidelines given in Box 15.1 (Taylor & Thomas 1997) used to monitor drug interaction.

◆ How would you propose to manage John's medication needs in the community?

After examining the options John agrees that a depot injection may be appropriate. When it comes to choosing which depot to use, there is very little choice, especially when trying to avoid side-effects. In general, flupenthixol decanoate (Depixol) is used with clients who are slightly depressed and withdrawn, whereas zuclopenthixol decanoate (Clopixol) has a calming effect, which will benefit agitated or aggressive clients.

◆ What is the purpose of a 'test dose' of depot injection?

This is used to test the acceptability to the client of the injection being administered. The test dose is usually small and the client is observed for side-effects. Very rarely, the oil vehicle used to suspend the drug can lead to systemic reactions (anaphylaxis).

◆ How could any actual or potential side-effects be monitored?

All practitioners should be prepared to undertake a systematic assessment of

Box 15.1 Guidelines for polypharmacy

1. Identify specific target symptoms for each drug use.
2. If possible, start with one drug and evaluate effectiveness before starting with another.
3. Be alert for adverse drug interactions.
4. Consider the effects of a second drug on the absorption and metabolism of the first drug.
5. Consider the possibility of additive side-effects.
6. Change the dose of only one drug at a time and evaluate the results.
7. Be aware of increased risk of medication errors and of increased cost of treatment.
8. Be aware of decreased client compliance in the aftercare setting when medication is complex.
9. In follow-up treatment, eliminate as many drugs as possible and establish the minimum effective dose of the drugs utilised.
10. Client education programmes regarding concomitant drug regimens must be clear, organised and effective.
11. Client follow-up contacts should be more frequent.

medication and its side-effects. The Abnormal Involuntary Movement Scale (AIMS) (Box 15.2) can help to detect tardive dyskinesia.

Clients themselves are also perfectly capable of monitoring for side-effects. A very useful self-rating scale is the LUNSERS Scale (Day et al 1995). It covers 51 side-effects, ten of which are red herrings, such as hair loss.

 Case study

Over the next 2 years John has three admissions to the hospital and the dose of zuclopenthixol decanoate has reached 1000 mg every 2 weeks. After this, it was felt that his mental state was little changed and LUNSERS and AIMS assessments identified distressing side-effects. He was transferred to a rehabilitation ward where it was decided to give him a trial of an atypical antipsychotic.

◆ Which atypical antipsychotic would you recommend? Give your reasons.

If a client fails to respond adequately to two conventional antipsychotics, at appropriate doses, for 6 weeks' duration each, then the patient is considered to be treatment refractory. Clozapine is the only antipsychotic to have been

Box 15.2 Abnormal Involuntary Movement Scale (AIMS)

Either before or after completing the examination procedure, observe the client unobtrusively at rest. The chair used for this experiment should be a hard firm one without arms.

Rate:

0----------------|----------------2----------------3----------------4
None   Minimal   Mild   Moderate   Severe

Ascertain from the client if there is anything in his/her mouth (if so ask them to remove it); ask them about their current dental condition – are dentures worn? Do teeth or dentures cause pain?

Do you experience any movement in your mouth, face, hands or feet? NO/YES – if yes, ask for a description. How much does it bother the client or interfere with activity?

Rate the client's movements whilst sitting on a chair with hands on knees, legs slightly apart, and feet flat on the floor.

0----------------|----------------2----------------3----------------4
None   Minimal   Mild   Moderate   Severe

Rate the client's movements whilst sitting on a chair with hands hanging unsupported (observe hands and other areas of the body)

0----------------|----------------2----------------3----------------4
None   Minimal   Mild   Moderate   Severe

Ask the client to open mouth (rate tongue in resting position)

0----------------|----------------2----------------3----------------4
None   Minimal   Mild   Moderate   Severe

Ask the client to protrude tongue (observe abnormalities of movement)

0----------------|----------------2----------------3----------------4
None   Minimal   Mild   Moderate   Severe

Ask the client to tap thumb with each finger as rapidly as possible – left and right (observe facial and leg movements)

0----------------|----------------2----------------3----------------4
None   Minimal   Mild   Moderate   Severe

Flex and extend the client's arms (one at a time)

0----------------|----------------2----------------3----------------4
None   Minimal   Mild   Moderate   Severe

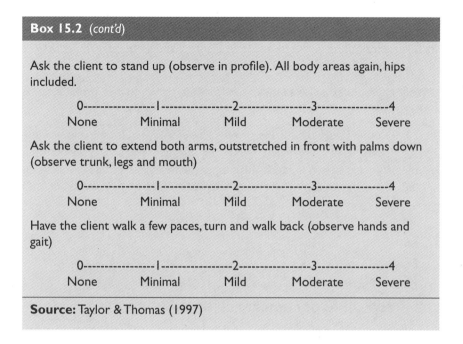

Box 15.2 *(cont'd)*

Ask the client to stand up (observe in profile). All body areas again, hips included.

0-----------------1-----------------2-----------------3-----------------4
None   Minimal   Mild   Moderate   Severe

Ask the client to extend both arms, outstretched in front with palms down (observe trunk, legs and mouth)

0-----------------1-----------------2-----------------3-----------------4
None   Minimal   Mild   Moderate   Severe

Have the client walk a few paces, turn and walk back (observe hands and gait)

0-----------------1-----------------2-----------------3-----------------4
None   Minimal   Mild   Moderate   Severe

Source: Taylor & Thomas (1997)

shown to be efficacious in treatment refractory patients. Therefore, clozapine offers John the best chance of relief from his symptoms.

◆ What side-effects would you anticipate and how would you help John to deal with this?

Clozapine is associated with a 1–3% risk of neutropenia, and haematological monitoring is a mandatory condition of treatment. John should be registered with the Clozaril Blood Monitoring Service and treatment should only proceed once the haematological results are green.

Other side-effects of clozapine are excess sedation, hypersalivation, postural hypotension, tachycardia, constipation, weight gain and seizure (usually after 600 mg/day). These side-effects are minimised if the dose of clozapine is titrated gradually upwards according to response.

Case study

John received drug A and his delusional ideas diminished substantially. He became pyrexial with a temperature of 38.2 °C and on examination he was found to have a chest infection. His full blood count showed a white cell count of 22 × 10⁹/L (reference = 4–10 × 10⁹/L) and his neutrophil count was 18.3 × 10⁹/L (reference = 2.2–7 × 10⁹/L).

◆ Should drug A be discontinued?

No, his neutrophil response to infection is intact and so the natural course of the infection will not be altered by clozapine.

◆ What alternatives are available if neutropenia proves to be a problem in the future?

There is no other antipsychotic with equivalent efficacy to clozapine at present. Other options that have been tried are augmentation of conventional neuroleptics with agents such as lithium, carbamazepine and a high dose of different depot injections. These regimens have little clinical evidence and use is often driven by desperation.

Key principles of compliance therapy

◆ Emphasis on personal choice and responsibility
◆ Non-blaming atmosphere
◆ Focus on eliciting the client's concern
◆ Express empathy
◆ Support self-efficacy

Phases of therapy

1. Elicit the patient's stance toward treatment:
◆ Review client's illness history
◆ Formulate client's stance toward treatment
◆ Link medication cessation to relapse
◆ Meet denial with gentle enquiry only
◆ Acknowledge negative treatment experiences

2. Explore ambivalence to treatment:
◆ Predict common misgivings about treatment
◆ Correct misconceptions
◆ Guide consideration of benefits and drawbacks of treatment
◆ Use metaphors, e.g. medication as a protective layer within stress vulnerability model
◆ Highlight indirect benefits of treatment
◆ Cautiously explore delusional resistance to medication

3. Work towards treatment maintenance:

◆ Encourage self-efficacy

◆ Medication as positive strategy to enhance quality of life

◆ Illness as a hand of cards life has dealt you

◆ Emphasise prevalence and well-known sufferers

◆ Analogy to physical illness needing long term maintenance treatment

◆ Predict consequences of stopping medication

◆ Identify characteristic prodromal symptoms

◆ Value of staying well to achieve goals

◆ Medication as insurance policy to stay well

Source: Adapted from Compliance therapy manual (Kemp, Hayward & David 1997)

CONCLUSIONS

There is now little doubt that chemicals produce their effects through acting on synaptic communication in the brain. Human beings have long been ingesting substances that can alter their mood and experience. It is not surprising that many licit and illicit psychoactive drugs are taken on a regular basis by clients suffering from schizophrenia in an attempt to alleviate symptoms. This brings into focus the relatively new issue of dual diagnosis, and the use of alcohol to relieve depression and other symptoms (see Ch. 12).

Psychopharmacology is concerned with finding medications that provide maximum benefit with regard to reducing symptoms with the minimum drawbacks with regard to side-effects. In reality, this is difficult. As the case study demonstrates, it is also individual and needs to be constantly assessed, from both a physical and a mental health remit.

Summary of practical strategies identified

◆ Medication treatment and management needs to be considered in the real world.

◆ In this real world, most people take some form of drug which is not regulated.

Summary of practical strategies identified (*cont'd*)

◆ Medication treatments need to be balanced in conjunction with feedback from client and carers.

◆ If medication is not effective it is best to consider a new medication rather than just increase the dose.

◆ All clients should have regular checks for side-effects.

◆ Good medication treatment is not simply about giving the medication, but about giving the client information to make an informed choice, listening and talking to them about their experiences with medication and acting on what they say.

◆ Medication, although important, is not the only treatment strategy.

◆ Mental Health pharmacists are an excellent source of professional advice.

◆ Professionals, clients and carers can call **020 7919 2999** 11am–5pm Monday to Friday for pharmacological advice from the UK Pharmacy Group.

References

Corrigan P W, Liberman R P, Engel J D 1990 From non-compliance to compliance in the treatment of schizophrenia. Hospital and Community Psychiatry 41:1203–1211

Day J, Wood G, Dewey M, Bentall R 1995 A self rating scale for measuring antipsychotic side effects. British Journal of Psychiatry 166: 650–653

Healy D 1997 Psychiatric drugs explained, 2nd edn. Mosby, London

Jordan S, Hardy B, Coleman M 1999 Medication management: an exploratory study of the role of community mental health nurses. Journal of Advanced Nursing 29(5):1068–1081

Kemp R, Hayward P, David A 1997 Compliance therapy manual. Maudsley Hospital, London

Lieberman J A 1993 Understanding the mechanism of action of atypical antipsychotic drugs. A review of compounds in use and development. British Journal of Psychiatry 163:7–18

Perkins R, Repper J 1998 Softly, softly. Mental Health Care 2(2):70

Rogers A, Pilgrim D, Lacey R 1993 Experiencing psychiatry: users' comments of services. Macmillan/Mind, London

Taylor D, Thomas B 1997 Psychopharmacology. In: Thomas B, Hardy S, Cutting P (eds) Stuart and Sundeen's principles and practices of mental health nursing. Mosby, London, pp 411–440

Winger G, Hofman F, Woods J 1992 A handbook on drug and alcohol abuse: the biomedical aspects. Oxford University Press, London

Annotated further reading

Day J, Bentall R P 1996 Neuroleptic medication and the psychosocial treatment of psychotic symptoms: some neglected issues. In: Haddock G, Slade P D (eds) Cognitive–behavioural interventions with psychotic disorders. Routledge, London, Ch. 12

For those who do not have a thorough understanding of psychopharmacology, this chapter presents a brief overview of the clinical literature on neuroleptics. It goes on to examine the adverse effects of medication and highlights the importance of learning from clients about their experiences of taking neuroleptics. Lastly, it draws together how neuroleptic medication and psychosocial interventions can work together to alleviate psychiatric disorders.

Healy B 1996 Psychiatric drugs explained, 2nd edn. Mosby-Wolfe, London

Do not be put off by the density of this book's text; its content is extremely useful and informative. It examines psychopharmacology and describes a range of problems for which neuroleptics are prescribed, such as schizophrenia, mania and anxiety disorders.

Taylor D, Thomas B 1997 Psychopharmacology. In: Thomas B, Hardy S, Cutting P (eds) Stuart and Sundeen's principles and practices of mental health nursing. Mosby-Wolfe, London, pp 411–440

This excellent chapter is focused towards nurses and their role in psychopharmacological treatments, such as assessing side-effects, providing education, promotion of adherence and the use of drugs in the control of behaviour. It also describes pharmacokinetics, problems of polypharmacy and drug interactions and contains some useful and clear diagrams.

Section 4

Considerations for effective practice

4

16

Serious mental illness: cross-cultural issues

Avie Luthra   Dinesh Bhugra

KEY ISSUES

◆ Culture shapes all aspects of our identity. In particular, culture affects how we see our own health and how we present to health services.

◆ In all cultures there is an interaction between an illness and its culture. This chapter examines depression and schizophrenia as examples.

◆ Epidemiology shows us the differences and similarities in incidence rates of schizophrenia across cultures. Significantly, outcome studies have shown a better outcome in developing rather than developed countries.

◆ Depression is more varied world-wide, with different cultures expressing different symptoms. Some studies have focused on defining this variability.

◆ When assessing a client from another culture it is important to take into account individual and general factors.

◆ Management of the client is complex. Planning should take into account the client's culture, the treatment setting and the family resources available.

◆ Physical treatments, psychotherapy and indigenous therapies are all possible options, but depend very much upon the treatment situation.

◆ Service provision is a key area for future development as it presents options for developing care tailored to the needs of specific ethnic minorities.

INTRODUCTION

Culture influences an individual's functioning in several ways. It defines the sick role and help seeking, and where individuals get support from. The role of culture is paramount in making diagnoses and planning treatments, especially if the patients and clinicians come from different backgrounds (Bhugra et al 1997a). As this volume deals with severe mental illness, this chapter highlights some of the key problems in diagnosing and managing these illnesses, illustrating some of the key points through describing schizophrenia and depressive illness.

WHAT IS CULTURE?

Culture refers to the many socially determined aspects of an individual's identity. It dictates not only the way people eat, sleep and function, but also how people think and behave. It forms values and beliefs. Understanding illness is very culturally dependent. By this, we mean it structures the way people perceive normal and abnormal health. It shapes how people appreciate the origins and mechanisms of illness, and how medical and psychiatric services are used and accessed.

The advantage of understanding a client's culture is not to explain away certain trends or behaviours as simply 'cultural'. Further understanding of 'culture' functions as the means by which the primary goal of better care can be achieved.

VARIATION OF ILLNESS ACROSS CULTURES

Studies have shown significant epidemiological differences across cultures (Sartorius et al 1983, World Health Organization 1973). Also, different generations of immigrant families have different levels of expressed illness within a given culture – so-called 'second generation' immigrants differ from the first generation (Bhugra et al 1998), and from refugees (Ager 1993). Each group therefore possesses its own characteristics that shape illness behaviour.

The following description of the research to date aims to discuss these differences, and their importance in the treatment and management of clients with serious mental illness.

Schizophrenia

One of the first key studies to ascertain whether schizophrenia exists across cultures, and what its symptomatology and outcome differences are, was the

International Pilot Study of Schizophrenia (IPSS) (WHO 1973). The main aim of the study was to establish whether such a study was possible across cultures.

Using nine centres around the world, WHO investigators were trained to a high level of inter-rater reliability. Several findings emerged highlighting cross-cultural differences. The key observation was that the core symptoms of schizophrenia (narrow definition schizophrenia S+, according to the CATEGO program of the Present State Examination) were broadly similar across cultures and the variation in rates was not very marked. The broad category of schizophrenia, on the other hand, showed marked differences – thereby suggesting that non-specific symptoms vary a lot. The outcomes at 2 years and 5 years were shown to be favourable in developing countries when compared with those in developed countries. The reasons for such a marked differential are many, and include family support, agricultural settings, low stigma, etc.

The second important study that looked at the incidence rates of schizophrenia and other social factors was the Determinants of Outcome of Severe Mental Disorder study (DOSMD) (Jablensky et al 1992). Having established the pattern in the IPSS, the WHO researchers then set out to study incidence rates in ten countries and 12 field centres (although, for purposes of carrying out incidence rates, Agra in North India, and Ibadan in Nigeria were excluded). The research instruments included PSE-9 (Wing, Cooper & Sartorius 1974), the Psychiatric and Personal History Schedule (PPHS), diagnostic and prognostic schedules and follow-up PPHS along with the Disability Assessment Schedule. In addition, some centres included additional substudies – for example, Expressed Emotion was measured in Chandigarh in North India, Aarhus and Rochester, and life events were measured in nine centres. Disability and impairment were assessed in six centres, and perceptions of illness in three centres. Not surprisingly, there were marked social–demographic differences across centres. Annual incidence rates for ages 15–54 varied from 0.7/10 000 population in Aarhus for narrow definition schizophrenia, to 1.4/10 000 in Nottingham. Rates of broad definition schizophrenia varied from 1.6 in Aarhus and Honolulu to 2.2 in Nottingham. By applying a uniform case definition and case-finding methodology, the study was able to demonstrate that there were no large differences in the manifestation rates of core schizophrenic disorders across cultures and geographical areas.

The WHO studies, however, have been criticised by Cohen (1992) as well as others. Cohen's key argument is · the emphasis by the researchers on similarities rather than differences – what the anthropologists would call the 'universalist view' rather than a relativist one. Better outcome in developing countries was shown to be the case and was attributed to low Expressed

Emotion, as shown in North India (Wig et al 1987). However, looking at differences across cultures can introduce a range of variables that may cloud the picture; hence it becomes important to study rates of schizophrenia in the same culture, but in different ethnic groups. From the early 1960s there have been several studies in the UK that have reported high rates of schizophrenia in African-Caribbeans when compared with whites or Asians. These differences have been startling (Leff 1988). Although some of the early studies had serious methodological flaws and sometimes relied on case note data, even the more recent methodologically sound studies have upheld these findings (Bhugra et al 1997c, Harrison et al 1988, Harrison et al 1997, King et al 1994). The finding that rates of schizophrenia among African-Caribbeans are much higher are robust and several possible explanations have been put forward (Harrison 1990). The rates of schizophrenia among Asians are not confirmed to be elevated. King et al (1994) reported that rates of all psychoses were raised among all migrant groups, although numbers in some of the groups were very small. Bhugra et al (1997c), on the other hand, found that overall rates of schizophrenia were not elevated among all Asians, but were so in the older females only.

The outcome of schizophrenia has been shown to be generally poor in African-Caribbeans, except in one study (McKenzie et al 1995). The reasons for poor outcome have been hypothesised to be poor compliance, poor experiences of psychiatric services, social and economic deprivation, etc. The answers on the long term follow-up are not yet fully clear, but what is apparent is that different ethnic groups have different outcomes.

Depression

Depression has been notoriously difficult to classify. Different theories of depression have yielded different approaches to 'low mood', producing different classification systems (Kendell 1976). There has been so much variability within specific Western cultures that it is easy to see why examining depression across cultures is fraught with difficulty.

The 'depression' equivalent of the WHO IPSS is a study performed by the WHO in 1983 (Sartorius et al 1983). This looked at depressive symptoms across five centres – Basle, Montreal, Nagasaki, Teheran and Tokyo. The study employed specific inclusion criteria and used a schedule that included an open-ended component for culture specific items. Overall, the most frequent symptoms seen were joylessness and sadness. Cultural differences included less suicidal ideas in Tokyo and Teheran, with more feelings of guilt and self-reproach in Basle and Montreal, and no psychotic depression recorded in Teheran.

Comparisons within countries are equally varied. The Indian subcontinent shows north and south differences in both prevalence rates and symptomatology

(Venkoba Rao 1987, Wig 1980). Biological features of depression such as sleep disturbance, low libido and poor appetite are more common in the south than in the north, where loss of energy, loss of confidence and low self-esteem are more prevalent (Singh 1979).

The colonial myth of low levels of depression within the 'happy savage' African population has been revealed for what it is (Rwegellera 1981, Wittkower 1969). Africa's complex mix of races and tribes, and the sheer size of the continent, opens the possibility of a wide range of presentations. A study from Ghana using the the same WHO schedule shows a similar symptom profile to the other countries (Majodina & Johnson 1983). Guilt and suicide have been reported to be low in Nigeria (Binite 1975), atypical presentations higher in Senegal (Colombb 1965) and hysterical symptoms more common in Zambia (Bhugra 1996).

Studies from the Middle East have been contradictory, and Far East studies reveal guilt to be as common amongst Japanese as amongst German Catholics (Bhugra 1996).

Finally, work in the UK shows differences between ethnic minority groups. African-Caribbean studies suggest first admission for affective disorders is slightly higher than in the white population (Hemsi 1967). This is more marked in the English-born rather than the Caribbean-born members of this group. Rates amongst Indians/Pakistanis are broadly similar to the white population. Correlates with depression in Asians include: length of time in the UK, speaking only another language, the experience of racial prejudice and the presence of children at home (Furnham & Li 1993). Refugees also suffer increased levels of depression when compared with the general population. The factors behind this have already been mentioned (Ager 1993).

Other conditions

Rates of bulimia are particularly high in Asian females, and this has been linked to severe emotional deprivation. Rates of alcohol abuse are low in Asians and African-Caribbeans. Subpopulations such as Sikhs, however, have a high reported rate of alcohol abuse (Bhugra 1998). Refugees have higher rates of post-traumatic stress disorder, which is linked to the experience of trauma (Ager 1993).

Having discussed the importance of culture to mental illness, we shall now look at both assessment and management of the cross-cultural client.

ASSESSMENT OF THE CROSS-CULTURAL CLIENT

The aim of assessment is to access the core of illness – that is, to peel away the layers of illness behaviour, and find the treatable centre. Those layers can be multiple and highly variable and are dependent upon both client and practitioner.

The factors considered are both individual factors and general cultural factors. These are not mutually exclusive categories, just a convenient way of dividing the processes involved in the assessment of the cross-cultural client.

Individual factors

Individual factors relate to the practitioner and to the client. Practitioners should be aware of their position, which is not only their cultural and racial backgrounds, but also their class, gender and professional roles. Identity is a shifting balance between these various elements, where at given times one aspect of identity is more relevant than another. Professional factors depend upon training and level of expertise. Important cultural factors include language and past experience of the other cultural group.

With respect to the patient, there are extra aspects to be considered. The practitioner observes not only the race/class/gender and culture of the client, but also the specific experiences, which can be very different from those of the practitioner – for example, racism, the process of seeking asylum, or linguistic difficulties. Appreciation of these can be tricky without direct first hand experience. A close relationship with the client is obviously highly beneficial, as is a good collaborative history. The family can often provide this history, acting as a rich source of cultural information (Bhugra 1997a).

General cultural factors

These factors are wider than the individual factors, but the two areas overlap.

'World view' is the means of understanding events and situations. It is a product of culture. North American world view is seen as individualistic rather than collaborative, focusing on self-actualisation and a linear interpretation of events. This generalisation is useful in providing practitioners with a background to the assumptions behind their own biomedical model – essential when treating clients from different cultures (Sue 1981).

It is also important to remember that cultures shift and change. A migrant culture such as Indian culture in the UK may be engaged in a process of acculturation, which differs from generation to generation. Their world view therefore shifts accordingly. Identity is chiselled through acculturation, and is shaped by family, peer groups, media and religion. The period since migration and the reasons behind migration are very important in shaping this process. As each patient's needs are so unique practitioners cannot expect to be experts in all these historical elements. Nevertheless, this broad principle should be kept in mind when working with the cross-cultural client.

The stigma attached to psychiatric illness depends very much on culture. This is one of the explanations put forward for somatisation, particularly within Asian culture. The expression of depression or anxiety as physical symptoms is less stigmatising in these cultures. Other explanations for somatisation exist. For instance that an internal psychological explanation of distress is an especially Western idiom, and non-Western cultures not based on such psychology prefer a physical model.

Non-verbal behaviour differs between cultures as much as language. Eye contact and gaze avoidance may seem appropriate in certain cultures, but threatening in others. The practitioner should always be aware of the power of such behavioural subtleties.

Finally, the standard mental state examination is open to much cultural shaping. The mental state examination investigates the signs and symptoms of the illness. Skills required include the non-verbal skills mentioned, interviewing skills and observation skills. Cultural points of view operate in all aspects: appearance and behaviours that seem unusual to the clinician may be of cultural significance; aggression and weeping are emotions especially sensitive to the client's cultural make-up; delusions and hallucinations are also very dependent upon culture. In the last, misinterpretation can have several cultural routes. It could be a result of language miscommunication, producing misclassification of given phenomena as the aforementioned. Or it could be the product of a lack of cultural knowledge. By definition, to understand a belief as delusional requires a knowledge of the mechanics of a culture. The explanation of an event as 'witchcraft' may be normal within Shona culture, but is likely to be delusional in the West. To rescue ideas from the cultural mist, the practitioner should draw from the well of information available surrounding the patient. This includes family, friends, but also voluntary groups, user groups and support groups. Recording the beliefs verbatim and relaying them to these experts in the patient's culture is the most effective method of preventing misclassification (Bhugra 1997a).

MANAGEMENT OF THE CROSS-CULTURAL CLIENT

The relationship between client and practitioner is the foundation of management. Trust has to be built for the client to follow mutual objectives towards therapeutic goals. Many of the cultural ingredients of this relationship have been discussed in the section dealing with assessment, and these carry through for management.

Migrant communities are heterogeneous in nature. Issues to do with access and treatment vary as much between generations as between migrant groups. This heterogeneity makes treatment plans more complex in this client group. Planning is essential, as failure to recognise this complexity can perpetuate a misunderstanding that destroys trust. Management plans should be context dependent – from inpatient, to outpatient, to community strategies. Therapeutic goals should be mutually understood within these contexts and, at a practical level, effort should be made to peel away specific cultural layers. For the practitioner this involves extra work – that is, finding interpreters and individuals to provide a cultural background and understanding details of cultural conflicts, ties and relationships. It should be remembered that any psychiatric assessment filtered through the perspective of a third party is fraught with difficulty. Third parties too close to the client (family or friends) can edit or sanitise for the ears of the professional. The converse – the use of interpreters unknown to the client – can bring out issues of sensitivity and confidentiality. It is easy to see why a client would not wish to reveal intimate personal information to a complete stranger for the purpose of translation (Bhugra 1997a).

The rest of this chapter will focus on three aspects of management: first, the use of physical treatments across cultures, secondly, the role of various therapies with the cross-cultural client and, thirdly, the special needs and services required by this client group.

Physical treatments

Physical treatments include pharmacological and electroconvulsive treatment (ECT). Perceptions of the use of medication generally, and the use of psychiatric medication specifically, are very much culturally bound. Beliefs in medication providing a quick response, poor communication of side-effects owing to linguistic barriers, and a lack of faith in the role of the practitioner per se, all contribute to poor compliance (Westermayer 1989).

Pharmacokinetics vary across cultures and races. This may be as much because of diet and social habits (smoking/drinking) as the physical make-up of the client. Specific examples abound (Bhugra 1997b): Asians and black patients have shown greater blood levels of neuroleptics per milligram than Caucasians. Asians develop extra pyramidal side-effects faster than do black or Caucasian patients. Asians have also less need for high doses of tricyclic antidepressants, as blood and peak levels are reached earlier. Lithium displays highly variable blood levels, even within a single ethnic group: Taiwanese blood levels are lower than Hong Kong patients, which are lower than Chinese.

ECT is a controversial therapy. This controversy lies not in its effectiveness

– which is undoubtedly proven – but in the negative image it carries. This applies very much cross-culturally, and much effort should be made to explain the value and importance of this treatment. Evidence that ECT is given more frequently to African-Caribbeans, and the stereotype of it being an oppressive treatment, can only do damage to the trust between practitioner and this client group. Good communication is one means of overcoming such cultural barriers to a potentially life-saving treatment (Westermayer 1989).

Specific therapies

Among the specific therapies we shall look at psychotherapies and indigenous therapies.

Individual psychotherapy is very culturally biased. Western therapy has been described as ego dependent, and so can be at odds with cultures where the individual functions as an extension of a social or family unit. Such psychotherapies are not necessarily ineffective outside of Western cultural groups. An initial assessment can be useful in defining the needs of the client, and whether or not psychotherapy will be effective.

Examining the specific therapies, psychoanalysis is the most obviously culturally specific. The Oedipal complex, and concept of the id, ego and superego, all have clear European roots. Also the processes of counter-transference and transference can be imbued with elements shaped by racism or language, adding a complexity when used cross-culturally that is not present with European clients.

Conversely, behavioural therapy is very adaptable cross-culturally. This is due to the practical nature of this therapy – it requires little interpreter time, the therapy is specific and the results are clear. Cognitive therapy is also potentially beneficial, but remains to be tested cross-culturally (Sue 1981).

Finally, intercultural therapy has been developed as a means of tackling these issues. Nasfiyat in North London is a good example of this. It is based on the psychoanalytical approach, and it involves challenging assumptions and assessing the patient's experience. The work deals with issues of race and the social consequences of racism, allowing discussion with both white and black therapists. A therapist of the same cultural or racial origin is not an essential element of the treatment, as therapeutic skills depend largely on the therapist. But for discussion of areas of sensitivity, such as racism, it is seen as beneficial. Thomas (1995) reports a 90% 'good outcome' from such therapy with a marked improvement in General Health Questionnaire (GHQ) score (Thomas 1995).

The use of indigenous therapies seems an appropriate way of bridging the cultural divide. This means drawing upon psychotherapies available in given cultures, and adapting them to the Western context. Such adaptation can be very difficult as it is full of possible misinterpretation and dilution of the original effective treatment. For example, Ayurvedic or Tibetan treatments of mental illness, which involve not only diet and herbal remedies but also a specific cultural–religious belief system, would require much reinventing to be transposed effectively to a Western city. Many reports exist, however, of specific therapies that have been adapted. Hatha yoga, meditation and acupuncture are widely available treatments for stress – though mainly as Western adaptations for predominately Western clients. Other effective examples of adaptation include cuento therapy in Puerto Rican children in New York, and Japanese morita therapy in other parts of America (Fernando 1991). The fact that cross-cultural clients use a number of religious and non-medical healers, alongside Western doctors, shows the desire for several therapists. This remains fertile ground for development in the management of such patients.

Service provision

Service provision for cross-cultural clients with mental health needs is an area of much discussion. The aim is to provide specialised services for ethnic minorities based on their specialised needs. This involves setting up services de novo, and modification of pre-existent services. Bhugra (1997b) proposes an approach that emphasises clients' explanation of their symptoms, taking the focus away from psychiatric diagnosis. This approach should be the starting point for action and development.

This is of value in all aspects of psychiatric care: inpatient, respite and long term. Input from members of the community, non-statutory agencies and advocacy services belonging to a given cultural group is valuable. This approach also applies to forensic and liaison services, where ethnic minorities are overrepresented in particular ways.

A final mention needs to be made of user groups and non-statutory agencies. The user movement has a variable influence on psychiatric practice worldwide. It is particularly significant in Japan and America, where it broadens the scope of psychiatric care. Though there is no national user group for black people in the UK, individual agencies at a local level provide valuable input. If the practitioner is to develop a service for a client, then listening to that client's voice is crucial (Sassoon & Lindow 1995).

The same applies to voluntary agencies attached to the care of ethnic minorities. In London these include the Chinese Mental Health Association, the Brixton Circle, and the African-Caribbean Mental Health Association. These agencies meet needs that cannot be met by statutory mental health services. Their position is both advantageous and unstable – the former because of their autonomy, the latter because of the variability of their funding.

Collaboration between the statutory and voluntary sectors has been patchy, and how they fit together has yet to be determined. However, the grassroots perspective supplied by voluntary groups is invaluable to the practitioner providing care for the cross-cultural client (Ahmed & Webb-Johnson 1995).

CONCLUSIONS

In this chapter we have discussed the key aspects of serious mental illness in the cross-cultural client. Culture is relevant to all illness behaviour and it clothes disease with different presentations. Not only does this 'clothing' vary with different cultures, but so too does the disease itself. These cultural differences have been discussed for schizophrenia and depression particularly.

In order to get beyond the covering provided by culture, practitioners must have an understanding of the basics of assessment. This involves being aware of their position relative to the patient. Individual and general cultural factors operate with the cross-cultural client. These include differences in world view, and changes in cultural identity, stigma and somatisation. The standard mental state must also be scrutinised if it is to be used appropriately.

Management of all clients involves planning and trust. These aspects are even more important in this group. The practitioner has to work hard to unpack the complexity provided by culture. This involves an awareness of how physical treatments and psychotherapies vary across cultures, and trying to adapt therapies for the client. A service for the cross-cultural client will be provided only if needs are assessed and measured, and then catered for. This means listening to the clients closely and using as many organisations as possible in the client's care – that is, voluntary groups and user groups.

References

Ager A 1993 Mental health issues in refugee population: a review. Project on international mental and behavioural health. Harvard Medical School, Department of Social Medicine

Ahmed T, Webb-Johnson A 1995 Voluntary groups. In: Fernando S (ed) Mental health in a multi-ethnic society. Routledge, New York, pp 74–88

Bhugra D 1996 Depression across cultures. Primary Care Psychiatry 2:155–165

Bhugra D, Bhui K 1997a Cross-cultural psychiatric assessment. Advances in Psychiatric Treatment 3:103–110

Bhugra D, Bhui K 1997b Clinical management of patients across cultures. Advances in Psychiatric Treatment 3:233–239

Bhugra D, Bhui K 1998 Transcultural psychiatry: do problems persist in the second generation? Hospital Medicine 59(2):126–129

References (cont'd)

Bhugra D, Leff J, Mallett R, Der G et al 1997c Incidence and outcome of schizophrenia in whites, African-Caribbeans and Asians in London. Psychological Medicine 27(4):791–798

Binite A 1975 A factor analysis study of depression across cultures. British Journal of Psychiatry 127:559–563

Cohen A 1992 Prognosis for schizophrenia in the third world. Culture, Medicine and Psychiatry 16:53–75

Colombb H 1965 Assistance psychiatrique en Afrique: experience Senegalaise. Psychopathologie Africaine 1:11

Fernando S 1991 Mental health, race and culture. Macmillan, London

Furnham A, Li Y H 1993 Gender, generational and social support correlates of mental health in Asian immigrants. International Journal of Social Psychiatry 39:22–33

Harrison G 1990 Searching for the causes of schizophrenia: the role of migrant studies. Schizophrenia Bulletin 16(4):663–671

Harrison G, Owens D, Holton A, Neilson D, Boot D 1988 A prospective study of severe mental disorder in Afro-Caribbean patients. Psychological Medicine 18(3):643–657

Harrison G, Glazebrook C, Brewin J et al 1997 Increased incidence of psychotic disorders in migrants from the Caribbean to the United Kingdom. Psychological Medicine 27(4):799–806

Hemsi L K 1967 Psychiatric morbidity of West Indian immigrants. Social Psychiatry 2:95–100

Jablensky A, Sartorius N, Emberg G et al 1992 Schizophrenia: manifestations, incidence and course in different cultures. A World Health Organization 10 country study. Psychological Medicine Monograph (suppl 20)

Kendell R 1976 The classifications of depressions: a review of contemporary confusion. British Journal of Psychiatry 129:15–29

King M, Coker E, Leavey G, Hoare A, Johnson-Sabine E 1994 Incidence of psychotic illness in London. British Medical Journal 309:1115–1119

Leff J 1988 Psychiatry around the globe: a transcultural view. Gaskell/Royal College of Psychiatrists, London

McKenzie K, Van-Os J, Fahy T, Jones P 1995 Psychosis with good prognosis in Afro-Caribbean people now living in the United Kingdom. British Medical Journal 311 (Nov. 18):1325–1328

Majodina M Z, Johnson A F W 1983 Standardised assessment of depressive disorder in Ghana. British Journal of Psychiatry 143:442–446

Rwegellera G G C 1981 Cultural aspects of depressive illness. Psychopathologie Africaine, 17:41–63

Sartorius N, Davidson H, Ernberg G et al 1983 Depressive disorders in different cultures. WHO, Geneva

Sassoon M, Lindow V 1995 Consulting and expanding black mental health system users. In: Fernando S (ed) Mental health in a multi-ethnic society. Routledge, New York, pp 89–106

Singh G 1979 Depression in India: a cross-cultural perspective. Indian Journal of Psychiatry 21:235

Sue D W 1981 Counselling the culturally different. Theory and method. Wiley, New York

Thomas L 1995 Psychotherapy in the context of race and culture. In: Fernando S (ed) Mental health in a multi-ethnic society. Routledge, New York, pp 172–192

References (cont'd)

Venkoba Rao A 1987 Depressive disease. ICMR, New Delhi

Westermayer J 1989 Psychiatric care of migrants: a clinical guide. APA, Washington DC

Wig N N 1980 Depressive illness in North India. In: Venkoba Rao A, Parvathi S (eds) Depressive illness. A V Rao, Madurai

Wig N N, Menon D K, Bedi H et al 1987 Expressed emotion and schizophrenia in north India. Distribution of expressed emotion components among relatives of schizophrenic patients in Aarhus and Chandigarh. British Journal of Psychiatry 151:160–165

Wing J K, Cooper J E, Sartorius N 1974 Measurement and classification of psychiatric symptoms. Cambridge University Press, London

Wittkower E D 1969 Perspectives in transcultural psychiatry. International Journal of Psychiatry 8:811–824

World Health Organization 1973 Report of the International Pilot Study of Schizophrenia, vol 1. WHO, Geneva

Annotated further reading

Bhugra D, Bahl V (eds) 1999 Ethnicity: an agenda for mental health. Gaskell, London

This book covers a range of theoretical and clinical issues on diagnosis and management across different ethnic groups.

Okpaku S O (ed) 1998 Clinical methods in transcultural psychiatry. APA, Washington, DC

From across the Atlantic this book provides an overview of diagnostic and clinical management issues and education and training for different ethnic groups in the USA.

Vaccaro J V, Clark G H (eds) 1996 Practicing psychiatry in the community. APA, Washington, DC

This book covers a range of clinical issues in community mental health. It is aimed at multidisciplinary teams.

17

Ethical considerations

Paula Morrison

KEY ISSUES

◆ Ethical decision making.
◆ Ethical theory: consequentialism, deontology, professional codes.
◆ Autonomy.
◆ Consent.
◆ Confidentiality.
◆ Non-maleficence and beneficence.
◆ Developing ethical practice.

Ethics (which contains the morality of decision making) is often perceived as the exclusive domain of philosophical thinkers and those who are searching for the 'meaning of life'. In truth, everyone wrestles with ethical decision making on a daily basis. All of us are faced with decisions and their consequences. All of us have to find answers to decisions such as: 'Should I buy this product as it pollutes the environment?', 'Should I take that job in the private sector?' or 'Should I drive my car or take public transport?'

Doubts and anxieties when faced with decisions can often make us uncomfortable. This is often compounded in professional practice as mental health care and treatment may, at times, infringe human freedom and dignity. Yet doubts and anxieties should not be feared but celebrated within our work, as it is from the subsequent reflection and analysis that ethical decisions are often made and practice enhanced.

So, what exactly *is* ethics? In a nutshell, ethics can be defined as the rightness or wrongness of human actions.

This chapter will introduce the reader to some of the main ethical theories.

It will discuss principles that stem from those theories, which need to be developed by individual practitioners. Developing ethical decision-making skills is a lifetime challenge and this chapter will highlight only some of the issues. The reader may find they have more questions than answers by the end of the chapter. As Barker & Davidson (1998) point out: 'ethics as a state of being involves confronting our childlike self who is constantly looking for absolute answers'. Since life rarely has absolute answers we find ourselves facing many dilemmas in practice.

ETHICAL THEORY

Beauchamp & Childress (1989) state that a well-developed ethical theory provides a framework of principles within which a person can determine moral actions. The two types of ethical theory most cited to inform clinical practice are consequentialist theory and deontological (derived from the Greek word 'deon' meaning 'duty') theory.

1. Consequentialism

This is the moral theory that actions are right or wrong according to their consequences rather than to any features they may have, such as telling the truth. The most prominent consequentialist theory is that of utilitarianism. David Hume (1711–1776), Jeremy Bentham (1748–1832) and John Stuart Mill (1806–1873) are most connected to this theory. Utilitarianism is often described in lay terms as 'the end justifies the means' and that we must 'promote the greatest good of the greatest number'. Alternately, we could say that 'what is right is what is the most useful'.

An example of utilitarian thinking would be that to achieve the greatest benefit from mental health resources these resources should be targeted at serious mental illness. This act would be justified under utilitarianism if it produces more good than any other action. However, those who require services but who are not seen as seriously mentally ill may feel that this targeting means they lose out as individuals. There are many debates regarding targeting in the NHS with people trying to decide what is the most moral way of apportioning resources to achieve the greatest benefit. The decisions are difficult and controversy often follows because particular groups often feel excluded. The ethical dilemma in Box 17.1 illustrates this.

2. Deontological

By contrast to consequentialist theory, deontological theories hold that some features of an act make it right or wrong for reasons other than its

---

Box 17.1 Ethical dilemma 1

You are employed by a large GP practice as an autonomous mental health professional. On assessing the case histories you realise that you can deal with all clients diagnosed with psychotic illness *or* all clients with obsessive compulsive disorders, but do not have the resources for both.

How would you decide who receives your service and who does not? What factors would influence this decision?

---

consequences. For many deontologists, deception is wrong independently of its consequences. An example of this would be giving a patient a placebo without their knowledge. Deontological thinking would suggest that this is a non-moral act because deception is involved. Immanuel Kant (1734–1804) is regarded as the first deontologist.

The need for guidance with regard to what is right or wrong is often crucial within this framework. Some writers in religious traditions appeal to divine revelation, for example, the Ten Commandments, whereas others appeal to Natural Law, which they believe can be known by human reason. For example, the Nuremburg Trials held that the holocaust was against Natural Law. The defence of 'obeying orders', given by those who carried out mass executions, was seen as indefensible because human reason would know that this was wrong and against humanity. In other words, the Natural Law was seen to be higher than any law of the land.

The ethical dilemma in Box 17.2 illustrates this.

One of the most prominent deontological theories in recent philosophy has been Rawls' Theory of Justice (1972). Rawls (1972) argued for the following principles of justice:

Box 17.2 Ethical dilemma 2

Let us say that you have specialist skills in a certain area of mental health care. A person comes to you who would benefit from your skills, but you know that this person is in an experimental control group and that to give active treatment would affect the research.

Do you see it as your duty to treat this person, or do you consider it your duty to support the research, which may help all people with this particular health issue? How do you decide this?

---

1. the principle of equal liberty
2. the difference principle, which permits inequality in the distribution of social and economic goods *only* if those inequalities will benefit everyone, especially the least advantaged
3. the principle of fair equality of opportunity.

Rawls' theory has led to the development of equal opportunities as we see them today.

PROFESSIONAL CODES

Together with these ethical theories, public policy, formal guidelines and codes of professional ethics, such as those developed by the United Kingdom Central Council for Nursing (UKCC 1992a, b, 1996, 1998), have been developed in an attempt to introduce guides to ethical practice. However, Beauchamp & Childress (1989) argue that one of the major defects in contemporary theory in ethics is that it is distanced from clinical practice. They state that some professional codes oversimplify moral requirements or claim more completeness than they are entitled to. As a consequence, professionals may think that they have satisfied all moral requirements if they have simply followed the rules of the code.

It is therefore essential for clinical practitioners to develop their understanding of ethical theory and how to apply this in their practice. This goes well beyond the requirements of professional ethical codes.

Ethics in care involves:

◆ obtaining relevant factual information
◆ assessing its reliability
◆ identifying moral problems and mapping out alternative solutions to problems that have been identified.

This mapping entails presenting and defending reasons in support of one's decisions, while at the same time analysing and assessing one's basic assumptions and commitments (Beauchamp & Childress, 1989) – for example, the assumption that people should be kept alive at all costs versus the commitment of a carer to relieving pain, which may also hasten death.

ETHICAL PRINCIPLES IN PRACTICE

As stated earlier, certain principles derived from ethical theory need to be developed in practice in order to care for people in a moral and human way. These principles are: respect for autonomy, non-maleficence and beneficence.

I. Principle of respect for autonomy

People are assumed to be self-determining, self-governing individuals who use reason and choice in their lives. This is described as 'autonomy' and professional ethics promote the idea of ensuring that people's autonomy is respected. Seedhouse (1988) describes autonomy as: 'a person's capacity to choose freely for himself, and to be able to direct his own life'.

This is sometimes questioned when applied to people with mental health problems as temporary constraints imposed on thinking owing to the illness can lead to diminished autonomy. However, even if someone has been determined as legally incompetent they may still be able to make autonomous decisions such as the right to refuse to see relatives or to permit any clinical information being given to carers.

Promoting client independence and autonomy and seeing this as a prerequisite to any care provided is *essential* in mental health care practice. This recognises a person's capacities to make choices and take action based on personal values and beliefs. Promoting autonomy also includes enabling people to act autonomously to the best of their capacity. But what does this mean in reality? Kohner (1996) argues that if we respect the idea of autonomy this would demand that the following imperatives are followed:

◆ discussing any proposed treatment and care with the client
◆ being aware of power inequalities in the professional/client relationship
◆ determining the client's priorities and needs
◆ communication and sharing of knowledge
◆ listening
◆ honesty
◆ confidentiality
◆ dignity and respect for the client and the client's situation
◆ consent.

Conflicts often arise because clients competently refuse treatment that professionals think would be of benefit, or some clients act autonomously, placing themselves or others at risk. Determining mental capacity for autonomous decision making in combination with risk assessment is therefore a skill to be developed. This has been addressed in previous chapters (see Chs 4 and 7).

Respecting the autonomy of others beside the client also needs consideration. Gillon (1994) describes respect for autonomy as: 'the moral obligation to respect the autonomy of others in so far as such respect is compatible with equal respect for the autonomy of all those potentially affected'. This is a difficult area in mental health where conflicts often arise between respecting both clients' and their families' autonomy. For example, clients may refuse to permit information about their illness to be disclosed to family members, even though the family members are affected by the illness but are none the less expected to carry on caring without any information. The balancing of need and duty in this situation is itself an ethical dilemma (see Ch. 11).

Consent

There are certain responsibilities in regard to obtaining consent that need to be followed in order for the autonomy of any client to be respected (Barker and Baldwin 1991, UKCC 1998):

1. that competence for consent is present
2. that information is disclosed and that the information is understood
3. that the consent is given voluntarily
4. that authorisation is given by the person to consent to treatment.

Assessing whether a client is competent depends on whether the client can understand and retain treatment information and can weigh it up to make an informed decision. This assessment of competence is an integral part of mental state examination, although rarely specified (see Ch. 4).

Assumptions are often made about the capacity to consent for those people with a serious mental illness. These assumptions detract from the autonomy of individuals. An example would be that clients are often given large doses of neuroleptic medication without the necessary information on side-effects or long term consequences. For this reason, consideration should be given to using trained advocates to assist clients in decision-making processes in order to protect their autonomy. This will be particularly important when clients' first language is not English or when they have other communication difficulties. Clear plans should exist on how these difficulties can be overcome such as using an interpreter.

Confidentiality

Confidentiality is another cornerstone of respecting client autonomy, which is generally accepted by professionals but widely ignored in practice. Consider what clients would think about the fact that sometimes over 20 people may see their clinical records. Clients may expect more rigorous standards and therefore the limits of confidentiality should be explained and reasons given for when that confidentiality will be broken. It is also important to explain the need to disclose to others in the team and what that entails. It is also generally accepted in mental health that confidentiality should be broken only in certain circumstances. Beauchamp & Childress (1989) state that breaking confidentiality should happen only when a higher obligation needs to be followed, such as to adhere to the law or to protect the client or the public.

2. The principles of non-maleficence and beneficence

Non-maleficence

The principle of non-maleficence is the maxim 'that above all do no harm' or 'one ought not to inflict evil or harm'. This is interpreted by Johsen, Siegler & Winslade (1986) as the moral requirement of health professionals:

◆ to strive to serve the well-being of their clients
◆ to promote standards of due care
◆ to carry out risk–benefit assessments that focus on risks of harm and determine detriment–benefit assessments that focus on the harms that occur at the time of procedure or benefit (see Ch. 7).

When considering 'doing no harm', omitting care is of prime importance. Many negligence claims are for *omissions* of treatment that subsequently caused harm. For instance, many public inquiries into crimes committed by people with mental health problems living in the community have stated omissions of care as one of the main reasons for the incidents happening.

Beneficence

The principle of beneficence proposes an obligation to help others to further their important values, beliefs and interests. It requires the provision of benefits and the balancing of benefits and harms. Therefore, promoting the welfare of clients, not merely avoiding harm, is the goal of health care (Beauchamp & Childress 1989).

However, beneficence confronts limited resources and controversies abound on policy decisions that limit beneficence. For example, three people need psychosocial interventions; however there are only two places, so how will the decision be made to be beneficent to all three clients?

When considering beneficence in mental health it is important to consider paternalism also. For instance, suppose that a client was suicidal and was deemed unable to make a reasoned decision on treatment. Professionals often act beneficently by protecting clients against the potentially harmful consequences of their own actions (e.g. not allowing the person to commit suicide) thus limiting clients' autonomy and acting paternalistically. The accepted wisdom on how to decide to act in a paternalistic fashion is accepted by professionals if:

◆ a client is at risk of injury or illness

◆ the risks of the paternalistic action to the patient are not substantial
◆ the benefits outweigh the risks
◆ there is no alternative to the paternalistic action
◆ infringement to autonomy is minimal.

DEVELOPING PRACTICE

Understanding the stress and vulnerability of a person's situation and insight into the ethical consequences of decisions made on behalf of the person is the prime development need for mental health care providers. Lutzen, Evertzon & Nordin (1997) have named this 'moral sensitivity'.

Moral sensitivity and the relationship with the client underlies all other mental health knowledge. Mental health practice in its widest sense as well as everyday interactions between clients and practitioners are in fact ethical; they happen in an environment of disproportionate power, especially that of the interpersonal relationship when the illness occurs (Pellegrino & Thomasma 1993). Clients rely on practitioners to make decisions that are in agreement with their value systems. The clinician, however, has the authority in some instances to make decisions for the client that may not always agree with the latter's value system (see Ch. 18).

Although trust is central in professional ethics, as well as being a basic ingredient in a therapeutic relationship, it can be either exploited or forfeited if patients do not understand or agree with decisions that are made on their behalf (Pellegrino & Thomasma 1993). Another characteristic of mental health ethics is the unpredictability and emergency of situations that can arise. There is no highway code of rules to adhere to; however, there are principles and guidelines such as those already discussed that clinicians can use to help in developing their ethical decision-making skills.

Lutzen, Evertzon & Nordin (1997) state that this sensitivity can be developed through the following means:

◆ building a trusting relationship
◆ reflection on finding moral reasons for actions
◆ expressing beneficence – doing good
◆ knowing when to limit autonomy and understanding why limits are imposed
◆ experience of ethical dilemmas
◆ confidence in clinical knowledge.

Many clinicians rarely have opportunities to reflect on their experiences from an ethical viewpoint. Formulating and debating the specifically moral questions raised by particular experiences can help clinicians develop their awareness of the moral dimension of their everyday practice, their confidence in addressing ethical issues and their ability to think in ethical terms (Kohner 1996).

Opportunities to reflect on and discuss experiences of ethical difficulty can be created formally or informally within a work setting. Using Johns (1993) model of structured reflection, for example, will guide practitioners through clinical experiences, their consequences, alternative approaches and the learning that has occurred. Debriefing sessions, case reviews, ward rounds, clinical supervision and CPA reviews already exist and can be used to discuss ethical issues, thus making the issues live, real and related to practice. Although classroom approaches can be useful to discuss philosophical theory and offer distance from the clinical area, which can be useful to reflect on what Kohner (1996) calls the moral maze of practice, it is in the practice arena where the biggest difference will be felt by clients.

It is also important to create opportunities to reflect on and discuss the ordinary events of practice, which are frequently ignored because of their ordinariness but which raise significant ethical issues. Clinical supervision, based on reflection and closely related to practice, offers an appropriate means of developing ethical thinking in a more sustained way around everyday events. Carlisle (1997) reports on a study carried out by Tower Hamlets Community Trust that showed 77% of all care providers experienced one or more ethical problems a week at work, with 93% of these discussing these with colleagues. The most commonly cited problems were client rights, client autonomy, treatment decisions, resource allocation, client competence, confidentiality and client quality of life. The Trust has now set up ethics discussion groups in practice in order to develop an ethical culture where ethics is part of everyday work.

CONCLUSIONS

Everyone in clinical practice wrestles with ethical decision making on a daily basis, which challenges us on choices of decisions and their consequences. Being able to walk a path through this decision making is a foundation stone for effective clinical practice in mental health. Everyday realities will produce ethical dilemmas. This chapter can be used to introduce clients and practitioners to ethical theory, principles of ethics and approaches to developing practice in ethical decision making so that more 'moral' or more 'right' decisions can be attempted.

References

Barker P J, Baldwin S (eds) 1991 Ethical issues in mental health. Chapman & Hall, London

Barker P J, Davidson B 1998 Psychiatric nursing – ethical strife. Arnold, London

Beauchamp T L, Childress J F 1989 Principles of biomedical ethics, 3rd edn. Oxford University Press, Oxford

Carlisle D 1997 Moral maze. Health Service Journal 3 April: 26–27

Gillon R 1994 Medical ethics: four principles plus attention to scope. British Medical Journal 309:184–188

Johns C 1993 Professional supervision. Journal of Nursing Management 1(1):9–18

Johsen A R, Siegler M, Winslade W J 1986 Clinical ethics, 2nd edn. Macmillan, New York

Kohner N 1996 The moral maze of practice – a stimulus for reflection and discussion. King's Fund, London

Lutzen K, Evertzon M, Nordin C 1997 Moral sensitivity in psychiatric practice. Nursing Ethics 4(6):472–482

Pellegrino E D, Thomasma D C 1993 The virtues in medical practice. Oxford University Press, Oxford

Rawls J 1972 A theory of justice. Oxford University Press, Oxford

Seedhouse D 1988 Ethics. The heart of health care. Wiley, Chichester

UKCC 1996 Guidelines for professional practice. United Kingdom Central Council for Nursing, Midwifery and Health Visiting, London

UKCC 1998 Guidelines for mental health and learning disabilities nursing. United Kingdom Central Council for Nursing, Midwifery and Health Visiting, London

UKCC 1992a Code of conduct for the nurse, midwife and health visitor. United Kingdom Central Council for Nursing, Midwifery and Health Visiting, London

UKCC 1992b The scope of professional practice. United Kingdom Central Council for Nursing, Midwifery and Health Visiting, London

Annotated further reading

Kohner N 1996 The moral maze of practice – a stimulus for reflection and discussion. King's Fund, London

Nurses, midwives and nurses and health visitors tell stories of their experiences of ethical difficulty in their everyday practice. The stories are offered as material for reflection, with suggested discussion points and commentary on four themes accepting and respecting the individuality and autonomy of the client/patient, the nurse/patient/client relationship, the nurse/family relationship and the role and responsibility of the nurse.

Annotated further reading (*cont'd*)

Beauchamp T L, Childress J F 1989 Principles of biomedical ethics, 3rd edn. Oxford University Press, Oxford

This book provides a thorough introduction to ethical theory for health professionals. Its practical purpose is a systematic analysis of the ethical principles that apply to biomedicine.

Barker P J, Davidson B (eds) 1998 Ethical strife – psychiatric nursing. Arnold, London

This book explores the philosophical background to ethical dilemmas, the individual strategies that they generate for practitioners and some of the ideological conflicts in mental health care.

Barker P J, Baldwin S (eds) 1991 Ethical issues in mental health. Chapman & Hall, London

This book explores some of the key ethical issues affecting mental health workers. An emphasis has been placed on autonomy, therapeutic ideologies, treatment and therapy in relation to people with mental illness, learning difficulties and ageing.

18

Professional considerations

Sharon Dennis

KEY ISSUES

◆ Practitioners create conditions for user empowerment.
◆ Personal sense of professional responsibility.
◆ Clear organisational structures to support and develop staff.
◆ Open communication and partnership working.

INTRODUCTION

Practitioners have an overriding professional responsibility which underpins the use of any treatment strategy. In order to implement identified interventions and achieve the best outcomes for clients, it is clear that practitioners must maintain their own health, be appropriately prepared and feel supported by the system within which they work.

This chapter aims to examine possible psychological and physical barriers to effective implementation of treatment and considers the implications for individual practitioners, teams, managers and organisations. As the author is a mental health nurse the examples used will mainly come from a nursing perspective. However, as all mental health professionals are required to adhere to policies and procedures laid down by organisations and their own codes of conduct, the outlined principles and experiences generally apply to all disciplines.

STRESS AND THE PRACTITIONER

There are many groups who contribute to mental health care. However, a recent review of staff roles has identified similarities between the skills of the various professionals (Duggan et al 1997). Irrespective of the discipline to which staff belong, the stressful nature of mental health work has long been recognised (Harper 1997). Working with people who are experiencing severe mental illness has rewards, but there are times, especially in today's underresourced mental health services, when these can be obscured by the many demands on the practitioner.

Having to cancel an appointment with a client in order to release the time to see another as a crisis has arisen is not unusual. The stress of responding to the original call is compounded with the stress of missing the appointment. In reality the situation creates difficulty for everyone concerned: the practitioners are under stress due to the unexpected change and apprehension about new priorities; the original clients because their needs may be undervalued and the emergency clients because those coming to deal with their issue are already stressed and possibly resentful of the situation.

For some practitioners the above is the norm rather than the exception. These workers are placed under stress by the systems they work within. The physical and psychological effects of too much stress are described as: anxiety, agitation, insomnia, irritability, low motivation, anger, frustration, poor concentration and difficulties in decision making (Thomas 1997). Associated with these symptoms are: lack of fulfilment at work or enjoyment in social activities, increased absenteeism, domestic conflict and increased caffeine, alcohol, drug or tobacco intake. Long term stress may also lead to burnout. Subsequently, those on the receiving end may experience a distant practitioner who avoids contact and lacks empathy. Although Figure 18.1 shows that there is a fine line between optimum performance and overload, many practitioners report symptoms of burnout described within the right hand side of the curve.

TEAMS AND STRESS

You have possibly observed the symptoms listed above in yourself and your colleagues at one time or another. Those of us who have had the privilege of working in a supportive team will know that it is possible to overcome these symptoms by: disseminating work responsibilities; taking time out; or discussing the prevailing issues and evaluating our interventions via group, peer or individual supervision. Those who do not have access to such systems

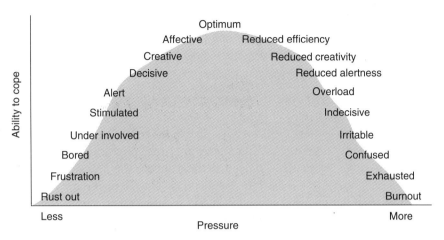

Figure 18.1 The pressure curve.

may find these symptoms further exacerbated if some members of a team decide to try and incorporate a new style of working (e.g. using psychosocial interventions) when other members do not understand or want to work in the same manner.

Interdisciplinary working is usually described in positive tones; the opportunity for clients to receive care influenced – and possibly provided – by many different professions is thought to improve the quality and diversity of the care offered. However, for this aim to be achieved many considerations have to addressed.

Considerations to be addressed

1. Understanding each other's roles

It is evident that most professional groups are ignorant of the skills base of their colleagues and the contribution they make to client care (Gijbels 1995). One way to address this issue would be to introduce interdisciplinary education (Jackson 1994). In addition, an explicit expression of the skills professionals contribute (including the philosophy underpinning these competencies) to everyday practice would go some way to reducing misconceptions and difficulties borne out of ignorance.

2. Power of professional groups

Price & Mullarkey (1996) suggest mental health nurses exercise three types of power:

- **expert**: by virtue of the role
- **legitimate**: as employees with certain responsibilities
- **referent**: as a result of identification (and self-disclosure) with the service user.

In spite of having this power, nurses sometimes feel they cannot access it due to working practices, roles of others, or structures within organisations. One advocated way to address this is to draw up explicit contracts with clients and promote greater information sharing with other professionals (Price & Mullarkey 1996, Sully 1996). Indeed if this concept was transferred to all professionals, there would be less likelihood of one group becoming more powerful than another and more likelihood of cooperation. An example of contracting within teams might be a psychologist contracted (either formally within the organisation or informally between the workers themselves) to provide supervision. This occurrence is usually due to the supervisor being perceived as having a skill that can penetrate team boundaries. Other examples of creative use of skills include pharmacists attending multidisciplinary review meetings with a clear remit to advise on medication.

Medical staff in particular are viewed as having 'expert' traditional power that is greater than other groups. The perceived power of the medic can be a double-edged sword as the psychiatrist may be cast in the role of arbitrator between, or decision maker for, the rest of the team. Either way, there is a potential that other professionals will envy this level of influence, which can lead to status conflicts and non-cooperation. Consequently, it is possible that either clients' needs are not appropriately addressed or imaginative care packages are 'watered down' to ensure the sensibilities of all professionals remain intact.

3. Negotiating between professionals

This is a complex process. Some clinical work has to be carried out by particular professionals whereas other responsibilities can be shared. Delegation of shared work may produce conflict between team members. Individuals may not participate if they feel undervalued or excluded and have not had the opportunity to air their views. In such situations, the ability to summarise one's views succinctly and appreciate the views and position of other team members is crucial, because every team member deliberates before volunteering support and cooperation. Common language and clear communication between professionals is the key to cooperative working practices. For example:

In addition to feeling valued, another influencing factor in accepting work is agreeing to take on roles that fit professional orientation (an occupational

Case example

A practitioner informally visits a client who is restless and pacing about. The practitioner thinks this could be a side-effect of the medication, so asks the doctor to review it. The request is perceived as a low priority because no other information is provided and so an outpatient appointment is arranged for 3 months' time. Consequently the practitioner feels her contribution has been ignored. Another practitioner is in agreement with the first. However, in this case they both meet the client formally and review the symptoms in depth. A full standardised assessment is completed. When reporting the evidence, they are able to stipulate that the inner restlessness and pacing that the client is experiencing is akathisia – a very unpleasant side-effect of medication and not anxiety based. The information is succinct and is presented in a language that the doctor understands. Subsequently, it is valued and perceived as a high priority. The client is seen by the doctor the next day and her antipsychotic medication is changed.

therapist carrying out an assessment of daily living activities, for example). Another influence is having the skills required. If the client needs cognitive–behavioural therapy a practitioner with these skills would feel prepared to take them on, irrespective of their original professional training.

4. Roles and clinical responsibilities

Practitioners are always aware of the demands of their current case load and need to review this when considering taking on more work as this may affect the quality of care they are providing. Responsibilities such as research, teaching, supervision or managerial duties will need to be balanced with clinical commitments. Such reviews are particularly important if practitioners intend to develop their role and commence on intensive, clinical programmes of study. Indeed, those with large case load sizes and staff/patient ratios in the workplace have been found to struggle and in some instances dropped out (Gamble 1997).

From all above points it is possible to conclude that, for stress in individuals and conflict within teams to be reduced, a number of components would need to be considered (Box 18.1).

DEVELOPING LINKS WITH USERS AND OTHER AGENCIES

Statutory mental health work is complemented by informal carers, the voluntary

---

Box 18.1 Stress reduction pointers

◆ Team members feel valued and able to identify with and exhibit loyalty to the team rather than their own discipline.

◆ Members openly acknowledge and are confident of each other's skills.

◆ Members recognise and support blurring and overlapping of roles.

◆ Team is freely able to discuss general management issues, their own group dynamics as well as the cases they are dealing with.

◆ Clients are allocated depending on their needs and the skills of the practitioner.

Source: Adapted from Headley & Moore (1996)

---

sector and other statutory agencies such as primary health care, housing and hostel workers. Professionals are becoming increasingly aware of the need to develop links with and spend time supporting the many groups whose services clients value highly.

User groups and the antipsychiatry movement have helped to influence professionals by highlighting the lack of power users have over their own care, treatment and self-determination. However, a power discrepancy remains. Practitioners are: aware of what services are available and have access to them, are privy to discussions that take place without the client, and have all the information contained in medical records at their disposal. Therefore, to dissipate power it is essential that information and choice on the pros and cons of each treatment option is provided. In addition, alternatives should also be supplied to facilitate informed decision making and empowerment. Access to independent advocacy services may be required to start to redress the power balance. Achieving a balance of power relies on a practitioner's willingness to create the conditions in which the service user can act autonomously.

On a macro level, consulting with user and carer organisations enhances advocacy. Professionals have the responsibility of developing consultancy mechanisms that allow users' and carers' views to be canvassed. They need to be imaginative and systematic in gathering information particularly when targeting users who do not join organisations, such as user groups. Therefore practitioners should be aiming for an equilibrium, as illustrated in position one of the 'power see-saw' (Fig. 18.2). However, Sully (1996) suggests that professionals who attempt to provide conditions where service users are empowered may encounter conflict from others who feel challenged by the service user exercising control. It is possible that positions two and three (in

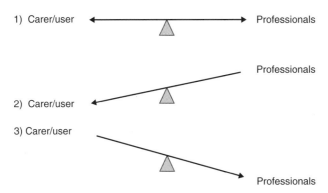

Figure 18.2 The 'power see-saw'.

Fig. 18.2) will occur. In these positions, one party exercises power over the other. Professional power has already been discussed, but in scenario three there is a likelihood that the carer and client may opt out as professionals are not perceived to have anything to offer.

BALANCING OBJECTIVITY WITH EMPATHY

Objectivity is required for practitioners to weigh the complex issues presented when considering personal freedom versus the safety of all. The level of involvement of the practitioner with the service user is one that needs to be considered. The presence of empathy is essential for the establishment and maintenance of a therapeutic relationship (see Ch. 8).

Balancing empathy with objectivity produces the correct level of practitioner involvement – that is, professional distance. This provides clarity by conveying to users that the practitioners' interest in them is one of a professional providing a service. Therefore the setting, maintaining and sometimes restating of boundaries is crucial in balancing appropriate intimacy with professionalism. Empathy, compassion, attachment and transference are related concepts (Kadner 1994) and link to intimacy, which involves trust, closeness, self-disclosure and reciprocity. However, being continually empathetic can be stressful, especially when practitioners are not able to achieve high standards of care (Brown et al 1994). In such circumstances, the danger for staff is that negative feelings borne from feeling helpless, transference or not being able to achieve negotiated goals (Watts & Morgan 1994) may lead to them to fail to engage with clients or afford them with the warmth and empathy they deserve. Pilette, Berck & Achber (1995) write: 'Nurses voluntarily and repeatedly subject themselves as witnesses to the pain and suffering of others'. If this continues with no resolution a further distancing from service users will occur (Brown et al 1994). Indeed, the nature of the work with this client group is usually slow and can lead to frustration (Watts & Morgan 1994). In these circumstances there is a need for staff to reflect together, and regular, skilfully facilitated 'awaydays' that provide space for team members to raise these concerns must be a part of any agenda.

LOOKING AFTER OURSELVES

Careful management, support and guidance for practitioners is crucial in facilitating the continuance of quality care. Therefore, one of the additional methods to address the aforementioned is clinical supervision. This is important, because it is an 'exchange between practising professionals to enable the development of professional skills' (Butterworth 1992). Clinical supervsion has been recommended by professional bodies such as the UKCC (1996) as a valuable means to reduce stress. In addition to developing professional skills, it can produce outcomes such as decreased staff sickness, lower stress and enhanced risk management (UKCC 1996). Robust research that supports these claims is currently unavailable, as reviews have tended to concentrate on the implementation of clinical supervision systems (Bulmer 1997, Butterworth 1997).

Barker (1992) writes: 'Supervision in psychiatric nursing has two main aims: to protect people in care from nurses and protect nurses from themselves'. From this, supervision can be seen as a monitoring process that aims to safeguard the client as well as support the practitioner. Barker's (1992) definition describes the latter two of the three stages of the clinical supervision. These are referred to as: formative/educative, normative/quality control and restorative/supportive (Everitt, Bradshaw & Butterworth 1996, Faugier 1994). Depending on their needs, balanced supervision occurs when practitioners have access to all three aspects (Table 18.1).

Table 18.1 Supervision

Aspects of supervision	Components
Formative/educative	◆ Learning new skills ◆ Consolidation of skills ◆ Learning through reflection
Normative/quality control	◆ Maintaining standards of care ◆ Auditing and evaluating practice ◆ Adhering to policies, procedures and professional guidelines
Restorative/supportive	◆ Dealing with stress ◆ Offloading ◆ Recharging batteries

Farrington (1995) reminds us that there are four elements present in clinical supervision: the supervisor, supervisee, client and work context. This means that the supervision process will always be dynamic and unique.

THE SUPPORTIVE ORGANISATION

A supportive organisation is one in which the views of staff and service users are taken into account. These have established appropriate, clear structures and procedures that enhance the effectiveness of the practitioner. Workplace issues must be reviewed regularly in light of new developments and consequently addressed to support individuals (Thomas 1997). This is underlined by the Department of Health (1998), which has set standards in relation to promoting the health and welfare of its workforce in recognition of the need to 'care for the carer'. Professionals must have access to supportive mechanisms which allow them to alleviate stress, take into account personal issues and allow them to develop.

MANAGERIAL CONSIDERATIONS

Working in teams can be a supportive and nurturing experience. Managers have an important role to play to ensure these conditions are created. They need to provide innovative, clear, uncomplicated structures and be able to recognise and subsequently utilise the skills of practitioners (Kanter 1988). Recent reviews of those who have undertaken the Thorn psychosocial interventions course, for example, have shown that they have found it difficult to implement the skills they have learned (Jackson 1998). Managers who second staff for any type of skills-based training need to consider the implications fully (time required per case versus overall case load, for example). Engaging in a dialogue with trainers and practitioners would help them to review the team's culture and orientation, thus enabling newly trained practitioners to deliver and implement care using their new skills.

Balancing a managerial role with working in a team is a must. The need to work independently and yet in conjunction with others is a fine balance that is learned over time. To be effective, managers must demonstrate openness with staff concerns as this contributes to staff cooperation and early identification of problems. Individual staff members have a duty to report instances when they are unable to carry out their roles effectively and managers should be prepared to work together with team members on resolving the situation.

Managers are often the filter for information to and from other parts of the organisation. Facilitating regular team meetings for information exchange is of vital importance in maintaining clinicians' sense of being part of a wider organisation and allowing them to communicate with and influence others. Systems such as the CPA (see Ch. 5) seek to provide a framework within which care is planned and delivered. Managers need to develop a working knowledge of such systems and ensure practitioners have the required level of knowledge to implement these while explaining these to service users and carers in a clear and unambiguous fashion. Indeed, the full and accurate recording of information has been criticised in recent reviews of mental health care. The need to document care given (and, where necessary, reasons for deciding not to provide care) and conversations regarding the client (and carer where appropriate) cannot be overemphasised. Indeed, the Sainsbury Centre's (1998) document outlines a strategic approach to working with clients who are difficult to engage in mental health services, which includes effective management and appropriate recruitment and training for staff.

CONCLUSIONS

Collaboration is the key to providing a comprehensive mental health service. Practitioners and managers must have strategies in place that will address the need for information and decision making at both individual and group level for service users and carers.

The responsibilities inherent in mental health work are such that staff must be supported by the employer with procedures that are workable and opportunities for development that fit service and individual needs. Furthermore, managers need to canvass and disseminate information to and on behalf of the team in order to represent views, monitor practice and ensure organisational standards are maintained. The professional is ultimately responsible for keeping up to date. By working together in an atmosphere of openness all parties can fully contribute to a service that delivers appropriate and effective care.

References

Barker P J 1998 Psychiatric nursing. In: Butterworth T, Faugier J, Burnard P (eds) Clinical supervision and mentorship in nursing, 3rd edn, Stanley Thornes, London, p 67

Barker P J, Baldwin S (eds) 1991 Ethical issues in mental health. Chapman & Hall, London, p 66

Brown D, Carson J, Fagin L, Bartlett H, Leary J 1994 Coping with caring. Nursing Times 90(45):53–55

Bulmer C 1997 Supervision: how it works. Nursing Times 93(48):53–54

References (cont'd)

Butterworth T 1992 Clinical supervision as an emerging idea in nursing. In: Butterworth T, Faugier J (eds) Clinical supervision and mentorship in nursing. Chapman & Hall, London, p 12

Butterworth T 1997 It's good to talk: an evaluation of clinical supervision and mentorship in England and Scotland. University of Manchester, Manchester

Department of Health 1998 Working together. DOH, Leeds

Duggan M et al 1997 Pulling together. Sainsbury Centre, London

Everitt J, Bradshaw T, Butterworth A 1996 Stress and clinical supervision in mental health care. Nursing Times 92(10):34–35

Farrington A 1995 Models of clinical supervision. British Journal of Nursing 4(15):876–878

Faugier J 1994 Thin on the ground. Nursing Times 90(20):64–65

Gamble C 1997 Thorn nursing practice: its present and future. Mental Health Care 1(3):95–97

Gijbels H 1995 Mental health nursing skills in an acute admission environment: perceptions of mental health nurses and other mental health professionals. Journal of Advanced Nursing 21:460–465

Harper H 1997 Pressures and rewards of working in community mental health teams. Mental Health Care 1(1):18–21

Headley M, Moore R 1996 Establishing a community service. In: Thompson T, Mathias P (eds) Lyttle's mental health and disorder. Baillière Tindall, London

Jackson C 1998 Thorn in a dilemma. Mental Health Care 2(3):86–87

Jackson S 1994 The case for shared training for nurses and doctors Nursing Times 92(26):40–41

Kadner K 1994 Therapeutic intimacy in nursing. Journal of Advanced Nursing 19:215–218

Kanter R M 1988 Change – master skills what it takes to be creative. In: Kuhn R (ed) Handbook for creative and innovative managers. McGraw-Hill, New York, Ch 11, pp 54–61

Pilette P C, Berck C B, Achber L C 1995 Therapeutic management of helping boundaries. Journal of Psychosocial Nursing 33:1

Price V, Mullarkey K 1996 Use and misuse of power in the psychotherapeutic relationship. Mental Health Nursing 16(1):16–17

Sainsbury Centre 1998 Keys to engagement. Sainsbury Centre, London

Sully P 1996 The impact of power in therapeutic relationships. Nursing Times 92(41):40–41

Thomas B 1997 Management strategies to tackle stress in mental health nursing. Mental Health Care 1(1):15–17

UKCC 1996 Position statement on clinical supervision for nursing and health visiting. UKCC, London

UKCC 1998a Guidelines for mental health and learning disability nursing. UKCC, London

UKCC 1998b Guidelines for records and record keeping. UKCC, London

Watts D, Morgan G 1994 Malignant alienation. British Journal of Psychiatry 164:11–15

Annotated further reading

Reynolds A, Thorncroft G 1999 Managing mental health services. Open University Press, Buckingham

NHS Executive 1995 Clincial supervision – a resource pack. Department of Health, Leeds

Index